Third Edition

ESSENTIALS OF ANESTHESIOLOGY

DAVID C. CHUNG, M.D.
Associate Professor (Clinical)
Department of Anesthesia
University of British Columbia
Vancouver, British Columbia, Canada

ARTHUR M. LAM, M.D.
Professor
Department of Anesthesiology
University of Washington
Seattle, Washington

W. B. SAUNDERS COMPANY
A Division of Harcourt Brace & Company
Philadelphia, London, Toronto, Montreal, Sydney, Tokyo

W. B. SAUNDERS COMPANY
A Division of Harcourt Brace & Company

The Curtis Center
Independence Square West
Philadelphia, Pennsylvania 19106

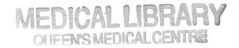
Library of Congress Cataloging-in-Publication Data

Chung, David C.
    Essentials of anesthesiology / David C. Chung, Arthur M. Lam—3rd
ed.
        p.   cm.
    Includes bibliographical references.
    ISBN 0–7216–6675–2
    1. Anesthesiology—Handbooks, manuals, etc.   I. Lam, Arthur M.
II. Title.
    [DNLM: 1. Anesthesia. 2. Anesthetics.   WO 200 C559e 1997]
    RD82.2.C48 1997
    617.9′6—dc20   1001397283
    DNLM/DLC   96-22873

ESSENTIALS OF ANESTHESIOLOGY   ISBN 0–7216–6675–2

Printed in the United States of America.

Last digit is the print number: 9   8   7   6   5   4   3   2

Preface
to the Third Edition

In this edition, we heeded the advice of our colleagues to consolidate *Essentials* as an introductory textbook on surgical anesthesia. To fulfill this goal, we have de-emphasized chapters dedicated to subspecialty areas and expanded on knowledge dealing with basic principles and practice. Two new chapters have been created to reflect current interest: one on the management of postoperative pain and the other, anesthesia for outpatient surgery. In addition, the chapter that was dedicated to tracheal intubation only in previous editions has been replaced by one on airway management, in which management of the difficult airway and use of the laryngeal mask and emergency airways are discussed in detail. Similarly, we have improved all the chapters on the pharmacology of anesthetic drugs, included detailed check-out procedures in chapters dealing with anesthestic equipment, and added a section on assessment of the airway in the chapter on assessment of the patient. No effort was spared and all chapters have been revised. Students of anesthesiology should be able to move on to specialty textbooks after reading *Essentials* and also keep it as a pocket companion in the wards and operating rooms.

Once again we would like to thank our students and colleagues for sharing their ideas with us. We are also indebted to Andrea Aikens, Vicky Earle, and Dale Northey for contributing to the new illustrations in this edition; to Intavent Research Ltd., Henley-on-Thames, U.K., Vitaid, Toronto, Ontario, Canada, and Gensia Inc., San Diego, California, U.S.A. for providing information on the Laryngeal Mask Airway; to Cook (Canada) Inc., Stouffville, Ontario, Canada for helping with the illustration of the cricothyrotomy airway; to *An-*

aesthesia, Anesthesia & Analgesia, Anesthesiology, British Journal of Anaesthesia and *Clinical Pharmacology and Therapeutics* for permission to reprint copyrighted material; to Berta Steiner of Bermedica Production, Ltd. for editorial assistance; and to Joan Sinclair of W. B. Saunders Company for supervising the production of this edition.

David C. Chung, M.D.
Arthur M. Lam, M.D.

Preface
to the Second Edition

When preparing this new edition, we were troubled with what should reasonably be included in an introductory textbook of anesthesiology. After all, the specialty has made progress in many areas: monitoring, new drugs, management of surgical pain, definition of standards of safe practice, quality assurance, and so forth. In the end we have included all these topics and revised others, but have increased the length of the text only slightly. We believe this edition retains the basic conciseness and comprehensiveness of the first edition. We trust it will continue to serve as a companion to our students; and again we welcome the opinion of our readers.

David C. Chung
Arthur M. Lam

Preface
to the First Edition

Anesthesia is a recognized subject in the curriculum of most medical teaching facilities, and many monographs have been published on the subject. However, we have had difficulty in recommending a basic textbook for our students. Indeed, there is more than one good introductory anesthesiology textbook on the market, but they are directed more to students at an intermediate level rather than to those being introduced to the specialty for the first time. The idea of writing this book was conceived to fill this need, and our students and colleagues urged us on.

Anesthetic procedures can be learned only in the operating room. The goal of this book is to provide the scientific basis of anesthesia, not to replace practical experience. In twenty-four chapters, anesthesia-related problems in the patient undergoing surgery are defined and the principles of safe anesthetic practice are discussed. Every attempt to be comprehensive and concise has been made so that the reader can easily acquire a firm foundation in anesthesiology. The student is encouraged to regard this book as his companion—to bring it with him to the ward and into the operating room; to read it; and to refer to it.

Anesthesiology is still a growing specialty. Many of our colleagues are practicing only in areas of special interest in the operating room—for example, in cardiovascular and thoracic surgery or neurosurgery; others are active in the emergency room, the intensive care unit, and the pain clinic. We have chosen to limit the scope of this book to the principles of surgical anesthesia and resuscitation. Other than the anesthetic management of obstetric, pediatric, geriatric, and ambulatory patients, areas of subspecialty are omitted by intention; we feel that the student should not be expected to be involved in these areas in an introductory course.

Although this book is written for clinical clerks, it should be a useful primer for all students of anesthesia. It should also be instructive for physicians, dental surgeons, nurses, and respiratory technicians who are involved in the care of the surgical patient. We trust this book will serve the needs of many, and we welcome the opinion of our readers.

David C. Chung
Arthur M. Lam

Contents

1
General Anesthesia—Basic Principles......................... 1

2
Intravenous Anesthetics 11

3
Inhalation Anesthetics... 28

4
Opioids.. 45

5
Muscle Relaxants 59

6
Local Anesthetics 79

7
The Anesthetic Machine and Accessories.................. 92

8
Anesthetic Circuits 109

9
Mechanical Ventilators... 119

10
Effect of Anesthesia on Respiratory Function............. 127

11
Anesthesia and Systemic Illness 137

12
**Preoperative Assessment and Preparation
of the Patient** 153

13
Airway Management in Anesthetized Patients 162

14
Monitoring Principles and Practice 188

15
Techniques of General Anesthesia 214

16
**Management of Complications
during Anesthesia** 223

17
Techniques of Local and Regional Anesthesia 237

18
Care of the Patient during Recovery 252

19
Management of Acute Postoperative Pain 262

20
Special Considerations in Surgical Outpatients 281

21
**Fluid and Electrolyte Requirements
of Surgical Patients** 290

22
Blood Transfusion in Surgical Patients........................ 299

23
**Anesthetic Mishaps, Quality Assurance, and
Risk Management**... 314

APPENDIX
I
Further Reading 321

Index... 327

General Anesthesia—Basic Principles

1

The noun *anesthesia* was coined by Oliver Wendell Holmes to describe the temporary and reversible state of "unawareness" induced by drugs to render surgery painless. Before the discovery of anesthetic drugs, surgery was largely limited to the excision of lesions on the body wall, the amputation of digits and limbs, and the extraction of teeth. Through the centuries, many methods have been tried to relieve the agony of surgery—including hypnosis, ingestion of alcohol or herbal concoctions, application of pressure to nerve trunks, and local hypothermia—but none was effective or reliable.

In 1823, Henry Hill Hickman, a physician-scientist from Shropshire, England, set out on a quest to find an inhaled anesthetic. Carbon dioxide attracted his attention because of its anesthetic-like properties at high concentrations. Unfortunately, carbon dioxide is not an anesthetic, and Hickman died young in 1830 with his dream unfulfilled. After him no others made deliberate attempts to find an anesthetic until some 20 years later, when American physicians and dentists discovered almost simultaneously the anesthetic properties of nitrous oxide and ether.

The discovery of nitrous oxide anesthesia came on December 10, 1844, when Horace Wells, a dentist from Hartford, Connecticut, attended an exhibition by Gardner Q. Colton, who prepared nitrous oxide and administered the gas to another audience member named Samuel A. Cooley. While he was intoxicated, Cooley accidently injured his leg but did not cry out in pain. Realizing the significance of what he observed, Wells decided to try out the effectiveness of this agent in obtunding the pain of dental surgery. The following day he arranged to have one of his own teeth extracted by an assistant while Colton gave him nitrous oxide. He felt no pain! Emboldened by this experience, Wells began to use nitrous oxide in his practice. In January 1845, he arranged a public demonstration of his technique at the Harvard Medical School in Boston, but the event turned into a fiasco and was declared a failure.

Although Wells and other dentists continued to use nitrous oxide in their practice, it took another 2 decades before nitrous oxide regained its rightful place as an effective anesthetic.

Whereas the discovery of nitrous oxide anesthesia was well recorded, the discovery of ether anesthesia is shrouded. There is evidence to show that William E. Clarke of Rochester, New York, gave his first and only ether anesthetic to a young woman for dental extraction as early as January 1842, but no personal record of this event was made. Crawford W. Long, a physician practicing in Jefferson, Georgia, gave the first recorded ether anesthetic on March 30, 1842. Subsequently he continued to administer ether anesthesia occasionally in his own practice, but he did not report his experience until 1849, when ether anesthesia was already being practiced worldwide. It was William T. G. Morton, a dental colleague of Wells, who successfully carried out a public demonstration of ether anesthesia on October 16, 1846, at the Massachusetts General Hospital in Boston. Within weeks of this event, ether anesthesia was practiced across the United States and Canada and met with equal enthusiasm in Great Britain, continental Europe, Australia, and South Africa. Arguably William T. G. Morton is regarded by some to be the forefather of anesthesia. The inscription on his tombstone reads:

> *Inventor and Revealer of Inhalation Anesthesia;*
> *Before Whom, in All Times, Surgery was Agony;*
> *By Whom, Pain in Surgery was Averted and Annulled;*
> *Since Whom, Science has Control of Pain.*

In the ensuing years the art and science of anesthesia developed rapidly. In 1847, James Simpson, a Scottish obstetrician, introduced chloroform as an alternative to ether; and in 1863, Gardner Q. Colton re-established nitrous oxide as an adjunct in anesthetic practice. During these early years of inhalation anesthesia, morphine quickly established itself as a preanesthetic medication and as an intraoperative supplement.

It is not surprising that the first anesthetics discovered were all given by inhalation. After all, the respiratory and the gastrointestinal tract were the only routes routinely used in the administration of medicinals. The parenteral route awaited the arrival of the hollow hypodermic needle and the syringe, which were not invented until the 1850s. The dawn of intravenous anesthesia came in 1873, when Pierrre-Cyprien Ore of Bordeaux, France, published his experience with intravenous chloral. Subsequent clinical trials were carried out also with hexobarbital (a short-acting oxybarbiturate), but the technique was not firmly established until 1935, when J. S. Lundy of the Mayo Clinic demonstrated the safe use of thiopental (an ultra-short-acting thiobarbiturate), still a popular induction agent in use today. Although the muscle relaxant curare had been used to treat spastic disorders for a number of years, it was not until 1942 that Griffith and Johnson of Montreal reported its use in surgical anesthesia.

Thus, the discovery of all four groups of anesthetic drugs used in modern practice (i.e., the intravenous anesthetics, inhaled agents, narcotic analgesics, and muscle relaxants) spanned 100 years. Since then, new members in each group have been introduced to meet specific needs. At the same time, the science and practice of anesthesia has developed into a well-recognized medical specialty called anesthesiology. The anesthesiologist is no longer just an averter and annuler of surgical pain. The anesthesiologist works hand in hand with surgeon and other medical colleagues in both evaluation and preparation of the patient before surgery, is the patient's primary care physician during the intraoperative period, and has direct input in the postoperative management of the patient. Using expertise gained in the operating room, the anesthesiologist has also become a significant contributor in other areas of health care, such as the intensive care unit and pain clinic. By training and by action, the anesthesiologist has earned his or her position as a medical consultant.

In English-speaking countries other than the United States, the anesthesiologist is commonly called an "anesthetist." This term, although perhaps confusing to American students, has an entirely reasonable basis: One who administers an anesthetic is an anesthetist. However, in the United States, only half the anesthetics given annually are administered by anesthesiologists (physician anesthetists); the other half are given by nurse anesthetists. Whereas the anesthesiologist is a graduate physician who has had 4 or more years of postgraduate training in the management of surgical patients both inside and outside the operating suite, of critically ill patients in intensive care and trauma units, and of patients with acute or chronic pain syndromes, the certified registered nurse anesthetist (CRNA) is a professional who has had 2 or 3 years of postgraduate training in surgical anesthesia after basic nursing education and acquiring work experience in critical care. In many hospitals and clinics, nurse anesthetists are integral members of the surgical team.

■ Molecular Mechanisms of Anesthetic Action

Anesthesia is a state of reversible loss of awareness and reflex reactions to noxious stimuli. A large number of agents, ranging from inert gases and volatile liquids to water-soluble and -insoluble organic compounds, can induce the general anesthetic state. The diversity of molecular species that can produce this state and the lack of a structure-activity relationship have eliminated a molecular mechanism of action that is common to all. Yet this diversity does not rule out a common target in their mode of action.

Action on Nerve Cell Membrane Ion Channels

In recent years a growing body of evidence has indicated that anesthetic drugs exert their effect through interference with the function of ion channels in nerve cell membrane. Whereas the nerve cell membrane is composed of a bimolecular layer of phospholipids, the ion channels (or ionophores) are formed by globular protein subunits (typically five such subunits) penetrating the full thickness of the membrane. These protein subunits have been designated α, β, γ, or δ according to their amino acid composition. Ion fluxes through these channels are responsible for impulse generation (neuronal excitation) and impulse transmission (axonal conduction). Three types of ion channels have been identified:

1. *Ligand-gated* (ligand-activated) channels have binding sites on the channel protein subunits. When molecules with agonist activity (*the ligand*) bind to these sites, the channel proteins undergo conformational changes and the channels open to allow the passage of specific ions. These ionophores have binding sites for drugs that can modulate the activities of the natural ligand. These modulator sites are adjacent to and distinct from receptor sites for the physiologic ligand. Examples of physiologic ligands are acetylcholine, gamma-aminobutyric acid (GABA), L-glutamate, and serotonin.

2. *Voltage-gated* (voltage-activated) channels can sense changes in the electrical potential across the nerve cell membrane. Changes in this potential change the conformation of the globular channel proteins and open the channels to the flux of specific ions. Some voltage-gated ionophores also have receptor sites for drugs that can modulate the behavior of the channel.

3. *Metabotropic receptor–gated* channels are indirectly activated by ligands. The binding of agonist molecules to receptor sites sends a signal that is transduced via a guanosine triphosphate–binding protein (G protein) to the channel protein subunits to open the channel. In addition to G protein, intracellular second messengers may be involved also in signal transduction.

Intravenous Anesthetics at GABA_A-Gated Channels

Many intravenous anesthetics depress central nervous system activity by enhancing inhibitory synaptic transmission.

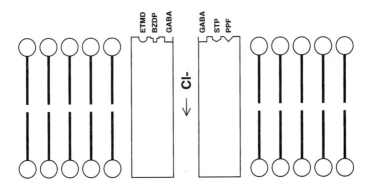

FIGURE 1–1. Illustration of a GABA$_A$-gated chloride channel in nerve cell membrane. Whereas the nerve cell membrane is a bimolecular layer of phospholipids, the ion channel is a pentameric structure made up of five protein subunits penetrating the full thickness of the membrane. The channel protein subunits contain binding sites for the natural ligand gamma-aminobutyric acid (GABA) as well as modulator sites for benzodiazepines (BZDP), thiopental (STP), etomidate (ETMD), and propofol (PPF). These modulator sites are adjacent to and distinct from the GABA sites and are unique for each drug. Occupation of GABA sites by the natural ligand causes conformation changes in the protein subunits, and the channel opens to allow negatively charged chloride ions to enter the neuron, leading to hyperpolarization of the nerve cell membrane and rendering the neuron less excitable. Occupation of the modulator sites by the respective drug molecules enhances the action of GABA.

The main inhibitory neurotransmitter in the central nervous system is gamma-aminobutyric acid. Two subtypes of GABA receptors have been identified Subtype A (GABA$_A$) receptors are found on postsynaptic neuronal membranes. Occupation of GABA$_A$ binding sites by the physiologic agonist GABA activates chloride channels (GABA-gated chloride channels). Negatively charged chloride ions entering the neuron through opened channels cause hyperpolarization of the nerve membrane (the resting membrane potential becomes more negatively charged), rendering the neuron less excitable.

Benzodiazepines, thiopental, etomidate, and propofol can occupy binding sites *adjacent* to and *distinct* from GABA$_A$ sites on the postsynaptic nerve cell channel protein subunits and enhance the inhibitory effect of GABA on postsynaptic neurons. Whereas the benzodiazepines achieve this positive modulation on GABA by increasing the frequency of opening of the chloride channels, thiopental achieves its effects by increasing the opening time of these channels. The binding sites on the postsynaptic nerve cell membrane are different among agents (Fig. 1–1).

Ketamine at NMDA-Gated Channels

Unlike the other intravenous anesthetics, ketamine depresses central nervous system activity by suppressing excitatory synaptic transmission mediated by L-glutamate. Binding of L-glutamate to channel protein sites on the postsynaptic nerve cell membrane activates calcium channels. The flux of positively charged calcium ions into the cell through these opened channels causes depolarization of the membrane potential and facilitates neuronal excitation. A subtype of glutamate receptors binds the agonist N-methyl-D-asparate (NMDA) selectively, and the ionophores associated with this subtype of receptors are called NMDA receptor channels. (NMDA is used to classify these glutamate-gated channels only; the natural ligand at these channels is L-glutamate.) Ketamine, a dissociative anesthetic (see "Ketamine" in Chapter 2), is a noncompetitive antagonist of L-glutamate at NMDA receptor sites and inhibits the postsynaptic excitatory action of L-glutamate. Ketamine binding sites are *adjacent* to and *distinct* from NMDA receptor sites.

Action of Inhalation Anesthetics

There is also convincing evidence that inhalation anesthetics depress central nervous system excitability through modulation of normal ion channel function. However, their site of action is less clear. At the turn of the century, Meyer and Overton observed a direct relationship between potency of inhalation anesthetics and their solubility in oil. More recently, it has been confirmed that the minimum alveolar concentration required to maintain anesthesia is lower for more lipid-soluble inhalation agents and vice versa (see "Minimum Alveolar Concentration" in Chapter 3). The Meyer-Overton rule implies that inhalation anesthetics act on the lipid environ of the brain, and nerve cell membranes of phospholipids have been suggested as their site of action. However, the lipid solubility of inhalation anesthetics does not rule out the action of these molecules on amphophilic pockets of channel protein subunits.

Lipid Solubility Hypothesis

There is more than one version of the hypothesis relating lipid solubility to action. The *volume expansion hypothesis* postulates that anesthetic drug molecules taken into the lipid matrix of nerve cell membrane cause expansion of these sites and increase lateral pressure on the protein units of ionic channels that penetrate the membrane. When a critical volume of expansion is reached, ionic flux through these channels is obstructed and neuronal excitability inhibited. This hypothesis is supported by the observation that exposure to high hydrostatic pressure, perhaps by restricting the expansion of the lipid matrix, can partially antagonize the effect of inhalation anesthetics in some animal species.

The *membrane fluidization hypothesis*, in contrast, proposes that the protein units forming the ion channels are embedded in a bilayer of phospholipid molecules arranged in an orderly way in the gel phase. The presence of anesthetic drugs increases the motility and disrupts the orderly arrangement of these lipid molecules—that is, a transition from the gel to the fluid phase occurs. As a result, the protein molecules forming

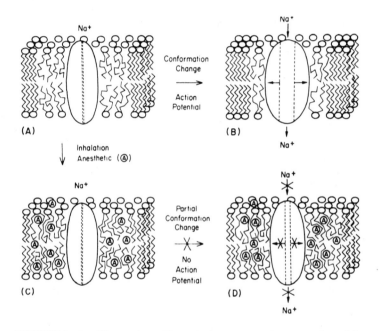

FIGURE 1–2. Illustration of lateral phase separation, a version of the lipid solubility hypothesis of the action of gaseous anesthetics. *A*, A closed ion channel in the axonal membrane is surrounded proximally by phospholipids in the fluid phase and farther laterally by those in the gel phase. *B*, During excitation, the channel springs open for passage of ions, a process facilitated by transforming some of the lipids from the high-volume fluid phase to the low-volume gel phase. *C*, In the presence of anesthetic molecules, some of the outlying gel-phase lipids become more fluid. *D*, These fluid-phase lipids fail to condense into the low-volume gel phase, so there will not be room for the ion channel to open on receiving an excitatory impulse. (From Trudell JR: A unitary theory of anesthesia based on lateral phase separations in nerve membrane. Anesthesiology 46:5, 1977; reprinted with permission.)

the ion channels lose their structural support and function. In a more elaborate version of the fluidization hypothesis, it is said that protein molecules of closed ion channels in nerve cell membrane are surrounded proximally by phospholipids in the fluid phase and further laterally by those in the gel phase (Fig. 1−2A). During excitation, these channel proteins undergo conformational changes to allow the passage of ions, a process facilitated by transforming some of the lipids from the high-volume fluid phase to the low-volume gel phase (Fig. 1−2B). In the presence of anesthetic molecules, some of the outlying gel-phase lipids become more fluid (Fig. 1−2C). Furthermore, these fluid-phase lipids fail to condense into the low-volume gel phase to make room for the conformation changes to take place in the channel protein units (Fig. 1−2D). Consequently these channels become obstructed and neuronal excitation is inhibited.

Protein Interaction Hypothesis

The most convincing evidence that fat-soluble inhalation anesthetic molecules can bind proteins come from studies in fireflies. In the lanterns of fireflies, the enzyme luciferase binds the substrate luciferin to emit light. Inhalation anesthetics, binding to luciferase, inhibit this light-producing reaction.

The protein interaction hypothesis postulates that inhalation anesthetic molecules, acting directly on amphophilic sites of channel proteins, modulate the gating mechanism of ion channels. For example, it has been shown that inhalation anesthetics can increase the opening time of $GABA_A$-gated chloride channels and enhance GABA-mediated inhibitory synaptic transmission—an action similar to that of thiopental described above. Inhalation anesthetics have been shown also to reduce the opening time of NMDA channels and inhibit L-glutamate−mediated excitatory synaptic transmission, an action similar to that of ketamine. This direct interaction with channel proteins implies a more direct and specific action of inhalation anesthetics on ion fluxes, whereas the lipid solubility hypothesis suggests a less direct mode of action.

■ Stages of Ether Anesthesia

Whereas knowledge of the mode of action of anesthetic drugs continues to expand, the clinical effects of these drugs have been described in detail since their discovery. Guedel described the progressive depression of the central nervous system by ether in four stages: analgesia, excitement, surgical anesthesia, and impending death. Although ether is no longer used in modern anesthesia practice, many of the signs of anesthesia described by Guedel are still in popular usage to describe the anesthetic state.

Analgesia (Stage I). The stage of analgesia lasts from onset of drowsiness to loss of eyelash reflex (blinking in response to stroking of the eyelash).

Excitement (Stage II). The stage of excitement is characterized by agitation and delirium. Respiration is irregular, and copious salivation can occur. Pupils are large and the eyes are divergent. Toward the end of this stage, respiration is again rhythmic (automatic respiration).

Surgical Anesthesia (Stage III). This stage is subdivided into four planes:

Plane 1   Respiration is rhythmic and rapid eye movement from side to side is seen

Plane 2   Lasts from cessation of rapid eye movement to onset of paresis of intercostal muscles

Plane 3   Lasts from onset of paresis of intercostal muscles to paralysis of these muscles

Plane 4   Lasts from paralysis of intercostal muscles to paralysis of the diaphragm; the patient ceases to breathe at the end of this plane

Impending Death (Stage IV). The stage of impending death lasts from onset of apnea to failure of the circulation and represents medullary depression.

■ Components of General Anesthesia

When ether is replaced by modern volatile inhalation agents, the stages of anesthesia described for ether remain more or less intact, although progression from consciousness to the surgical planes is rapid and landmarks between stages are less obvious. Concurrent use of intravenous anesthetics, opioids, and muscle relaxants, in contrast, can obscure all the stages and signs of anesthesia observed with inhalation anesthetics. Rees and Gray therefore described the state of general anesthesia in terms of three basic components—the triad of unconsciousness (hypnosis), analgesia (areflexia), and muscle relaxation.

Unconscious (Hypnosis). With development of unconsciousness, the patient is oblivious of all sensation, but somatic and autonomic reflexes to pain and noxious stimuli can still occur.

Analgesia (Areflexia). Withdrawal of a limb or flight (somatic reflexes) and hypertension, tachycardia, and sweating (autonomatic reflexes) are part of the subconscious reaction to pain. These potent reflexes must be subdued during anesthesia.

Muscle Relaxation. The degree of muscle relaxation required varies according to the operation. In general, only a mild degree of muscle relaxation is necessary for superficial operations on the body wall or extremities, but moderate to profound muscle relaxation is required for operations within body cavities.

Anesthetic Drugs

In the past, the triad of general anesthesia was obtained by progressive depression of the central nervous system with ether or chloroform alone. In current practice, a multiplicity of agents with specific actions are used to provide unconsciousness, analgesia, and muscle relaxation. These include intravenous anesthetics, inhalation anesthetics, narcotic analgesics, and muscle relaxants. The pharmacology of these agents is discussed in the next four chapters.

Intravenous Anesthetics

2

The intravenous route is a popular method for administration of drugs used in anesthetic practice. Injection of a drug directly into the circulation allows rapid distribution to the site of action and quick onset of pharmacologic effects. By giving the drug in small increments, dose can be titrated against observed effects. Once the desired actions are achieved, they can be maintained by repeated bolus injections or continuous infusion.

The intravenous route is not without drawbacks. Once the drug is injected, its effect cannot be reversed readily and there is potential for catastrophe. Side effects can be unexpectedly severe as a result of the high, although transient, plasma concentration attained following rapid intravenous injection, and the danger of anaphylaxis is ever present. In addition, phlebitis and thrombophlebitis are relatively common problems. Unless sterile technique is followed, the intravenous route can become the gateway for bacteria, pyrogens, and other foreign bodies to enter the circulation. Last but not least, there is the risk of fluid overload and air embolism.

Pharmacokinetics

When plasma concentration of an intravenous anesthetic (e.g., thiopental) is plotted on a logarithmic scale against time after it is given intravenously as a bolus, the curve thus obtained has three distinct features (Fig. 2–1). An initial peak is followed by a phase of rapid decline in plasma level (the distribution phase) and a later phase of slower decline (the elimination phase).

Peak Concentration

Following a bolus injection, plasma concentration peaks within one or two circulations of the drug in the body. The

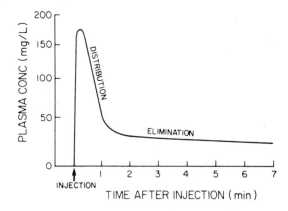

FIGURE 2-1. The rise and fall in plasma concentration of an intravenous anesthetic following injection of a bolus. The concentration rises to a peak following injection, then falls at a rapid rate in the distribution or α-phase, when the drug is distributed to and taken up by tissues. During the elimination or β-phase, when the drug is being metabolized and/or excreted, the rate at which the plasma concentration falls is considerably more gradual.

drug-laden blood circulates most rapidly to the vessel-rich group of organs, where the drug is taken up instantaneously (see "Tissue Blood Flow and Tissue Mass" below). This period of peak plasma concentration is only transient. As tissue uptake progresses, plasma concentration falls.

Distribution

The initial phase of relatively rapid decline in plasma level is known as the *distribution phase* (α *phase*). During this period, decline in plasma level is almost solely the result of distribution and redistribution of drug to and uptake of drug by various organs. The pharmacologic effect of intravenous anesthetics is determined by drug concentration in brain tissue, which is largely related to blood level. Therefore, the rate at which the plasma level falls determines the duration of action after a single bolus injection of intravenous anesthetic. The rate of this decline (i.e., the slope of the distribution phase) is determined by tissue uptake. Several factors act independently to influence tissue uptake and therefore this decline: protein binding, physical characteristics of the drug, and tissue blood flow and tissue mass.

Protein Binding

In the circulation, all intravenous anesthetics are bound to plasma protein (usually albumin), but the degree of binding varies according to the agent used. Because only free, non-protein-bound drugs can diffuse across cell membranes, protein binding decreases tissue uptake and drug action at tissue sites. These binding sites are nonspecific, so many foreign compounds can compete for them. In the presence of such a substance or in the event of a decreased plasma concentration of albumin (e.g., in liver disease), more of the drug will be present in the unbound form after intravenous injection of a usual dose. Because unbound drugs are pharmacologically active, this higher concentration of free drug can be the cause of an unexpected overdose.

Physical Characteristics of the Drug

Some physical characteristics of the drug itself are major determinants of how rapidly it is taken up by tissues. These include lipid solubility, molecular size, and the state of ionization.

Of these, *lipid solubility* is the most important. Highly lipid-soluble drugs (e.g., all intravenous anesthetics) are taken up rapidly by tissues. Lipid-soluble drugs also pass readily into "special circulations" (e.g., brain and placenta).

With water-soluble agents, *molecular size* is an important determinant of diffusibility across plasma membranes. The smaller the molecule, the more easily it can cross into tissue. With highly lipid-soluble agents, molecular weight plays little role in influencing diffusibility.

For drugs that are ionizable, the *state of ionization* greatly affects how rapidly they enter tissues. Only nonionized molecules diffuse across tissue barriers readily. As equilibrium exists across plasma membranes only for the nonionized form of a drug, so the total drug concentration (the ionized plus the nonionized fractions) on either side of the membrane can be very different. The pK_a of a drug is the pH at which 50% of the drug is ionized. The degree of ionization is determined by this value and the ambient pH, according to the Henderson-Hasselbalch equation:

$$pK_a - pH = \log \frac{[\text{acid form of drug}]}{[\text{base form of drug}]}$$

This equation can be rearranged for convenience as follows:

$$\frac{[\text{acid form of drug}]}{[\text{base form of drug}]} = \text{antilog}(pK_a - pH)$$

There is more acid form than base form of the drug when the difference between pK_a and pH is positive; there is more base form when the difference is negative. A drug is an acid if it is a donor of protons; it is a base if it is an acceptor of protons. Depending on the particular drug, the ionized fraction can be either a base or an acid. For example, the ionized fraction of sodium thiopental (NaTP) is a base. It can accept a proton according to the formulas:

$$\underset{\text{(sodium salt)}}{\text{NaTP}} \;\rightleftharpoons\; \text{Na}^+ + \underset{\text{(ionized base)}}{\text{TP}^-}$$

$$\underset{\text{(ionized base)}}{\text{TP}^-} + \underset{\text{(proton)}}{\text{H}^+} \;\rightleftharpoons\; \underset{\text{(nonionized acid)}}{\text{HTP}}$$

Conversely, the ionized fraction of lidocaine hydrochloride (XHCl) is an acid. It can donate a proton according to the formulas

$$\underset{\text{(hydrochloride salt)}}{\text{XHCl}} \;\rightleftharpoons\; \underset{\text{(ionized acid)}}{\text{XH}^+} + \text{Cl}^-$$

$$\underset{\text{(ionized acid)}}{\text{XH}^+} \;\rightleftharpoons\; \underset{\text{(nonionized base)}}{\text{X}} + \underset{\text{(proton)}}{\text{H}^+}$$

Ion trapping is a phenomenon related to this pH-dependent ionization of many molecules when there is a pH difference across tissue barriers. It is the cause of increase in urinary excretion of salicylate with alkalinization of urine. Sodium salicylate (NaS) can exist as an ionized base or a nonionized acid, according to the formulas

$$\underset{\text{(sodium salt)}}{\text{NaS}} \;\rightleftharpoons\; \text{Na}^+ + \underset{\text{(ionized base)}}{\text{S}^-}$$

$$\underset{\text{(ionized base)}}{\text{S}^-} + \underset{\text{(proton)}}{\text{H}^+} \;\rightleftharpoons\; \underset{\text{(nonionized acid)}}{\text{HS}}$$

After the nonionized acid has crossed into the lumen of renal tubules, a highly alkaline urine (i.e., urine abundant in hydroxyl ions) favors the equilibrium heavily to the right of the equation

$$\underset{\text{(nonionized acid)}}{\text{HS}} + \underset{\text{(hydroxyl ion)}}{\text{OH}^-} \;\rightleftharpoons\; \underset{\text{(ionized base)}}{\text{S}^-} + \text{H}_2\text{O}$$

Therefore, most of the salicylate will exist as negatively charged ions "trapped" in the tubular lumen. They cannot be reabsorbed from the urine and are excreted.

Tissue Blood Flow and Tissue Mass

All intravenous anesthetics are highly soluble in lipid; they are taken up readily by most tissues. The major factors influencing tissue uptake are tissue blood flow and tissue mass.

The tissues of the body can be divided into four groups according to their regional blood flow. Approximately 70% of the cardiac output goes to vessel-rich viscera (brain, heart, liver, kidneys), 25% to lean body mass (muscle), 4% to fat, and only 1% to the vessel-poor group (skin, cartilage, bone). Following bolus injection, a drug is first distributed to tissues receiving the greatest portion of cardiac output. Distribution to the vessel-poor group usually can be ignored.

Distribution of thiopental among the plasma pool and other tissues after a single injection is illustrated in Figure 2–2. As the fraction in the plasma falls, it is first taken up by the brain and other visceral organs, which account for only 10% of body weight. The fraction taken up by this vessel-rich group of tissues peaks at 30 seconds to 1 minute after injection. As time goes on, the fraction taken up by skeletal muscle, which accounts for approximately 50% of total body weight and has a relatively good blood supply, becomes more significant. This fraction surpasses that in the viscera by 5 minutes and peaks at approximately 20 minutes, while the fraction accumulated in brain and viscera falls. It is this redistribution of thiopental from brain to lean body mass that accounts for emergence from anesthesia after a single injection of this agent. Fat accounts for nearly 20% of body weight and has a high affinity for fat-soluble agents, but its blood supply is poor. For this reason, the fraction of thiopental taken up by fat plays no role in the emergence from thiopental anesthesia after an induction dose. This physiologic pharmacokinetic model of thiopental uptake and

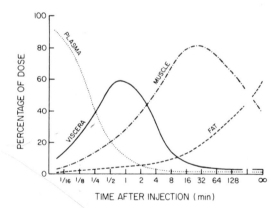

FIGURE 2–2. The distribution of thiopental among the plasma pool, viscera, muscle, and fat following an intravenous bolus. As the fraction of the dose in the plasma pool falls, the fraction taken up by viscera (brain, heart, liver, kidneys) peaks while that taken up by muscle continues to increase. Subsequently the fraction taken up by viscera falls and that taken up by muscle peaks. That is, there is first a distribution of the injected drug to viscera and then a redistribution of the drug from viscera to muscle. The fraction of the dose taken up by fat rises only slowly. (From Price HL, Kovnat PJ, Safer JN et al: The uptake of thiopental by body tissues and its relation to the duration of narcosis. Clin Pharmacol Ther 1:16, 1960; reprinted by permission.)

distribution also applies to the other intravenous anesthetic drugs.

Elimination

The phase of slower decline in plasma level represented by the latter portion of the graph in Figure 2–1 is the *elimination phase* (β *phase*). It is the result of elimination clearance of the intravenous anesthetic from the body by metabolism and biliary and renal excretion. Elimination starts immediately after a bolus injection is given for induction of anesthesia, but the rapid decline in plasma level and emergence from anesthesia that follow are due to redistribution of drug to lean body mass. Elimination plays no role in emergence from anesthesia after a single induction dose. However, elimination is important in other clinical settings:

1. After regaining consciousness following a single induction dose of an intravenous anesthetic, the residual sedative effect seen is due to a low level of drug in plasma that is in equilibrium with lean body tissue. The termination of this residual effect is quicker for drugs with a faster rate of elimination and slower for drugs with a slower rate of elimination.

2. After a large dose of an intravenous anesthetic drug has been given by multiple dosing or continuous infusion, the role played by elimination in terminating the anesthetic effect increases. If the dose is large enough to saturate the lean body depot, then elimination becomes the sole determinant of recovery from anesthesia. In these situations, time to awakening is shorter for drugs with a faster rate of elimination and vice versa.

Note: The emergence phase of anesthesia begins with discontinuation of anesthetic drugs and ends with awakening of the patient. The recovery phase begins with regaining of consciousness and ends with recovery from the residual effects of anesthetic drugs.

Hepatic Clearance

With few exceptions, intravenous anesthetics are cleared (removed) by the liver via biotransformation and biliary excretion. The capacity of the liver to extract a drug from the combined hepatic arterial and portal venous inflow can be expressed as a ratio known as the *hepatic extraction ratio* (HER) for that drug:

$$\text{HER} = \frac{\text{Hepatic arterial \& portal venous drug concentration} - \text{Hepatic venous drug concentration}}{\text{Hepatic arterial \& portal venous drug concentration}}$$

The product of this ratio and hepatic blood flow determines the rate of hepatic clearance of that drug according to the formula

Hepatic extraction ratio × hepatic blood flow = hepatic clearance

The maximum value of the hepatic extraction ratio is 1. Hepatic clearance is faster for drugs with high extraction ratios and slower for those with small extraction ratios.

Intravenous anesthetic drugs have hepatic extraction ratios ranging from 0.15 to 1. Because of their fast rate of hepatic elimination, intravenous anesthetics with high hepatic extraction ratios cause less residual sedation after a single induction dose and may be used for continuous infusion to maintain anesthesia. Drugs with a low hepatic extraction ratio can cause prolonged residual sedation even after a single bolus dose and can cause delayed emergence from anesthesia when used as a continuous infusion.

Renal Clearance

The kidneys are not a major depot for drug metabolism. Instead, renal clearance of drugs involves (1) the passive glomerular filtration of the non-protein-bound fraction and (2) an energy-dependent, carrier-mediated secretion of both the bound and unbound fractions by cells in the proximal tubules. After excretion, drugs may be reabsorbed in the distal tubules to a varying degree. This tubular reabsorption is dependent on the same physical characteristics discussed earlier: lipid solubility enhances reabsorption and delays excretion, whereas ionization impedes reabsorption and enhances excretion. Occasionally, specific transport mechanisms are also involved in reabsorption. With few exceptions, only a minute fraction of the given dose of lipid-soluble intravenous anesthetic drugs is excreted unchanged by the kidneys, although their water-soluble metabolites are.

■ Specific Agents

Intravenous anesthetics have a rapid onset and short duration of action. They are commonly given in a bolus for induction of anesthesia. Agents that are eliminated rapidly are sometimes given repeatedly or infused slowly to maintain anesthesia.

Barbiturates

Thiopental

Thiopental, a derivative of barbituric acid, is an ultra-short-acting barbiturate. It has been in use for induction of general anesthesia for 6 decades. Although its popularity is being challenged by propofol, it remains a commonly used induction agent in modern anesthetic practice. Its anesthetic action is obvious within one arm-to-brain circulation time. Induction of anesthesia with thiopental is pleasant. The induction dose is 3–5 mg/kg, which should be given slowly over 30–60 seconds so that the dose can be titrated against observed effects.

Thiopental has a pK_a of 7.6. Almost 60% of the molecules are in the nonionized form at normal body pH. In the presence of acidemia, even more becomes nonionized. This drug is also highly soluble in lipids, and approximately 70% of an injected dose is bound to plasma albumin. Decrease in plasma albumin concentration (e.g., in hepatic disease) or presence of substances competing for binding sites on these protein molecules (e.g., acetylsalicylic acid) may result in unexpectedly severe effects following the administration of a usual clinical dose.

The duration of anesthetic action following an induction dose is approximately 5 minutes. This ultra-short action is a result of rapid redistribution of the drug from brain to muscle. It is broken down in the liver by oxidative metabolism to a carboxylic acid derivative via the cytochrome P450 system. The hepatic extraction ratio of thiopental is only 0.15, and less than 1% of an injected dose is excreted unchanged in urine. This slow rate of elimination is responsible for the residual sedative effect seen with thiopental during recovery. It also makes thiopental unsuitable for maintaining anesthesia by repeated dosing or continuous infusion. (Continuous infusion of thiopental is used clinically for induction of barbiturate coma and cerebral protection but not for maintenance of anesthesia.)

Thiopental for injection is prepared as a 2.5% (25-mg/ml) aqueous solution of the sodium salt. It contains 6% anhydrous sodium carbonate as a buffer and has a pH of 10.8. Whereas extravascular injection of such an alkaline solution can produce tissue necrosis, intra-arterial injection will cause severe arterial spasm that may result in ischemic necrosis of tissues supplied by the artery. Therefore, sodium thiopental should be given only via a secure and freely running intravenous line.

The effect of thiopental on the central nervous system is complex. It generally depresses cerebral cortical function and is an effective anticonvulsant. By itself, thiopental has no analgesic properties. In fact, it is said to be antianalgesic because it appears to increase the subjective feeling of pain at subanesthetic doses. Following induction of anesthesia, there is a fall in cerebral metabolic rate for oxygen accompanied by a similar fall in cerebral blood flow. Intracranial pressure also declines. On this basis it has been suggested that thiopental may protect the brain from hypoxic or ischemic insults. The principle forms the basis for the induction of barbiturate coma in patients with cerebrovascular accidents and head injuries. Recent evidence suggests that it is not useful in global hypoxia or ischemia but can offer protection when given before the occurrence of focal ischemic events.

Thiopental depresses the vasomotor center of the brain stem, depresses the myocardium, and encourages peripheral vascular pooling, all of which can combine to produce hypotension. It must be given with extreme caution to patients with hypovolemia or myocardial disease.

The action of thiopental on the respiratory center at the brain stem is biphasic. Following a normal induction dose, it is not unusual to observe a big yawn or a brief period of hyperventilation (two to three large breaths) followed by transient apnea that can last for 30 seconds or more. Therefore, thiopental should not be given in the absence of resuscitative equipment and is contraindicated when a patient's airway or ventilation cannot be guaranteed following induction of anesthesia. In addition, thiopental can increase airway irritability, leading to laryngospasm or bronchospasm. This is seen soon after induction of anesthesia and is associated with premature instrumentation in the airway (e.g., insertion of an oropharyngeal airway immediately following loss of consciousness), which should be avoided.

Injection of thiopental into a vein can produce wheals and flares along the course of the vein as well as a characteristic mottled erythematous flush over the upper chest and neck. Both phenomena are related to the release of histamine. An increased incidence of bronchospasm in asthmatics following administration of thiopental is also attributed to this histamine-releasing property. It is absolutely contraindicated in patients acutely ill with asthma, and it is relatively contraindicated in those whose disease is in remission.

Like other barbiturates, thiopental can precipitate an acute crisis in patients who have porphyria, and so is contraindicated for them. Other contraindications include hypothyroidism and a history of hypersensitivity to other barbiturates.

Thiamylal

Like thiopental, thiamylal is also a thiobarbiturate. These two compounds are comparable in potency and action. Thiamylal injection is a 2% (20-mg/ml) aqueous solution buffered with anhydrous sodium carbonate. The induction dose is 3–5 mg/kg.

Methohexital

Methohexital is another ultra-short-acting barbiturate frequently used for the induction of anesthesia. Its pharmacologic action is similar to that of thiopental but, unlike thiopental, it is an oxybarbiturate. It is prepared as a 1% (10-mg/ml) aqueous solution with anhydrous sodium carbonate added but not a preservative. The induction dose is 1–2 mg/kg.

Methohexital has a hepatic extraction ratio that varies between 0.5 and 0.85. This faster rate of hepatic clearance imparts to it two major advantages over thiopental: less residual drowsiness during recovery and less cumulative effect with repeated injections. However, induction of anesthesia with methohexital is associated with a higher incidence of excitatory phenomena (cough, hiccup, and other myoclonic movements). It is also associated with a transient but unpleasant ache at the site of injection.

Alkylphenols

Several alkylphenol derivatives have hypnotic properties, but propofol is the only one useful in clinical anesthesia.

Propofol

Propofol is the newest intravenous anesthetic introduced into clinical practice. The induction dose is 1.5–3 mg/kg. Following an intravenous bolus, plasma concentration peaks and then falls off at a much faster rate than thiopental during the distribution phase because of extensive tissue uptake. It is metabolized primarily to water-soluble glucuronides and sulfates, which are excreted in urine. Less than 1% of a given dose is excreted unchanged by the kidneys. The hepatic extraction ratio of propofol is estimated to be 1. Therefore, the rate of hepatic clearance is equal in magnitude to hepatic blood flow of 1500 ml/min (see equation under "Hepatic Clearance" above). However, the rate of total body clearance of propofol is as high as 2200 ml/min, suggesting extensive extrahepatic metabolism. The site of extrahepatic clearance has not yet been identified. Because of its rapid redistribution and elimination, recovery from anesthesia following an induction dose of propofol is more rapid than that following other intravenous agents. This property makes it the most popular agent used in outpatient anesthesia. Its rapid elimination and lack of cumulative effect have also made it ideal for use in a continuous infusion to maintain anesthesia in the so-called total intravenous anesthesia (TIVA) technique.

Because propofol is water insoluble, it is formulated as a 1% (10-mg/ml) milky-white aqueous emulsion containing 10% soybean oil, 1.2% egg phosphatide, and 2.25% glycerol. Despite the presence of egg phosphatide in its formulation, it is safe in patients with a history of egg allergy because the allergen in these instances is egg albumin.

The pharmacologic action of propofol is similar to that of thiopental, but there are differences:

1. Propofol does not have antianalgesic activity. The incidence of nausea and vomiting after propofol is very low. It actually has clinically useful antiemetic properties.

2. Propofol causes a smaller fall in cerebral metabolic rate for oxygen than a comparable dose of thiopental. The latter is a better choice for cerebral protection in focal ischemia.

3. Like thiopental, propofol is an anticonvulsant. Yet cases of convulsion following the administration of propofol have been reported. Myoclonus can occur following induction of anesthesia using propofol. The incidence of these involuntary movements is more frequent, and the intensity more severe, in children than in adults.

4. An induction dose of propofol causes a larger drop in blood pressure than an equivalent dose of thiopental. This fall in blood pressure is not accompanied by a significant increase in heart rate. It is largely the result of a fall in systemic vascular resistance. Other factors contributing to hypotension include myocardial depression, venous pooling, and impaired baroreceptor reflex. (When the baroreceptor reflex is impaired, tachycardia in response to hypotension is depressed.)

5. An induction dose of propofol causes transient apnea in approximately 30% of inductions. This period of apnea is longer after propofol than after an equipotent dose of thiopental. However, propofol does not increase airway irritability, and instrumentation of the upper airway (e.g., insertion of laryngeal mask) is well tolerated immediately following loss of consciousness. Propofol does not cause bronchospasm and is not contraindicated in asthmatic patients. It may even have bronchodilating properties, but this effect is not as potent as that with ketamine.

6. When propofol is used for induction of anesthesia, some degree of pain occurs at the site of injection in all patients. This can be minimized by avoiding using small veins in the hand or by adding 40 mg of lidocaine to each 20-ml ampule of propofol.

7. Vivid dreams and sexual fantasies during emergence from propofol anesthesia have been reported. These episodes are different from the hallucinations and dysphoria seen during emergence from ketamine anesthesia. A careful explanation of the situation is usually enough to alleviate anxiety.

Benzodiazepines

The benzodiazepines are members of a large family of structurally related compounds classified pharmacologically as minor tranquilizers. They have found widespread use in anesthesia practice as nighttime and preanesthesia sedatives and for sedation during local anesthesia. Two of them, diazepam and midazolam, are also used for induction of general anesthesia. Flumazenil, a competitive antagonist, can bind benzodiazepine receptor sites and reverse all the central nervous system effects of agonist compounds.

All benzodiazepines have anticonvulsant, anxiolytic, sedative, amnesic, hypnotic, and mild muscle relaxant properties. The relaxant effect on skeletal muscles is probably mediated by inhibition of spinal reflexes. Following induction of general anesthesia with diazepam or midazolam, the cerebral metabolic rate for oxygen falls together with cerebral blood flow. The benzodiazepines have been shown in animal studies to protect the brain against ischemic insults, but the degree of protection is less than that by pentobarbital and they are not used clinically for this purpose. Diazepam and midazolam are promoted for induction of anesthesia in cardiac and critically ill patients because of their modest cardiovascular side effects. Nevertheless, hypotension similar in magnitude to that from an equipotent dose of thiopental is not uncommon, particularly when opioids are also used during induction. Like the barbituates, the benzodiazepines (particularly midazolam) depress activities of the respiratory centers in the brain stem. The incidence of apnea following equipotent doses of midazolam and thiopental is similar.

Diazepam

When diazepam is used to induce general anesthesia, the onset of action is gradual (2–3 minutes), and a wide variation in dose requirement is observed (0.2–0.6 mg/kg). Therefore, the dose should be titrated against the desired effect.

Whereas midazolam is considered a short-acting benzodiazepine, diazepam is intermediate to long acting. After an intravenous bolus, the duration of action of both, as with other intravenous anesthetics, depends on redistribution to lean body mass. This rate of redistribution is slower for diazepam than for midazolam, thus accounting for its longer duration of action.

Diazepam is broken down in the liver, yielding two active metabolites: oxazepam and N-desmethyldiazepam. The hepatic extraction ratio is less than 0.05. Over 70% of its metabolites are excreted in urine, and approximately 10% in feces. Because of the low hepatic extraction and the presence of active metabolites, the residual sedative effect of diazepam is prolonged during recovery from anesthesia and the effect of repeated or continuous dosing is cumulative.

Valium injection is prepared as a 0.5% (5-mg/ml) solution in an organic solvent of mixed composition (40% propylene glycol and 8% ethyl alcohol together with 1.6% benzyl alcohol as preservative, sodium benzoate and benzoic acid as buffers, and sodium hydroxide to adjust the pH). It becomes cloudy when mixed with aqueous intravenous solutions, but there is no apparent loss of potency. Pain at the site of injection is common when it is given intravenously, and the incidence of phlebitis is high. **Diazemuls** is a 0.5% (5-mg/kg) injectable emulsion of diazepam prepared in purified soybean oil, acetylated monoglycerides, purified egg phospholipids, and glycerol, with sodium hydroxide added to adjust the pH to 8. This latter preparation is less irritating to veins.

Midazolam

Midazolam is a water-soluble benzodiazepine. The injectable preparation comes either as a 0.1% (1-mg/ml) or a 0.5% (5-mg/ml) solution with disodium edetate and benzyl alcohol added as preservatives, together with hydrochloric acid or sodium hydroxide added to adjust the pH to 4 or less. As much as 95% of an injected dose is bound to plasma protein, mainly albumin. It is transformed to hydroxymidazolams in the liver, which are then conjugated and subsequently excreted in urine. The hepatic extraction ratio is 0.5. Compared to the parent compound, the pharmacologic activity of the hydroxyl metabolites is insignificant.

Midazolam has all the pharmacologic actions of diazepam and is associated with a higher frequency of anterograde amnesia. It is two to three times more potent than diazepam, causes little venous irritation, and is more reliably absorbed after intramuscular injection. The induction dose is variable (0.15–0.4 mg/kg) and the onset of action gradual. Although its duration of anesthetic action is less than that of diazepam, it is two to three times as long as that of thiopental.

Flumazenil

Flumazenil is a benzodiazepine with high affinity for benzodiazepine receptors but no agonist activities. It is capable of competitively antagonizing the central nervous system depressant effects of agonist benzodiazepines, including their anticonvulsant, anxiolytic, sedative, amnesic, and hypnotic properties. Like other benzodiazepines, it is metabolized in the liver to *N*-desmethylflumazenil, *N*-desmethylflumazenil acid, and flumazenil acid. Subsequently these metabolites are conjugated to form water-soluble glucuronides, which are then excreted in urine. The hepatic extraction ratio is near 1.

Flumazenil injection is an aqueous solution containing flumazenil 0.1 mg/ml. Acetic acid, disodium edetate, methylparaben, and propylparaben are added for preservation, and hydrochloric acid or sodium hydroxide to adjust the pH to 4. The recommended dose to antagonize the anesthetic effect of diazepam or midazolam is 0.2 mg intravenously initially and 0.1 mg every 60 seconds thereafter to a maximum of 1 mg to obtain the desired effect. Because the spectrum of central nervous system depression, from anxiolysis to sedation to hypnosis, by agonist benzodiapines increases with the population of receptors occupied, it is possible to titrate the dose of flumazenil to obtain the desired degree of reversal. (The population of receptors occupied is directly related to the dose given.) For example, a small dose of flumazenil will decrease the population of receptors occupied by the agonist and rouse the patient from unconsciousness but spare the anxiolytic effects. Because of its rapid hepatic clearance, the effect of flumazenil is short lived and sedation and hypnosis can recur. In this instance, an intravenous infusion of 0.1–0.4 mg/hr is useful.

Phencyclidines

Both phencyclidine and cyclohexamine (a congener) antedate ketamine as intravenous anesthetic agents, but both produced severe psychotic side effects and were removed from clinical practice.

Ketamine

Ketamine is a derivative of cyclohexanone. It produces a dissociative mental state characterized by catalepsy, sedation, amnesia, and analgesia. Analgesic effect accompanies subanesthetic doses, and this property is unique among intravenous anesthetic drugs.

Ketamine for injection is prepared either as a 1% (10-mg/ml) or 5% (50-mg/ml) aqueous solution. Both contain 1:10,000 benzethonium chloride as a preservative. Approximately 30% of an injected dose is protein bound. It is metabolized by the cytochrome P450 system in the liver first to norketamine, which has 20–30% of the potency of the parent compound. Subsequently norketamine is hydroxylated to hydroxynorketamines, which are then conjugated to form glucuronides. The hepatic extraction ratio is approximately 0.8. More than 90% of the water-soluble glucuronide metabolites are excreted by the kidneys, and less than 3% in feces.

Ketamine can be given intravenously or intramuscularly. The normal dose is 1–2 mg/kg intravenously over 1 minute or 6.5–13 mg/kg intramuscularly. The duration of action is 5–10 minutes after an intravenous dose and 15–25 minutes after an intramuscular injection. It has found application in pediatric diagnostic procedures, in burn surgery, and in critically ill patients.

In anesthetic doses, ketamine produces a seizure-like electroencephalogram (EEG) pattern in humans without the associated convulsive muscular activity. It also causes increases in intracranial pressure, cerebral metabolic rate for oxygen, and cerebral blood flow. Part of the increase in cerebral blood flow may be attributed to hypercapnia resulting from respiratory depression. Because the increase in cerebral metabolism is matched by the increase in blood flow, cerebral oxygen demand and supply remain in balance in normal subjects. Although the effect of ketamine on intracranial pressure would seem to make it unsuitable for patients who have intracranial hypertension or who are at risk of developing cerebral ischemia, there are studies suggesting that ketamine has cerebral protective effects because it depresses central nervous system activities by suppressing excitatory synaptic transmission mediated by L-glutamate at NMDA-gated channels.

Patients under ketamine anesthesia usually retain the laryngeal reflex and can maintain a patent upper airway without assistance, although aspiration and airway obstruction sometimes occur. These properties make ketamine a safer agent when anesthesia is required under primitive conditions, as at the scene of an accident. The effect of ketamine on the cardiovascular system is stimulatory; a rise in blood pressure of 20—40 mm Hg and an increase in heart rate of 30—40 beats per minute are usual. As a result, myocardial work is increased, so ketamine is contraindicated in hypertensive patients and in patients with ischemic heart disease. However, it is useful for induction of anesthesia in patients who are hypovolemic when the operation is urgent. Because it is a potent bronchodilator, it is also useful for induction of anesthesia in asthmatic patients.

Ketamine is related to the hallucinogens. Emergence from ketamine anesthesia is frequently associated with bad dreams and dysphoria. Patients should be allowed to recover undisturbed in a quiet, dark area. The administration of 5—10 mg of diazepam intravenously can reduce the incidence of emergence delirium without prolonging recovery.

Imidazoles

Etomidate

Etomidate is the only imidazole derivative that is used in clinical anesthesia. It exists both as positive and negative isomers, but only the positive form has anesthetic properties. As an intravenous anesthetic, it has an onset and duration of action similar to those of thiopental. It is water insoluble and is formulated as a 0.2% (2-mg/ml) solution in a solvent containing 35% propylene glycol. The induction dose is 0.2—0.4 mg/kg. About 75% of an injected dose is protein bound. It is hydrolyzed in the liver by esterases, and the hepatic extraction ratio is 0.9%. Extrahepatic breakdown by plasma esterases is also reported. Approximately 75% of a given dose is recoverable from urine as water-soluble metabolites, and another 15% from feces. Because of its rapid elimination, the residual sedative effect following emergence from anesthesia and the cumulative effect from repeated dosing or continuous infusion are short lived.

Like thiopental, etomidate decreases cerebral metabolic rate for oxygen, cerebral blood flow, and intracranial pressure; unlike thiopental, it causes only minor respiratory depression, little change in circulatory function, and no histamine release. Therefore, it can be used safely in hypovolemic, cardiac, and asthmatic patients. However, it is associated with a high incidence of pain at the site of injection, myoclonic jerks and hiccups (a facilitatory phenomenon not accompanied by epileptiform EEG patterns), and postoperative nausea and vomiting. Because a single dose of etomidate can suppress adrenocortical function for several hours, prolonged infusion to maintain sedation (e.g., in the intensive care unit) is discouraged, but its use as an induction agent is not contraindicated.

Butyrophenones

The butyrophenones are major tranquilizers. Whereas haloperidol is a popular antipsychotic drug, droperidol is used in anesthesia for both sedation and hypnosis.

Droperidol

Droperidol can produce a neuroleptic state of cognitive dissociation. It is also a useful antiemetic that acts directly on the chemoreceptor trigger zone in the medulla. The injectable preparation comes as a 0.25% (2.5-mg/ml) aqueous solution with lactic acid added to adjust the pH to 3.0–3.8. **Innovar** is an aqueous solution containing droperidol 2.5 mg and fentanyl (an opioid) 50 μg/ml.

Although droperidol itself has no analgesic properties, it is used in neuroleptanalgesia, a technique in which it is combined with a narcotic analgesic (usually fentanyl). This technique has been used to supplement regional anesthesia and to sedate patients during invasive diagnostic procedures. Together with fentanyl, nitrous oxide, and a muscle relaxant, droperidol is also used to induce and maintain neuroleptanesthesia. The neuroleptanalgesic dose in healthy adults is 2.5–5 mg of droperidol together with 50–100 μg of fentanyl. To induce neuroleptanesthesia, the dose is 15–25 mg of droperidol and 300–600 μg of fentanyl.

Droperidol has several noteworthy adverse side effects. It has some alpha-blocking properties that can cause hypotension when large doses are given. It can cause an anxious, agitated state (dysphoria) in some patients when it is given alone. Occasionally extrapyramidal dyskinesia and parkinsonian rigidity are seen because droperidol interferes with dopaminergic transmission in the central nervous system.

Inhalation Anesthetics

3

The first anesthetics introduced into clinical practice were inhalation agents (nitrous oxide, ether, chloroform). They were used for both induction and maintenance of anesthesia. Since the introduction of thiopental in 1934, however, the use of intravenous agents for induction has largely superseded the use of inhalation agents. Nevertheless, induction of anesthesia with inhalation anesthetics is still popular in children and in patients in whom intravenous agents are contraindicated. Unlike that with ether, induction with modern inhalation agents is both pleasant for the patient and rapid in onset. Except for transient agitation and irregularity of breathing, the second stage described for ether anesthesia is seldom obvious.

Definition of Commonly Used Terms

Administration of a drug via the respiratory tract to act on a distant target organ is unique to the practice of anesthesia. Before reviewing alveolar and tissue uptake of inhalation agents, it is necessary to define the *concentration, partial pressure*, and *minimum alveolar concentration* (MAC) of these agents. These terms apply to both gases and vapors.

Concentration

The fraction of a gas in a mixture is equal to the volume of that gas divided by the total volume of the mixture, and the concentration of this gas in the mixture is this fraction expressed as a percentage. For example, the concentration of nitrous oxide in a mixture of 7 liters of nitrous oxide and 3 liters of oxygen is 70%; a 10-liter mixture of oxygen, nitrous oxide, and 1% isoflurane has 100 ml of isoflurane vapor (not the liquid). Concentration is a convenient way of describing the composition of an anesthetic mixture. However, concentration gra-

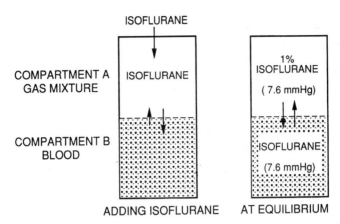

FIGURE 3–1. The movement of isoflurane across a gas-blood interface. At equilibrium, partial pressures of isoflurane in both compartments are equal.

dient is not the force behind the movement of gas molecules between a gas-liquid or a liquid-liquid interface.

Consider the example in Figure 3–1, in which a gas mixture in compartment A is separated by a semipermeable membrane from blood in compartment B. If isoflurane is added to compartment A so that its final concentration is 1%, some of the isoflurane molecules will cross into the blood in compartment B. With time, an equilibrium will be established, and the number of molecules crossing from compartment A into compartment B will equal those crossing from compartment B into compartment A. That is, the net movement of isoflurane molecules is zero. The force behind this movement of isoflurane molecules and the eventual state of equilibrium is partial pressure. If compartment B is, in turn, separated by another semipermeable membrane from a compartment C containing tissue fluid, as in Figure 3–2, isoflurane molecules will also cross into compartment C until equilibrium is established. At equilibrium, the partial pressures of isoflurane in all three compartments are equal.

Partial Pressure

Gas molecules are in constant motion, whether they are in a mixture or in solution. Molecules in a gas mixture are constantly bombarding the walls of their container; those in solution are always leaping into the atmosphere above the liquid they are dissolved in or are crossing the boundary of a liquid-

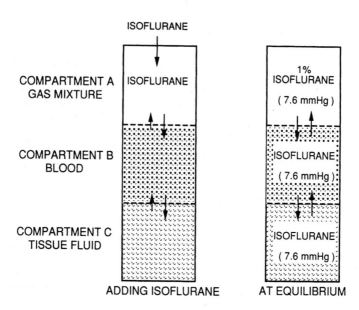

FIGURE 3–2. The movement of isoflurane across a gas-blood and a blood–tissue fluid interface. At equilibrium, partial pressures in all three compartments are equal.

liquid interface. Partial pressure (also called *tension*) may be regarded as a measure of these activities.

By definition, the partial pressure of a component gas in a mixture is equal to the fraction it contributes toward total pressure. That is,

$$\text{Partial pressure of component gas} = \text{Total pressure of mixture} \times \text{Concentration of component gas}$$

In the example in Figure 3–2, the partial pressure of isoflurane in compartment A is 1% of the atmospheric pressure (760 mm Hg), or 7.6 mm Hg.

When a gas is in solution, its partial pressure can be deduced from the composition of the gas mixture with which the solvent is in equilibrium. At steady state, the partial pressure of the gas in both phases is equal. In the example in Figure 3–2, the partial pressure of isoflurane in the blood of compartment B is equal to that in compartment A, 7.6 mm Hg. Similarly, the partial pressure of isoflurane in the tissue fluid of compartment C is 7.6 mm Hg. It should be noted that this example also describes gas exchange between alveolar gas and pulmonary blood, and between blood and tissue fluid.

Minimum Alveolar Concentration

The MAC of an inhalation agent is the concentration of that agent in alveolar gas necessary to prevent movement in 50% of patients when a standard incision is made. Because the MAC is in effect the median effective dose (ED_{50}) of an inhalation agent, it follows that an alveolar concentration higher than MAC will be required to retain immobility in the remaining 50% of patients when the same standard stimulus is used. Normally immobility can be achieved in 95% of patients when the alveolar concentration of the anesthetic is 30% above its MAC value.

Alveolar concentration is a convenient method of quantifying the dose of an inhalation agent a patient receives because it can easily be translated into partial pressure. At equilibrium, the partial pressure of the agent in alveolar gas equals that in blood as well as that in the brain (the site of action). The setting of the vaporizer is not a true reflection of the dose received because some of the anesthetic is lost to the tubing of the anesthetic circuit or to the surrounding atmosphere before it reaches the respiratory tract. Nor is the inspired concentration, measured at the upper respiratory tract, an accurate reflection of this dose, because a gradient exists between alveolar and inspired concentrations during the course of a normal anesthetic procedure (see "Alveolar Uptake" below). This dose can be monitored only by measuring end-tidal concentration of the vapor using an anesthetic vapor analyzer (see "Nitrous Oxide and Anesthetic Vapor Monitors" in Chapter 14).

The MACs of commonly used inhalation agents are listed in Table 3–1. For convenience, the alveolar concentration of an inhalation agent is commonly expressed as a multiple or a fraction of its MAC; for example, an alveolar concentration of 2.3% isoflurane is expressed as 2 MACs of isoflurane and an alveolar concentration of 0.85% enflurane as 0.5 MAC of enflurane. In general, the anesthetic effects and the MACs of inhalation

TABLE 3–1. Minimum Alveolar Concentration (MAC) of Inhalation Anesthetics

AGENTS (IN ORDER OF DECREASING POTENCY)	MAC (%)
Halothane	0.77
Isoflurane	1.15
Enflurane	1.70
Sevoflurane	2.05
Desflurane	6.0
Nitrous oxide	104.0

agents used in combination are more or less additive. That is, an alveolar concentration of 70% nitrous oxide (0.7 MAC) and an alveolar concentration of 0.57% enflurane (0.3 MAC) will keep 50% of patients immobile when they are subjected to the standard stimulus.

This definition of MAC has made it possible to compare the potency of inhalation anesthetics. An agent that has a lower MAC value is more potent than one with a larger MAC value (see Table 3–1). Similarly, the definition of MAC allows comparison of side effects of different agents at equipotent anesthetic doses.

There are many factors that will increase or decrease the MAC of an inhalation agent. Pyrexia and the administration of a central nervous system stimulant (e.g., dextroamphetamine, a drug that promotes the release of catecholamine in the central nervous system) increase MAC. Advancing age, hypothermia, and administration of a central nervous system depressant (narcotic analgesics, tranquilizers, and barbiturates) all decrease MAC. Other factors that decrease MAC include severe hypercapnia (arterial carbon dioxide tension [P_aCO_2] > 90 mm Hg), severe hypoxemia (arterial oxygen tension [P_aO_2] < 40 mm Hg), and severe anemia (hematocrit < 10%). In contrast, mild hypercapnia, profound hypocapnia, mild hypoxemia, mild anemia, circadian rhythms, hyperthyroidism, hypothyroidism, and the duration of anesthesia have no discernible effect on MAC.

Alveolar Uptake

As pointed out in the previous section, the alveolar concentration of an inhalation agent must be raised to a certain level in order to achieve anesthesia. At equilibrium, the partial pressure of the anesthetic agent in the alveoli equals that in blood and brain. In practice, the anesthetic is delivered to the upper respiratory tract, from which it is inhaled. The rate of alveolar uptake is gradual and follows an exponential growth pattern illustrated by the curves in Figure 3–3. Equilibration between alveolar concentration and inspired concentration occurs only at infinity and is not reached within the course of an anesthetic procedure.

The rate of alveolar uptake is determined by three different factors: *inspired concentration*, *washout of alveolar gas*, and *uptake by pulmonary blood*. However, both washout of alveolar gas and uptake by pulmonary blood are influenced by other independent factors. Those that affect alveolar washout are *alveolar ventilation* and *functional residual capacity*, and those that influence uptake by pulmonary blood are *solubility* of the agent in blood, *cardiac output*, and *alveolar–mixed venous tension gradient*.

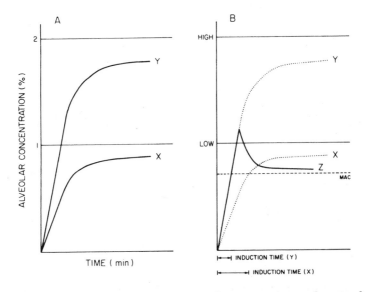

FIGURE 3–3. The influence of inspired concentration on the rate of alveolar uptake of an inhalation anesthetic and on induction time. *A*, When the inspired concentration is 1%, the alveolar uptake curve follows *X*; when the inspired concentration is doubled to 2%, the alveolar uptake curve follows *Y*. The faster rate of rise in alveolar concentration in *Y* (the slope of the curve) is obvious. *B*, When inspired concentration is higher, induction time is shorter because of the faster rate of rise in alveolar concentration.

Inspired Concentration

It is not surprising that the rate of rise in the alveolar concentration of an anesthetic agent is faster if more of it is delivered in the inspired gas mixture. Curve *X* in Figure 3–3*A* represents the exponential growth in alveolar concentration of a volatile anesthetic when the inspired concentration is 1%. When inspired concentration is doubled to 2%, alveolar concentration will grow along curve *Y*. The more rapid rate of rise in alveolar concentration when inspired concentration is increased is obvious. This effect is seen with both insoluble and soluble agents.

When pulmonary capillary blood takes up anesthetic vapor molecules from alveolar gas, the vapor concentration in the alveolar gas mixture falls. Therefore, the solution of a soluble agent in pulmonary capillary blood tends to reduce the rate at which its alveolar concentration increases. This retardant effect on the rate of rise decreases as the inspired concentration increases. This phenomenon is called the *concentration effect*. It is an additional factor that contributes to increasing the rate of alveolar uptake of soluble agents at higher inspired concentrations. The importance of this factor increases with the solubility of the agent. Because all volatile agents currently in use are relatively insoluble, the influence of concentration effect on the alveolar uptake of these agents can be regarded as minimal.

A practical application of increasing inspired concentration on alveolar uptake is found in inhalation induction. In Figure 3–3B, alveolar uptake follows curve X when a low inspired concentration of inhalation anesthetic is given, but it follows curve Y when the inspired concentration is increased. The consequence of giving a higher inspired concentration during induction is a shorter induction time. Once anesthesia is established, the inspired concentration can be adjusted to lower values for maintenance (curve Z).

Alveolar Ventilation

Because inhalation anesthetics are delivered only to the upper airway, from which they are inhaled, hyperventilation increases the rate of alveolar uptake and hypoventilation decreases it.

Functional Residual Capacity

Functional residual capacity (FRC) is the volume of gases in the lungs at the end of a normal expiration; it acts as a buffer to changes in the composition of alveolar gas. The time required to complete 63% of alveolar uptake (the *time constant*) is related to FRC and alveolar ventilation per minute ($\dot{V}_A$) by the following formula:

$$\text{Time constant} = \frac{\text{FRC}}{\dot{V}_A}$$

Thus the rate of rise in alveolar concentration is fast (short time constant) when FRC is small or alveolar minute ventilation large, and the rate of rise is slow (long time constant) when FRC is large or alveolar minute ventilation small.

Solubility of Anesthetic Agent

The solubility of an inhalation agent in blood is defined as the amount of anesthetic agent required to saturate a unit volume of blood at a given temperature, and can be expressed as the blood-gas partition coefficient. The relative solubility of agents in clinical use and their blood-gas partition coefficients are: desflurane (0.42) < nitrous oxide (0.47) < sevoflurane (0.65) < isoflurane (1.4) < enflurane (1.8) < halothane (2.3) < methoxyflurane (13.0). The more soluble the agent, the greater is the amount that will be carried away by blood in the pulmonary capillaries during uptake. Thus the rate of increase in the alveolar uptake curve is slowed. In contrast, the alveolar concentration of a relatively insoluble agent increases faster. In practical terms, the solubility of the inhalation agent in blood is the most important single factor in determining the speed of induction and of recovery in individual patients. Induction and recovery are fast with highly insoluble agents and slow with soluble ones.

Cardiac Output

Gases in the alveoli are in equilibrium with blood in the pulmonary capillaries. Therefore, how much anesthetic is removed from the lungs by pulmonary blood depends not only on the solubility of the agent but also on pulmonary blood flow. Alveolar anesthetic concentration rises slowly when cardiac output (pulmonary blood flow) is high. Cerebral blood flow usually remains normal in high cardiac output states, and most of the increase in flow is distributed to other tissues. Therefore, the slower rise in alveolar anesthetic concentration will slow the induction of anesthesia. Conversely, a low cardiac output will allow a faster rise in alveolar concentration and will speed up induction, provided cerebral blood flow is maintained.

Alveolar–Mixed Venous Tension Gradient

At the beginning of the alveolar uptake curve, the difference between the tension (partial pressure) of the anesthetic agent in alveolar gas and that in mixed venous blood is large. This gradient enhances the uptake of anesthetic by pulmonary blood and tends to slow the increase in alveolar concentration. As tissues and blood take up more anesthetic, this gradient decreases, and the effect of the alveolar–mixed venous tension gradient on uptake is less obvious.

Second Gas Effect

In previous sections it has been assumed that the volatile anesthetic is delivered to the airway in oxygen only. If a high concentration of nitrous oxide is also added to the inspired mixture, the uptake of a large amount of this agent into blood will decrease the volume of the mixture in the alveoli, increase the alveolar concentration of the volatile agent, and "draw in" more anesthetic mixture from the upper airway. This phenomenon, called the second gas effect, is an additional factor that contributes to increasing the rate of alveolar uptake of a volatile agent whenever nitrous oxide is used.

Practical Implications

Of the factors mentioned, inspired concentration, alveolar ventilation, solubility in blood, and the second gas effect can be manipulated to promote alveolar uptake and increase the speed of induction. The inspired concentration can be set high initially, ventilation can be enhanced with assistance, and nitrous oxide can be added to the anesthetic mixture. Choosing a less soluble agent is attractive, but the choice is often limited by other considerations (e.g., unwanted side effects).

■ Distribution and Tissue Uptake

Once an inhalation anesthetic is taken up by pulmonary blood, it is distributed to tissues of the body according to regional blood flow (see "Tissue Blood Flow and Tissue Mass" in Chapter 2). Tissues with the richest blood supply (brain, heart, liver, kidneys) take up the anesthetic rapidly. This rapid uptake of anesthetic by the brain means that its anesthetic partial pressure will very quickly come into equilibrium with that in the alveoli. This accounts for the efficiency of the respiratory tract as a route for administration of these inhaled anesthetic drugs.

■ Elimination

Excretion

Most of the inhalation agents are exhaled unchanged by the lungs. The fall in alveolar concentration follows an exponential decay curve (Fig. 3–4). The factors that influence this decay in alveolar concentration are exactly those that influence uptake, but the direction of the changes is reversed. Hyperventilation, a small FRC, a low solubility, a low cardiac output, or a large mixed venous–alveolar tension gradient increases the rate of

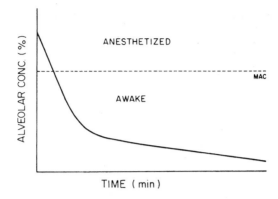

FIGURE 3–4. The fall in alveolar concentration of an inhalation anesthetic during emergence. It is an exponential decay curve, exactly the reverse of the exponential uptake curve that describes the rise in alveolar concentration during induction (Refer to text for details.)

decay. (Notice that "venous-alveolar" gradient instead of "alveolar-venous" gradient is used in describing excretion). Hypoventilation, a large FRC, a high solubility, a large cardiac output, or a small mixed venous–alveolar tension gradient decreases the rate of this decay. Because the inspired concentration of the agent is near zero during excretion, this factor has no influence on the rate of alveolar decay.

Metabolism

Until the mid-1960s, it was believed that all inhalation anesthetics were exhaled unchanged. Since then, it has been observed that a significant portion of these inhaled agents is metabolized by mixed-function oxidases (the cytochrome P450 system) in the liver. The degree of biotransformation varies according to the agent, and most of the water-soluble organic and inorganic metabolites are excreted by the kidneys. The significance of these findings for individual agents is discussed in the following section.

Specific Agents

Nitrous Oxide

Nitrous oxide is a colorless, odorless, and nonflammable gas approximately 1.5 times as heavy as air. It exists as a gas at room temperature and atmospheric pressure, but it can be compressed into a liquid unless its temperature is above 36.5° C. Medical-grade nitrous oxide is stored in cylinders as a liquid at room temperature under a pressure of 750 pounds per square inch (psi), or 50 atmospheres.

This agent is a weak anesthetic. Its MAC is 104%, a value that can be achieved only in the hyperbaric chamber. Normally no more than 70% nitrous oxide is administered in clinical practice, the other 30% being oxygen. After induction of anesthesia with an intravenous agent, it is given with a narcotic analgesic and a muscle relaxant to maintain anesthesia in the so-called balanced anesthesia technique. It is also used in combination with the more potent volatile agents. Because the MACs of nitrous oxide and other inhalation agents are additive (see "Minimum Alveolar Concentration" above), the use of nitrous oxide will reduce both the requirement of these agents and their side effects. In contradistinction to its weak anesthetic property, nitrous oxide is a good analgesic. Premixed 50% nitrous oxide in oxygen (Entonox and Nitronox) is used for pain relief in obstetrics and in dental surgery.

Few side effects are attributed to nitrous oxide. It does depress respiratory and myocardial function, but the degree of depression is small. It is also a cerebral vasodilator, particularly when it is used in combination with other volatile agents. Teratogenic effects have been observed in rats, and an increased incidence of spontaneous abortion has been reported in women who are chronically exposed to traces of nitrous oxide (e.g., operating room nurses and dental assistants). Administration of nitrous oxide for several days to patients during treatment of tetanus and poliomyelitis has also resulted in bone marrow depression and agranulocytosis.

Nitrous oxide is the only inorganic gas used in anesthesia today. It is not metabolized to any significant extent in the body.

Isoflurane

Isoflurane is a volatile, colorless, nonflammable liquid with a somewhat pungent odor. It is a halogenated ether and a prototypic agent, with pharmacologic properties qualitatively similar to those of the other volatile anesthetics.

Like the others, it causes a dose-related depression of the central nervous system. At anesthetic and subanesthetic concentrations, it reduces the cerebral metabolic rate for oxygen but increases cerebral blood flow and intracranial pressure. Changes in cerebral blood flow and intracranial pressure are only small in magnitude. Because cerebrovascular response to P_aCO_2 is preserved, its vasodilating action on cerebral blood vessels is effectively blocked by simultaneous hyperventilation. (Hyperventilation decreases P_aCO_2. Hypocapnia decreases cerebral blood flow.)

Respiratory depression is a major side effect of volatile anesthetics. Both the central chemoreceptor reflex (increase in ventilation in response to hypercapnia) and the peripheral chemoreceptor reflex (increase in ventilation in response to hypoxemia) are depressed. Patients anesthetized with volatile anesthetics breathe with a distinct pattern that is fast but shallow, but the increase in respiratory frequency with isoflurane is only slight. As a result, $PaCO_2$ is elevated but severe hypercapnia is seldom a problem. Like halothane and enflurane, isoflurane causes bronchodilation and has been used successfully to treat patients with acute asthma.

Isoflurane has only a mild myocardial depressant action. The drop in blood pressure seen in patients anesthetized with this agent is largely accounted for by a similar decrease in peripheral vascular resistance with little change in cardiac output. This property has made it nearly a perfect agent for inducing "controlled hypotension." It does not increase ventricular irritability and is compatible with infiltration of the surgical site with epinephrine (see "Halothane" below). Isoflurane would have been the agent of choice for patients who have coronary artery disease, except for the observation that it can shunt coronary blood flow away from collateral-dependent ischemic regions (a phenomenon known as coronary steal). However, there is no clear evidence that it does precipitate myocardial ischemia in these patients.

Another important side effect of isoflurane is its action on the gravid uterus. It can cause uterine relaxation, decrease the response of uterine muscle to oxytocin, and increase the incidence and severity of postpartum hemorrhage. Nevertheless, 1% isoflurane has been used during operative deliveries to prevent maternal awareness without increasing blood loss. With respect to its effect on skeletal muscles, it is arguable whether isoflurane has an intrinsic muscle-relaxant property, but it certainly potentiates the action of nondepolarizing muscle relaxants at the myoneural junction. When isoflurane is used to maintain anesthesia, the dose of the nondepolarizing muscle relaxant can be reduced by one third.

Although a newer agent, isoflurane has superseded halothane and enflurane as the most popular inhalation anesthetic. Its MAC is 1.15 and its blood-gas partition coefficient is 1.4. It is both potent and relatively insoluble in blood. Therefore, induction of and emergence from anesthesia is relatively rapid. It is more resistant to metabolic breakdown than halothane or enflurane. Less than 1% of the dose taken up by the body is metabolized. No clear evidence of hepatoxicity or nephrotoxicity attributable to isoflurane has been reported to date.

Halothane

Halothane is the most established inhalation agent in use today. Whereas all the other inhalation anesthetics in clinical use are halogenated ethers, halothane is a halogenated ethane. Its physical and pharmacologic properties are qualitatively similar to those of isoflurane, but there are major differences:

1. It is more potent than isoflurane; the MAC is 0.77. With a blood-gas partition coefficient of 2.3, it is more soluble in blood than isoflurane. Therefore, induction of and emergence from halothane anesthesia is slower (see "Solubility of Anesthetic Agent" above).

2. It is a more potent cerebral vasodilator than isoflurane, which cannot be easily counteracted by hyperventilation. It also causes a larger increase in intracranial pressure than isoflurane, making it less suitable for neurosurgical procedures.

3. The two agents cause similar respiratory depression, but patients under halothane anesthesia breathe with a distinct pattern that is fast and shallow. Like isoflurane, it is a useful bronchodilator.

4. It has a pleasant odor and is less irritating to the airway than isoflurane—properties that make the task of inhalation induction of anesthesia easier.

5. Nodal rhythm and a fall in arterial blood pressure are commonly seen during halothane anesthesia. Hypotension is particularly marked when halothane is given together with d-tubocurarine. The mechanism of its hypotensive effect is probably a combination of peripheral vasodilation, myocardial depression, depression of the vasomotor center, sympathetic ganglionic blockade, and inhibition of the baroreceptor reflex. (When baroreceptor reflex is depressed, vasoconstriction and increase in heart rate in response to a fall in blood pressure are inhibited.)

6. Another prominent cardiac side effect of halothane is ventricular irritability. This problem is especially serious if the surgical field is infiltrated with epinephrine for hemostasis. It is recommended that the dose of epinephrine be limited to 10 ml of a 1:100,000 concentration in short procedures or to 30 ml of the same concentration in 1 hour during halothane anesthesia. Other factors that increase the incidence of ventricular arrhythmias during halothane anesthesia are surgical stimulation and hypercapnia. This increase in ventricular excitability can usually be controlled by an adequate depth of anesthesia and analgesia, by replacing part of the halothane with nitrous oxide, and by assisting the patient's ventilation. If the ventricular arrhythmia remains troublesome despite the above remedies, halothane should be replaced with one of the other volatile agents.

7. In equipotent concentrations, halothane and isoflurane have an equal relaxant effect on the gravid uterus. No more than 0.5% should be used in obstetric patients for operative deliveries, except when relaxation of the uterus is desirable (e.g., for external version or delivery of retained placenta.)

8. Approximately 20% of the dose taken up by the body is metabolized in the liver in humans; the rest is exhaled unchanged. The water-soluble metabolites (bromide, chloride, and trifluoroacetic acid) are excreted in urine.

9. Halothane is associated with a rare and somewhat ill-defined complication known as *halothane hepatitis*, a syndrome characterized by postoperative fever, eosinophilia, and hepatic dysfunction with or without jaundice. The incidence is said to be higher with repeated exposures, particularly when they are close in time. It is recommended that patients not be exposed to halothane again for at least *3 months* after a halothane anesthetic.

Enflurane

Enflurane, like isoflurane, is a halogenated ether. It was introduced into anesthesia practice after halothane but before isoflurane and gained popularity because of the concern over halothane hepatitis following repeated exposure. Pharmacologically, it is distinguishable from both isoflurane and halothane by the following qualities:

1. Enflurane is not as potent as isoflurane, its MAC being 1.7. Its blood-gas partition coefficient of 1.8 is less than that of halothane and closer to that of isoflurane. So induction of and emergence from anesthesia are slightly more rapid with enflurane than with halothane.

2. Under enflurane anesthesia, approximately 2% of patients exhibit EEG patterns of seizure activity with or without muscle twitches, particularly in the presence of hypocapnia. The significance of these findings is unclear, but enflurane is not contraindicated in epilepsy patients.

3. The cerebrovascular dilation action of enflurane is between that of isoflurane and halothane. Intracranial pressure increases to a lesser extent under enflurane anesthesia than under halothane anesthesia.

4. Enflurane has a considerably more potent respiratory depressant effect than halothane and isoflurane at equivalent anesthetic concentrations. It has a pleasant odor, but it is slightly more irritating to the upper airway than halothane.

5. Enflurane has a somewhat more potent circulatory depressant effect than halothane and isoflurane. Ventricular arrhythmias are much less common with enflurane than with halothane, and interaction with epinephrine is highly variable.

Infiltration of the surgical site with epinephrine in patients under enflurane anesthesia is not contraindicated, but caution is required.

6. The muscle relaxant property of enflurane is more potent than that of halothane and similar to that of isoflurane.

7. Enflurane 1% does not increase blood loss in patients undergoing operative deliveries.

8. Only 2−4% of enflurane taken up by the human body is metabolized. Metabolism results in a low serum concentration of inorganic fluoride, which is potentially nephrotoxic. This is of little clinical significance except in patients whose renal function is already impaired.

Desflurane

Desflurane is a new halogenated ether with a molecular structure similar to that of isoflurane. These two agents share many common pharmacologic properties, but desflurane also has certain unique qualities:

1. Of all the inhalation agents, desflurane is the most volatile. Its boiling point of 23.5° C almost equals room temperature. It must be dispensed like a gas from a pressurized heated vaporizer.

2. It is the least potent inhalation agent in clinical use, its MAC being 6%.

3. Its blood-gas partition coefficient of 0.42 is even lower than the 0.47 of nitrous oxide. It is the most insoluble inhalation agent in use and is compatible with rapid induction and recovery.

4. It has sympathomimetic properties. Rapid increase in desflurane concentration during inhalation induction can lead to tachycardia and hypertension.

5. It is more resistant to biodegradation than any of the other halogenated inhalation anesthetics, giving it little potential for systemic toxicity.

Sevoflurane

Sevoflurane is a halogenated ether approved for general clinical use in North America in 1995. Compared to isoflurane, it has the following clinical profile:

1. Its MAC of 2.05% is almost twice that of isoflurane (see Table 3−1).

2. With a blood-gas partition coefficient of 0.65, it is almost as insoluble in blood as nitrous oxide and desflurane. Thus

induction of and recovery from sevoflurane anesthesia are more rapid than those associated with isoflurane anesthesia. Its low blood solubility also makes rapid adjustment of anesthetic depth possible.

3. Its smell is nonpungent and it does not irritate the respiratory tract. Together with its low blood solubility, these properties make it pleasant for inhalation induction. It is associated with a dose-dependent depression of respiratory function. Like isoflurane, sevoflurane depresses both central and peripheral chemoreceptor reflexes.

4. The cardiovascular effects of sevoflurane are comparable to those of isoflurane: blood pressure, peripheral vascular resistance, and cardiac output are well maintained; risk of spontaneous ventricular arrhythmias is minimal; and sensitization of the myocardium to the arrhythmogenic effects of epinephrine is not seen.

5. The central nervous system effects of sevoflurane are similar to those of isoflurane: central nervous system depression is dose related, cerebral metabolic rate for oxygen is reduced, cerebral blood flow and intracranial pressure are elevated, but cerebrovascular responsiveness to P_aCO_2 is preserved.

6. Like isoflurane, no hepatotoxicity has been associated with sevoflurane.

7. Although less than 5% of sevoflurane taken up by the body is metabolized, plasma inorganic fluoride levels of 50 μmol/L and higher have been reported. Plasma fluoride levels this high have been associated with methoxyflurane nephrotoxicity, but such is not the case with sevoflurane. (Methoxyflurane is a halogenated ether that has been removed from clinical use because of nephrotoxicity.) Most investigators do not even find biochemical or subclinical signs of altered renal function in patients who have high plasma fluoride levels associated with sevoflurane anesthesia. Sevoflurane is spared from being nephrotoxic partly because of its insolubility in blood and tissues. It is eliminated rapidly from the body following emergence from anesthesia. Although plasma fluoride concentration peaks at a high level, this level is not sustained. Methoxyflurane, in contrast, is highly soluble in blood and tissues, its blood-gas partition coefficient being 13.0. As much as 50% of the methoxyflurane taken up by the body is metabolized. Following emergence from methoxyflurane anesthesia, much of this agent remains in tissue depots, and the plasma fluoride level is kept high through its gradual breakdown. Furthermore, human kidneys metabolize methoxyflurane much more avidly than sevoflurane, yielding intrarenally generated fluoride and other metabolites. This may be a second reason why methoxyflurane is nephrotoxic and sevoflurane is not, despite the fact that both can yield high levels of plasma inorganic fluoride levels.

8. Unlike isoflurane, sevoflurane can react with carbon dioxide absorbents (soda lime and Baralyme) to yield five poten-

tial breakdown products. Compound A, a fluorinated vinyl ether, is consistently found in clinical settings when sevoflurane is used in combination with the circle system (see "The Circle System" in Chapter 8). Compound A production is higher with Baralyme than soda lime and increases with low fresh gas flow and high absorbent temperature. Because low-flow anesthesia and high absorbent temperature come hand in hand, fresh gas flow rates below 2 L/min are not recommended. Compound A is a nephrotoxin in laboratory rats, and toxicity is dose related, but there is no evidence of clinical or subclinical nephrotoxicity and hepatotoxocity in humans following sevoflurane anesthesia.

Opioids

4

The opioids are narcotic analgesics; their main application in the practice of anesthesia today is to relieve pain, either during surgery or in the postoperative period. Since the 1970s, large doses of opioids (mainly morphine and the fentanyls) have also been used to induce and maintain anesthesia in patients undergoing cardiac operations and in those who are critically ill.

Mechanism of Action

The discovery of opioid receptors in the early 1970s has expanded our knowledge of pain and its treatment. These opioid receptors are widely scattered throughout the entire central nervous system, but they are more concentrated in the limbic system, the thalamus and hypothalamus, the striatum, the reticular activating system in the midbrain, and the substantia gelatinosa of the spinal cord. They are also found in nerve plexuses of intestines. Opioid molecules interact with these receptors to produce all the observed effects described in this chapter. There are endogenous polypeptides that can interact with these receptors to produce effects not unlike those of morphine-like drugs; these are the enkephalins, beta-endorphin, and the dynorphins. Five species of opioid receptors have been identified: the mu (μ), the delta (δ), the kappa (κ), the sigma (σ), and the epsilon (ϵ). Furthermore, two subtypes of μ and three subtypes of κ receptors exist. The major pharmacologic actions mediated by these receptors are listed in Table 4–1.

There are a supraspinal and a spinal mechanism of analgesic action. In the supraspinal system, the sites of action are the periacqueductal and periventricular gray areas; in the spinal mechanism, the site of action is receptors in the substantia gelatinosa region of the spinal cord (see "Pain and Pain Control Pathways" in Chapter 19).

Morphine, an *agonist*, acts primarily on the μ-receptors and, to a lesser extent, on the κ receptors. Some compounds bind these receptors and exert only limited morphine-like actions; they are *partial agonists*. Other compounds compete with mor-

TABLE 4–1. Major Pharmacologic Actions Mediated by
Opioid Receptors

RECEPTOR	SUBTYPE	PHARMACOLOGIC ACTIONS
μ	μ₁	Supraspinal analgesia, sedation
	μ₂	Spinal analgesia, respiratory depression, euphoria, physical dependence
δ		Spinal analgesia
κ	κ₁	Spinal analgesia
	κ₂	Unknown
	κ₃	Supraspinal analgesia
σ		Dysphoria, hallucination, cardiac stimulation
ε		Hormonal response

phine for these receptors but exert no morphine-like actions; they are *competitive antagonists.* Still others exert antagonist-like or weak agonist-like actions at the μ receptors and agonist-like actions at the κ and σ receptors; they are *agonist-antagonists.*

■ Morphine

Systemic Effects

Crude opium has been used as medicine since biblical times, mainly for its antidiarrheal effect. Morphine, a pure alkaloid, was not isolated until 1803 and has been exploited since for its antidiarrheal, antitussive, and analgesic properties. Morphine is a prototypic agonist; its pharmacologic actions are common to all other agonists.

Central Nervous System

The effects of morphine on the central nervous system are both depressive and stimulatory. Depression leads to analgesia, sedation, mood changes, and alveolar hypoventilation. Stimulation leads to pupillary constriction, nausea and vomiting, hyperactive spinal reflexes, and convulsions.

Many central nervous system depressants can produce a state of analgesia, but only together with gross impairment of intellectual function or unconsciousness. Morphine and other opioid agonists, in contrast, are selective analgesics because they can produce profound analgesia with no effects on other sensory modalities. After an analgesic dose of morphine, most patients who are experiencing pain will feel relaxed, tranquil, and drowsy, provided nausea or vomiting is not a problem. However, morphine alone has poor amnestic properties and is not a complete anesthetic; many patients who had even ultra-high doses of morphine for anesthesia could recall intraoperative events vividly.

Alveolar hypoventilation is a result of the direct action of morphine on respiratory centers at the brain stem. The degree of respiratory depression is dose related. Death from an overdose is invariably caused by respiratory failure. Even after a therapeutic dose, responsiveness of the respiratory centers to a rise in P_aCO_2 is obtunded. Although tidal volume remains relatively unchanged, respiratory rate is diminished and minute volume is reduced. Suppression of the cough reflex and a decrease in the frequency of sighing are also part of this depression. Maximum respiratory effects occur between 5 and 10 minutes after an intravenous dose and between 30 and 60 minutes after an intramuscular dose. Therefore, morphine is contraindicated in patients with respiratory insufficiency, unless artificial ventilation is instituted.

Pupillary constriction is an unmistakable side effect of morphine, and pinpoint pupils are the hallmark of an overdose. Miosis is due to stimulation of the parasympathetic component of the third cranial (oculomotor) nerve nucleus. Morphine also stimulates the chemoreceptor trigger zone at the medulla directly, causing nausea and vomiting. This unpleasant side effect is often delayed and is potentiated by ambulation. Truncal rigidity, a result of hyperactive spinal reflexes, is seen occasionally following intravenous administration of morphine and frequently following administration of fentanyl, but convulsion occurs with extremely high doses only.

Cardiovascular System

Morphine produces a dose-dependent bradycardia by direct stimulation of the vagal nucleus, but it does not depress myocardial contractility. Therapeutic doses of morphine have little effect on hemodynamic function in young, healthy adults when they are lying supine. However, morphine is a potent dilator of resistance and capacitance vessels (arterioles and veins), and orthostatic hypotension is a common side effect in ambulatory patients. Its peripheral action is largely the result of histamine release.

Respiratory System

Besides its effects on the control of breathing (see "Central Nervous System" above), morphine can induce bronchial constriction, caused in part by histamine release. Although this is of no consequence in healthy persons, morphine is contraindicated in patients with asthma or bronchitis who are having an acute attack of bronchospasm. It should also be used cautiously in those who have chronic airway obstruction.

Gastrointestinal Tract

Morphine stimulates the smooth muscle of the gastrointestinal tract, but propulsive peristalsis is diminished and segmental tonic contraction is increased. The consequence is an increase in bowel transit time and constipation. Owing to spasm of Oddi's sphincter, pressure in the biliary tree can rise substantially after the administration of morphine. Many patients with gallbladder disease will develop biliary colic after a therapeutic dose of morphine; this phenomenon can occur even years after cholecystectomy. The sudden onset of pain in these patients may be confused with acute myocardial ischemia. This spasm can be reversed with the administration of naloxone or nitroglycerine, but only partially with the administration of atropine. Whereas naloxone will relieve morphine-induced biliary colic but not the pain of myocardial ischemia, nitroglycerine will relieve both. These differential actions can be used to distinguish colic from angina.

Genitourinary Tract

Therapeutic doses of morphine increase contractions of the lower third of the ureter, but this is of little clinical significance. However, spasm of the bladder sphincter can lead to urinary retention.

Other Effects

Morphine has no direct effects on cerebral circulation. However, hypercapnia following a therapeutic dose of morphine can increase cerebral blood flow to cause a rise in intracranial pressure in patients with intracranial space-occupying lesions. Furthermore, the sedative and pupillary effects of morphine can interfere with assessment of neurologic functions in these patients. Therefore, morphine and morphine-like opioids should be used with caution in neurosurgery.

It is said that therapeutic doses of morphine stimulate the release of antidiuretic hormone (ADH) and inhibit the stress-induced release of adrenocorticotropic hormone (ACTH). These observations are of little clinical significance.

Tolerance and Addiction

Tolerance to a drug is characterized by the need for increasing doses to obtain the same therapeutic effect after repeated exposure. Tolerance to morphine is obvious only with its depressant effects (e.g., analgesia and respiratory depression) and not with its excitatory effects (e.g., pupillary constriction and constipation). Tolerance to morphine is a reversible phenomenon, and sensitivity to a therapeutic dose will return to normal after an abstinence of 1–2 weeks. Despite differences in molecular structure, cross-tolerance occurs between morphine and other opioid agonists. The mechanism of both tolerance and cross-tolerance is unclear.

Addiction is a state of psychological and physical dependence that manifests itself in the withdrawal syndrome. Mild physical dependence can occur as early as 24 hours after the first dose of morphine if it is given regularly (e.g., for pain in the immediate postoperative period). In long-term addicts, signs of withdrawal usually appear approximately 8 hours after the last dose. They are mild at first and the patient appears anxious and restless. The syndrome progresses over the next several hours, reaches a peak in 48–72 hours, and runs its course in 5–10 days. It is characterized by lacrimation, rhinorrhea, diaphoresis, vomiting and diarrhea, incessant yawning, gooseflesh, dilated pupils, hypertension, tachycardia, abdominal cramps, and muscle aches. Cross-dependence between morphine and other opioid agonists can occur. The administration of an opioid antagonist or agonist-antagonist to patients addicted to morphine or other agonists will precipitate this syndrome. The mechanism of addition, like that of tolerance, is not known.

Drug Interaction

Phenothiazines counteract the emetic effect of morphine but potentiate its analgesic, sedative, and respiratory depressant effects. Similarly, the depressive effects on respiratory centers caused by opioid agonists and those caused by intravenous and inhalation anesthetics are additive.

Allergy and Idiosyncrasy

Allergic reactions to morphine are rare. Wheals and itch at the site of injection are local reactions to histamine release and should not be considered signs of true allergy. Many patients regard nausea and vomiting following morphine injection as an allergic manifestation. Careful questioning will reveal details of the event so that these reactions can be confirmed to be mere side effects.

Uptake, Distribution, and Elimination

Morphine is given subcutaneously, intramuscularly, or intravenously in anesthetic practice and intrathecally or epidurally as well in the management of postoperative pain. The absorption half-life of a dose is approximately 30 minutes after subcutaneous injection and around 8 minutes after intramuscular injection. (The absorption half-life is the time required for 50% of the dose given to be absorbed from the subcutaneous or intramuscular depot.) After absorption, approximately one third of the drug appearing in plasma is protein bound (mainly to albumin). At physiologic pH, only 10% of it exists in the nonionized form. In addition, because morphine is relatively lipid insoluble, only a small fraction of a given dose crosses the blood-brain barrier to act on opioid receptors (see "Protein Binding" and "Physical Characteristics of the Drug" in Chapter 2).

Following intravenous injection of a bolus of morphine, plasma concentration rises and falls in a manner similar to that seen after the administration of an intravenous anesthetic (see "Peak Concentration" and "Distribution" in Chapter 2). Decline in plasma concentration during the distribution phase is rapid because of uptake into lean body mass.

The major pathways for elimination of morphine from the body are conjugation in the liver with glucuronic acid and excretion of the water-soluble metabolite by the kidneys. The hepatic extraction ratio approaches 1. Nearly 90% of an injected dose is recovered in urine within 24 hours. The other 10% is excreted in bile and appears in feces.

Applications in Anesthetic Practice

Morphine is still a popular opioid used in all aspects of anesthetic care of the surgical patient. In combination with a parasympatholytic agent (e.g., atropine or hyoscine) or a phenothiazine (e.g., chlorpromazine or prochlorperazine), it is useful as a preanesthetic sedative. In the operating room, it is given intravenously as an analgesic adjuvant to supplement general anesthesia. Large doses of morphine or one of the fentanyls have also been used as a primary anesthetic in cardiac and critically ill patients. Although these opioids can replace the volatile inhalation anesthetics and reduce their MAC by 60−80% in a dose-related fashion, there is a *ceiling effect* beyond which further increases in the dose of opioids cause no further reduction in MAC. Therefore, these narcotic analgesic agents should not be regarded as reliable total anesthetics. When an opioid is used as the main anesthetic, small doses of a benzodiazepine or low concentrations of a volatile agent should be added as an adjuvant when required.

By far the most popular use of morphine in surgical patients is to relieve pain. In this respect, morphine is prescribed on the basis that it is given only when necessary. For pain of moderate intensity, a dose of 10−15 mg given subcutaneously or intramuscularly every 4 hours is usually adequate in adults. If pain is severe, the intravenous route is recommended; increments of 1−2 mg may be given as required. Other methods include intrathecal or epidural injection. These methods are discussed in detail in Chapter 19. It must be stressed that the analgesic dose of opioids varies according to the intensity of pain; dose should be titrated against effect. (Oxymorphone and hydromorphone are semisynthetic derivatives of morphine. Their pharmacologic actions are similar to those of the parent compound, but they are 8−10 times more potent.)

Other Agonists

Papaveretum

Papaveretum is a mixture of purified opium alkaloids, of which 50% is morphine. Its actions and fate are similar to those of its major component. Satisfactory pain relief can be obtained with a dose of 10−20 mg given subcutaneously or intramuscularly every 4 hours or 2−4 mg intravenously when necessary.

Meperidine

Meperidine is a synthetic agent whose molecular formula is quite different from that of morphine. However, the actions and side effects of these two agents are quite similar, except that

1. Meperidine has atropine-like effects that include dry mouth and blurred vision.
2. Fewer patients given meperidine are troubled with constipation. Its spasmogenic effect on the biliary tract and Oddi's sphincter is also less.
3. Pupillary constriction following an equianalgesic dose of meperidine is not as marked as that after morphine.
4. It is the most effective agent in stopping postoperative shivering, for which a dose of 20−25 mg is given intravenously.
5. Unlike morphine, large doses of meperidine have a discernible depressant effect on myocardial function. An increase in heart rate following intravenous injection of meperidine is also common.

6. The duration of action of meperidine is shorter than that of morphine.

Meperidine is much more lipid soluble than morphine. Also, more of it is bound to plasma protein—mainly glycoprotein and, to a lesser extent, albumin. It is transformed in the liver by hydrolysis, conjugation, and demthylation. The hepatic extraction ratio is slightly less than that of morphine. The products of hepatic detoxification are excreted in urine. Very little meperidine is excreted unchanged, but excretion of the unchanged fraction can be increased by acidification of urine (see discussion of ion trapping under "Physical Characteristics of the Drug" in Chapter 2).

Meperidine is only one tenth as potent as morphine. For analgesia, a dose of 75−125 mg is given intramuscularly every 3−4 hours, or 15−25 mg intravenously when necessary. Because meperidine can cause local irritation, it is not given subcutaneously.

Fentanyl and its Congeners

Fentanyl

Fentanyl, a synthetic agent related to meperidine, is 100 times more potent than morphine. It is even more lipid soluble than meperidine and crosses tissue barriers with ease. Following an intravenous bolus, the uptake and distribution of fentanyl is qualitatively similar to that of morphine, but a large fraction may be sequestered by the lungs during its first pass through this organ, before it reaches the systemic circulation. The rapid fall in plasma concentration during the distribution phase is due to tissue uptake, including that by fat. It is metabolized in the liver by N-dealkylation and hydroxylation, and the metabolites are excreted in urine. The hepatic extraction ratio approaches 1.

The degree and duration of respiratory depression following fentanyl are dose related, but the respiratory depressant effect may last longer than its analgesic action. Truncal rigidity following intravenous administration of large doses is a common observation, but signs of histamine release are rare. This opioid is free of circulatory depressant effects, although bradycardia can occur with very large doses.

The duration of analgesic action after a single intravenous dose of fentanyl, 1.5 μg/kg, is approximately 30 minutes. Owing to this short duration of action, fentanyl by injection is not useful for treatment of pain that is persistent; it is more useful either as an analgesic supplement during surgery or as a principle anesthetic in cardiac surgery. As the former, 1−3 μg/kg is given initially at the beginning and 25−50 μg subsequently every 30 minutes when required. As the latter, 50−150 μg/kg is given slowly for induction and maintenance of anesthesia. Intraoperative awareness has not been reported with doses larger than 120 μg/kg, but hypertension in reaction to surgical stimulation can still occur. Therefore, fentanyl should not be regarded as a total anesthetic. Even when high-dose fentanyl is used, the practitioner should be prepared to add small doses of a benzodiazepine or a low concentration of a volatile anesthetic to ensure amnesia and hypnosis. A common problem seen with induction doses of fentanyl is the development of truncal rigidity before loss of consciousness. This reaction can be abolished by giving a small dose of muscle relaxant and instituting manual ventilation of the lungs.

Sufentanil

Sufentanil and its parent compound fentanyl have similar lipid solubility and uptake and distribution characteristics, but uptake into tissue stores is less. It is broken down in the liver by oxidative dealkylation into inactive metabolites that are excreted in urine and feces. Like fentanyl, its hepatic extraction ratio approaches 1. Because accumulation in tissue stores is limited, recovery is faster from sufentanil than from fentanyl.

The pharmacologic properties of the two congeners are similar, but sufentanil appears to have a more pronounced negative chronotropic effect on the heart. It is also a more potent respiratory depressant, and instances of patients remaining apneic after regaining consciousness have been observed. Being 5−10 times as potent as fentanyl, sufentanil is more effective than the parent compound in blocking the pressor response to noxious stimuli, but it is still not a complete anesthetic.

Sufentanil is seldom used in operations that last less than 1 hour. To supplement anesthesia, 0.4−0.7 μg/kg is given at the beginning of surgery, to be followed by increments of 10−15 μg when required. In cardiac surgery, 10−30 μg/kg is given slowly during induction, but an anesthetic adjuvant (benzodiazepine or inhalation agent) should be added when necessary to prevent awareness.

Alfentanil

Alfentanil is another congener that is only one fifth to one third as potent as fentanyl. However, it is associated with a higher incidence of nausea and vomiting. It is extensively metabolized in the liver and small intestine. Although its rate of clearance is only half that of fentanyl, it is eliminated from the body faster because of very limited accumulation in body stores. Times to awakening, orientation, and ambulation following a therapeutic dose of alfentanil are significantly shorter than those following an equipotent dose of fentanyl or sufentanil. It is given in incremental doses to supplement inhalational anesthesia or in a continuous infusion together with an intravenous anesthetic in total intravenous anesthesia (TIVA). When the operation is not expected to exceed 30 minutes, 5–20 μg/kg should be given initially, to be followed by increments of 2.5 μg/kg as required. The total dose should be limited to 5–40 μg/kg. When surgery is expected to last between 30 and 60 minutes, 20–50 μg/kg should be given at the beginning, to be followed by increments of 5–15 μg/kg when indicated. The total dose should not exceed 75 μg/kg. When a continuous infusion is contemplated for operations longer than 45 minutes, a loading dose of 50–75 μg/kg should be given at the beginning, to be followed by an infusion of 0.5–1.5 μg/kg/min. In the last two instances, endotracheal intubation together with controlled ventilation are recommended.

Remifentanil

Remifentanil, a new congener being investigated for use in anesthesia practice, has a potency between that of fentanyl and sufentanil. Its molecule has an ester side chain that is easily hydrolyzed by blood and tissue esterases to yield metabolites that have only weak agonist actions. The elimination half-life of the parent compound is about 12 minutes. Its potency and rapid elimination make it well suited for titration of dose and continuous infusion.

> **Precautions:** Fentanyl and all its congeners are potent respiratory depressants. Transient apnea requiring assisted ventilation is not uncommon when incremental doses are given to patients who are breathing spontaneously. When anesthetic doses are used, controlled ventilation may have to be continued well into the postoperative period until the patient has recovered from the respiratory depressant effect.

Codeine

Codeine is another naturally occurring opium alkaloid. When given parenterally, its analgesic potency is only one sixth to one tenth that of morphine. However, it is widely used as an oral analgesic because only a relatively small fraction of codeine in portal venous blood is cleared by the liver immediately following enteric absorption (relatively low first-pass hepatic clearance). In fact, part of the codeine in portal venous blood is converted to morphine in the liver. Eventually elimination of codeine is by conjugation in the liver and by excretion of water-soluble metabolites in urine.

An analgesic dose of codeine has little effect on mental state, pupil size, and respiration. This lack of side effects is a distinct advantage in neurological and ambulatory patients. Otherwise use of codeine parenterally for analgesia is not popular. Usually a dose of 30−60 mg is given subcutaneously or intramuscularly every 3−4 hours for the treatment of pain following surgery. This dose can also be given orally for minor pain. (Oxycodone and hydrocodone are semisynthetic derivatives of codeine. Whereas oxycodone is formulated with acetylsalicylate or acetaminophen and used as an oral analgesic, hydrocodone is only employed in antitussive medications.)

Alphaprodine

Alphaprodine is another synthetic agent resembling meperidine in pharmacologic actions, but it has an even shorter duration of action (1−2 hours following subcutaneous injection). Usually a dose of 5−10 mg is given intravenously when necessary to supplement general anesthesia.

Agonist-Antagonists and Partial Agonists

Pentazocine

Pentazocine was synthesized in the 1960s during a search for a potent analgesic without addicting properties. It is an agonist-antagonist with potent agonist but mild antagonist actions. This agent differs from morphine in the following ways:

1. The degree of respiratory depression produced by an analgesic dose of pentazocine is similar to that produced by an equianalgesic dose of morphine, but increasing the dose of pentazocine does not produce further respiratory depression. This ceiling effect on respiratory depression is seen also with the agonist-antagonists nalbuphine and butorphanol and the partial agonist buprenorphine.

2. In general, the stimulatory actions of pentazocine on smooth muscle of the gastrointestinal tract are much milder than those of morphine.

3. Unlike morphine, pentazocine given intravenously can produce a rise in systemic and pulmonary arterial pressures as well as elevation of left ventricular end-diastolic pressure. Its circulatory depressant effect is particularly obvious in patients with heart disease.

4. Being an agent with mild antagonist actions, pentazocine can precipitate the withdrawal syndrome in patients addicted to morphine or other opioids.

5. Dysphoria is a frequent side effect of pentazocine.

6. The potential for abuse of pentazocine is low, but psychological and physical dependence in emotionally unstable patients has been reported.

Because of its low potential for abuse, the main application of pentazocine is in the treatment of chronic pain. It has also been used for premedication and for pain relief in the postoperative period. A dose of 30–60 mg is given subcutaneously or intramuscularly every 3–4 hours. It is also effective in the treatment of minor surgical pain when given orally; the usual adult dose is 50 mg every 4 hours after meals.

Nalbuphine

Nalbuphine is structurally related to oxycodone (an agonist) and naloxone (an antagonist). A ceiling effect is seen with both its respiratory depressant and analgesic effects. It can precipitate a withdrawal reaction in patients addicted to morphine-like drugs. It is used in anesthesia practice for postoperative pain relief, the dose being 10–20 mg subcutaneously or intramuscularly every 3–6 hours as required. It is also used to antagonize the respiratory depressant effect and relieve the pruritis associated with epidural or spinal opioids given for pain relief. The dose should be titrated carefully to obtain the desired effect without affecting analgesia.

Butorphanol

The analgesic potency of butorphanol is five times that of morphine. Like other agents of its class, it has a ceiling effect on respiratory depression. It can be given transnasally as a spray for pain relief. The dose is 1–2 mg every 3–4 hours as required.

Buprenorphine

Buprenorphine is a partial agonist that has a strong affinity for μ receptors. Once bound, buprenorphine dissociates from these receptors very slowly. This receptor affinity has given buprenorphine some unique properties:

1. If buprenorphine is given first, it can block the action or decrease the potency of other μ receptor agonists that have weaker receptor affinity (e.g., morphine).

2. Naloxone, an antagonist (see "Antagonists" below), can block the respiratory depressant action of buprenorphine if naloxone is given first, but naloxone may have difficulty reversing buprenorphine-induced respiratory depression that is already established.

3. During abstinence, patients addicted to buprenorphine will develop the withdrawal syndrome, but it can take days to 2 weeks to express itself.

Buprenorphine can be given intramuscularly or slowly intravenously. The dose is 0.3−0.6 mg every 4−6 hours.

■ Antagonists

Naloxone

The original "antagonists" used in anesthetic practice were nalorphine and levallorphan. They are in fact agonist-antagonists. Naloxone, in contrast, is a pure opioid antagonist. Although it is devoid of morphine-like agonist activities, it will promptly reverse the morphine-like actions of all opioids and will precipitate a full-blown withdrawal syndrome in addicts. Following administration of naloxone to patients who have received a therapeutic dose of morphine, respiratory rate increases, drowsiness disappears, pupils dilate, Oddi's sphincter relaxes, and blood pressure, if depressed, returns to normal. Likewise, naloxone reverses the agonist actions of pentazocine, butorphanol, and nalbuphine. In addition to these specific antagonist actions, naloxone also has a mild, nonspecific action on the central nervous system and partially reverses the depressant effects of pentobarbital and diazepam. This agent is poorly absorbed via the gastrointestinal tract and must be given by injection. It is metabolized in the liver, chiefly by conjugation with glucuronic acid.

The major indication for naloxone in the practice of anesthesia is to treat excessive respiratory depression induced by opioids. The dose is 100 μg to be given intravenously and repeated when necessary. Its effect is obvious within 1−2 minutes following injection. With careful titration, it is possible to reverse excessive respiratory depression without depriving the patient of adequate analgesia. If the dose of naloxone is excessive, an "overshoot" phenomenon characterized by hyperpnea, agitation, and hypertension is seen. Therefore, careful titration is mandatory. Because the duration of action of most opioids will outlast that of a single intravenous dose of nalox-one, patients should be observed until the effect of the agonist has worn off.

Naltrexone

This long-acting antagonist is active following oral adminis-tration. It is given to addicts to discourage their habit by block-ing the euphoric effect of opioids. Otherwise it has found little application in anesthesia practice.

Muscle Relaxants 5

All resting muscles have tone. There is a tendency for them to resist being stretched because small groups of muscle fibers are contracting at random; in fact they contract when stretched. If conduction of impulses in a motor nerve is interrupted, the muscle it innervates becomes flaccid. In the practice of anesthesia, muscle relaxation refers to the suppression of this resting muscle tone and stretch reflex. Usually only a mild degree of relaxation is required for operations on the body wall and extremities, but profound relaxation is required for operations within body cavities.

In the era of ether anesthesia, profound relaxation suitable for upper abdominal operations was obtained by increasing the depth of anesthesia to Plane 2 or 3 of Stage III (see "Stages of Ether Anesthesia" in Chapter 1). In current practice, use of muscle relaxants has allowed the anesthesiologist to obtain the desired degree of muscle relaxation without resorting to dangerous depression of the central nervous system. Since the introduction of curare more than 5 decades ago, many compounds of diverse origin have been found to possess muscle-relaxant properties. These compounds block the transmission of neural impulses between motor nerve endings and muscle fibers. In order to understand the mechanism of their action, it is necessary to review the sequence of events during normal neuromuscular transmission.

Neuromuscular Transmission

Anatomy of the neuromuscular junction and the physiology of neuromuscular transmission are summarized in Figure 5–1. Each motor nerve fiber (motor neuron) innervates several muscle fibers (muscle cells). Together they form a functional entity called the *motor unit*. Before it approaches these muscle fibers, the nerve fiber sheds its myelin sheath and divides into a number of terminal buttons. Each of these buttons synapses with a muscle fiber at the motor end-plate—a thickened area of muscle cell membrane thrown into folds. The synaptic gap or cleft is $0.02-0.05$ μm in width and the chemical messenger traversing it is acetylcholine. It is the product of acetylation of choline, a process catalyzed by the enzyme choline acetyltransferase. This transmitter substance is stored in clear vesicles, each of which contains 5000–10,000 acetylcholine molecules and is called a quantum of acetylcholine. Approximately 20% of these vesicles are easily mobilized for release; the rest act as a depot from which the readily available store is replenished.

On arrival of an impulse at the motor nerve ending, a fixed number of quanta (vesicles) of acetylcholine are released into the neuromuscular cleft by exocytosis (reverse pinocystosis). This process is facilitated by the influx of calcium ions during depolarization of the motor nerve. Following release, acetylcholine diffuses rapidly across the synaptic cleft to bind stereospecific receptor sites at the entrance of acetylcholine-gated ion channels in the muscle end-plate membrane.

> **Note:** The definitions of ligand-gated and voltage-gated channels apply equally to nerve and muscle fibers. Please review these definitions under "Action on Nerve Cell Membrane Ion Channels" in Chapter 1 before going on to the next sections.

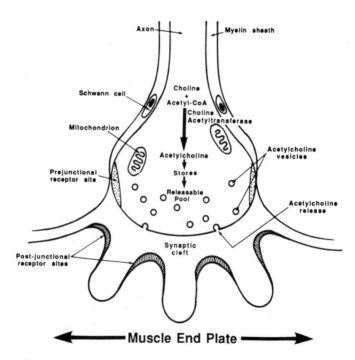

FIGURE 5–1. An illustration of the neuromuscular junction with presynaptic and postsynaptic acetylcholine receptor sites. (Refer to text for details.)

Structurally, each of these acetylcholine-gated nonselective channels for cations (positively charged ions) is formed by two α, one β, one δ, and one γ protein subunits penetrating the full thickness of the muscle end-plate membrane as illustrated in Figure 5–2A. Binding of two acetylcholine molecules simultaneously, each to a site on the α subunits, causes conformational changes in the channel proteins and opens the channel to sodium ions. Sodium ions moving intracellularly along their concentration and electrical gradients generate a depolarizing current called the *end-plate potential*. The height of this end-plate potential is directly proportional to the quanta of acetylcholine released, the number of postjunctional receptors occupied, and the number of channels opened. If the end-plate potential reaches a critical value known as the *threshold potential*, voltage-gated sodium channels become activated and more positively charged sodium ions enter the cell (Fig. 5–2B). As a result, the magnitude of the depolarizing current increases and propagates to the adjacent muscle cell membrane as an

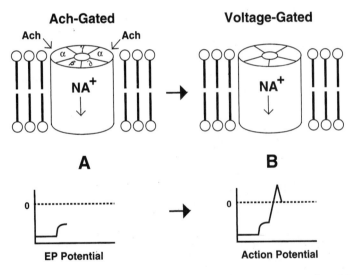

FIGURE 5–2. An illustration of two different types of ion channels in the membrane of skeletal muscle fibers. *A*, The acetylcholine-gated (Ach-gated) nonselective channel for cations is a pentameric structure of two α, one β, one δ, and one γ protein subunits. Occupation of a stereospecific site at each of the two α subunits by an acetylcholine molecule (Ach) simultaneously will activate the channel and allow the influx of positively charged sodium ions into the muscle fiber to generate an end-plate (EP) potential. *B*, When the end-plate potential reaches a threshold value, voltage-gated sodium channels are activated, generating an action potential that travels up and down the entire length of the muscle fiber.

action potential. This wave of action potential travels up and down the entire length of the muscle fiber, and muscle contraction ensues through the mechanisms of excitation-contraction coupling. Subsequently the released acetylcholine is hydrolyzed by acetylcholinesterase present within the folds of the end-plate, the sodium channels close, and the muscle fiber returns to its inactive state (repolarized).

In addition to postjunctional acetylcholine receptors on the motor end-plate, there are prejunctional acetylcholine receptors on the nerve membrane. When released acetylcholine molecules bind with these prejunctional receptors, mobilization of acetylcholine from the depot to join the readily available pool is facilitated. This function ensures a steady supply of acetylcholine for release during sustained tetanic contractions.

■ Neuromuscular Blockade

Although there is evidence indicating that muscle relaxants act on many sites at the neuromuscular junction to block impulse transmission, the major site of action is the cholinergic-nicotinic receptors on the motor end-plate. These agents are divided into two subgroups according to whether their mode of action is a nondepolarizing neuromuscular blockade or a depolarizing neuromuscular blockade.

Nondepolarizing Neuromuscular Blockade

Nondepolarizing muscle relaxants are acetylcholine analogues. They are capable of competing with acetylcholine and binding reversibly with the postjunctional cholinergic-nicotinic site on the α protein subunits without opening the acetylcholine-gated nonselective cationic channels. Occupation of the site at only one of the two α-protein subunits is enough to inactivate the ion channel. As the concentration of relaxant molecules increases, the population of functioning receptors and their associated ion channels declines. Consequently, the amplitude of the end-plate potential generated by the quanta of acetylcholine released by each nerve impulse falls. (The amplitude of the end-plate potential is directly proportional to the quanta of acetylcholine released and the number of functioning receptors accessible to acetylcholine.) If the end-plate potential falls below the threshold potential that activates the voltage-gated sodium channels, no action potential will be propagated and the muscle fiber will fail to contract in response to an incoming motor nerve impulse.

Animal studies have shown that individual muscle is composed of muscle fibers with varying susceptibility to nondepolarizing neuromuscular blockade. Some will fail to propagate an action potential when 75% of the receptors are occupied by relaxant molecules, the majority will fail when 80–90% of the receptors are occupied, and all will fail when 90–95% of the receptors are occupied. At this high level of receptor occupancy by nondepolarizing relaxant molecules, neuromuscular transmission fails completely and the muscle remains flaccid. The method of evaluating the degree of nondepolarizing neuromuscular blockade is discussed in Chapter 14 (see "Monitoring Neuromuscular Function").

Nondepolarizing muscle relaxants also can interfere with muscle contraction by their action on prejunctional receptors. Even in subparalyzing doses, these agents can block the access of acetylcholine molecules to prejunctional receptors competitively, interfering with mobilization of acetylcholine from storage depots and replenishment of the readily available pool. As a result, a steady demand for continuous release of acetylcholine cannot be sustained and tetanic contractions will fade.

These actions of nondepolarizing relaxants can be reversed with anticholinesterases, which inhibit the hydrolysis of acetylcholine by acetylcholinesterase. Following administration of an anticholinesterase, the concentration of acetylcholine molecules at the neuromuscular junction rises. Because a higher concentration of acetylcholine can compete more effectively against relaxant molecules at both postjunctional and prejunctional receptor sites, neuromuscular transmission will return toward normal and tetanic contraction can be sustained once again. In practice, it is recommended that an anticholinesterase be given only after some spontaneous return of neuromuscular function is obvious; otherwise reversal of neuromuscular blockade may not be satisfactory.

Depolarizing Neuromuscular Blockade

Depolarizing muscle relaxants are also acetylcholine analogues but, unlike nondepolarizing agents, they have agonist activities. Binding of these molecules to postjunctional cholinergic-nicotinic sites on the α protein subunits opens the ligand-gated nonselective channels to sodium ions and depolarizes the motor end-plate, which in turn activates the voltage-gated sodium channels and depolarizes the muscle fiber. Consequently the muscle contracts, although the contraction is not sustained. However, as long as the receptors are occupied by these molecules, depolarization of the motor end-plates persists, neuromuscular transmission is interrupted, and the muscle remains flaccid. This is the Phase I depolarizing block. The hallmark of a depolarizing neuromuscular blockade is random contraction of motor units, seen as muscle fasciculations, followed by paralysis. The electromechanical characteristics of the Phase I depolarizing block are discussed in Chapter 14 (see "Peripheral Nerve Stimulation"). During Phase I block, mobilization of depot acetylcholine remains normal and no fade occurs during tetanic contraction.

Recovery from Phase I block depends on washout of relaxant molecules from the junctional area and their elimination from the body. Compared with nondepolarizing muscle relaxants, depolarizing agents are eliminated from the body more rapidly and their action at the neuromuscular junction is short lived.

If Phase I block is maintained with continuous infusion or repeated injections of a depolarizing agent, both postjunctional and prejunctional receptors may become insensitive to the normal action of acetylcholine even after the relaxant molecules are removed from the junctional area. This is Phase II block (also known as dual block or desensitization block). Phase II block has all the electromechanical characteristics of the nondepolarizing block (see "Peripheral Nerve Stimulation" in Chapter 14). Like the nondepolarizing block, a fully developed Phase II block can be reversed with anticholinesterases. The mode of action in producing Phase II block is unclear. Sensitivity of the receptors to acetylcholine usually returns with time.

■ Nondepolarizing Muscle Relaxants

Most nondepolarizing muscle relaxant molecules have either a benzylisoquinolinium or a steroidal structure. Whereas *d*-tubocurarine, metocurine, atracurium, doxacurium, and mivacurium are benzylisoquinolinium compounds, pancuronium, vecuronium, pipecuronium, and rocuronium are nonmetabolic steroids. In contrast, gallamine is a phenolic ether and alcuronium is a toxiferine derivative. These compounds have varying properties and duration of action, but *d*-tubocurarine is still a standard to which all others are compared.

Long-Acting Agents

d-*Tubocurarine*

After intravenous injection, the action of *d*-tubocurarine reaches a peak in 4 minutes and lasts approximately 30–45 minutes. Adequate muscle relaxation can be obtained with a loading dose of 0.4 mg/kg and maintained with increments of 0.1 mg/kg when necessary.

> **Note:** Nondepolarizing blocks are potentiated by succinylcholine given to facilitate tracheal intubation and by volatile agents given concurrently. The doses of nondepolarizing muscle relaxants recommended are average doses based on these assumptions. if a nondepolarizing muscle relaxant is used to facilitate tracheal intubation, the loading dose may have to be increased by 20–30%. As with other anesthetic agents, the dose should be titrated against effect.

A significant amount of circulating *d*-tubocurarine is bound to plasma protein, more to globulin than albumin. Approximately 40% of an injected dose is recoverable in urine within 24 hours, a small amount is taken up by tissues, and the rest is eliminated via biliary excretion.

The most obvious side effect of *d*-tubocurarine is arterial hypotension. The degree of hypotension is particularly severe in the elderly, in patients who are hypovolemic, and in those under halothane anesthesia. The fall in blood pressure is related chiefly to histamine release from tissue depots and partly to sympathetic ganglionic blockade.

Owing to its hypotensive side effect and histamine-releasing property, care should be exercised in the administration of *d*-turbocurarine to the elderly, to hypovolemic patients, and to those with asthma and bronchitis. Otherwise there are few contraindications to the use of *d*-tubocurarine, provided artificial ventilation of the lungs is instituted.

Pancuronium

Pancuronium is five times as potent as *d*-tubocurarine and has a slightly longer duration of action. Maximum muscle relaxation is seen within 2 minutes following intravenous injection. The recommended loading dose is 0.08 mg/kg. Increments of 0.015 mg/kg can be given when necessary.

A considerable amount of pancuronium is bound to plasma protein. Compared with *d*-tubocurarine, this agent is more dependent on renal excretion for elimination. As much as 80% of an injected dose is recoverable from the urine of laboratory animals; the rest is metabolized and excreted by the liver. Hepatic metabolism produces active but less potent metabolites that are of little clinical importance.

Sinus tachycardia with or without an increase in blood pressure is a common side effect following the injection of a bolus of pancuronium. This pressor response is the result partly of a parasympatholytic action on the cardiac vagus nerve and partly of the inhibition of catecholamine reuptake by sympathetic nerves. Unlike *d*-tubocurarine, pancuronium has no significant effect on autonomic ganglia and causes little histamine release.

Metocurine

Metocurine is twice as potent as *d*-tubocurarine but has a similar duration of action. Optimum muscle relaxation can be obtained with a loading dose of 0.2 mg/kg and maintained with increments of 0.05 mg/kg when necessary. It has no effect on the sympathetic ganglia and is devoid of histamine-releasing properties, but it still can cause arterial hypotension in a significant number of patients. It is largely dependent on renal excretion for elimination and should be avoided in patients with impaired renal function.

Pipecuronium

Pipecuronium, a derivative of pancuronium, is 30% more potent but has minimal cardiovascular side effects. Both agents have a similar duration of action. The recommended loading dose of pipecuronium is 0.05 mg/kg and the maintenance dose 0.01 mg/kg when required. It is excreted largely unchanged in urine and to a lesser extent in bile.

Doxacurium

Doxacurium, another muscle relaxant with minimal cardiovascular side effects, is 20 times as potent as *d*-tubocurarine. It is slightly longer acting than pancuronium or pipecuronium, and the recommended doses are 0.02 mg/kg for loading and 0.005 mg/kg for maintenance. Although it is an ester of succinic acid, doxacurium is not hydrolyzed by plasma cholinesterase. Most of it is excreted unchanged in urine and a small portion in bile.

Alcuronium

Alcuronium, a long-acting muscle relaxant 2.5 times as potent as *d*-tubocurarine, is used mainly outside North America. Its cardiovascular side effects are limited to a small increase in heart rate and an insignificant fall in blood pressure. The recommended doses are 0.15 mg/kg for loading and 0.05 mg/kg for maintenance. No histamine release is associated with these clinical doses. Most of a given dose is excreted in urine, and a small amount in bile.

Intermediate-Acting Agents

Gallamine

Gallamine is one fifth as potent as *d*-tubocurarine. After intravenous injection, action reaches a peak at between 2 and 3 minutes, with a duration of action approaching 30 minutes. The recommended loading dose and increment for maintenance are 2 mg/kg and 0.5 mg/kg, respectively. Histamine release is considerably less with gallamine than with *d*-tubocurarine. The most prominent side effect is sinus tachycardia—a result of cardiac vagal blockade. This agent is totally dependent on renal excretion for elimination and is absolutely contraindicated in patients in renal failure.

Atracurium

Atracurium is as potent as *d*-tubocurarine. A loading dose of 0.4 mg/kg should be given initially, to be followed by increments of 0.1 mg/kg for maintenance when necessary. Peak action is reached within 2−5 minutes after a bolus and total paralysis lasts 20−35 minutes. Because of its relatively short duration of action and lack of cumulative effect, atracurium is given as a continuous infusion as well at a rate of 8 μg/kg/min. Histamine release causing hypotension has been reported occasionally, but this usually occurs after a very large bolus.

Less than 10% of a given dose is dependent on renal excretion for elimination. Approximately 60% of a dose is broken down in plasma by nonspecific esterases and 30% by a nonenzymatic chemical process known as Hoffman elimination. The Hoffman reaction occurs at normal body pH and temperature. If the patient's body temperature falls below 34° C, the action of atracurium may be prolonged. One of the products of degradation is laudanosine, a neurotoxin with convulsant properties. However, the plasma level of laudanosine reached, even after major operations lasting several hours, is clinically insignificant.

Cis-atracurium, a pure stereoisomer of atracurium, is now available for clinical use. It is five times as potent as *d*-tubocurarine, does not release histamine in clinical doses, and is associated with more hemodynamic stability.

Vecuronium

Like pancuronium, vecuronium is five times as potent as *d*-tubocurarine but it has a duration of action of only 25−40 minutes. The initial loading dose is 0.08 mg/kg, to be followed by increments of 0.015 mg/kg for maintenance as required.

Vecuronium does not release histamine, nor does it cause hypotension or tachycardia. It is metabolized in the liver to deacetylated products. The major metabolite, 3-deacetylated vecuronium, is almost as potent as the parent compound and is dependent on biliary and renal excretion for elimination. Hence the duration of action of vecuronium may be prolonged in patients who have liver cirrhosis or renal failure.

Rocuronium

Rocuronium has a potency similar to that of *d*-tubocurarine but a faster onset of action than any of the depolarizing muscle relaxants mentioned before. Its duration of action is similar to that of vecuronium, and the loading dose is 0.5 mg/kg, to be followed by 0.15 mg/kg as required for maintenance. It does not cause histamine release or hypotension but may cause a small increase in heart rate as a result of a mild vagolytic effect. It is secreted both in bile and in urine; no metabolic products have yet been identified.

Short-Acting Agents

Mivacurium

Mivacurium is the only short-acting nondepolarizing muscle relaxant introduced into clinical practice recently. Its duration of action is approximately 15 minutes (approximately three times that of succinylcholine), but an unexpectedly long duration of neuromuscular blockade has been reported. Mivacurium has no significant effects on the cardiac vagus nerve or sympathetic ganglia but can cause hypotension as a result of histamine release. The recommended loading dose is 0.15 mg/kg, to be followed by 0.05 mg/kg for maintenance as required.

The mivacurium molecule has two ester bonds susceptible to hydrolysis by plasma cholinesterase, which constitutes its major pathway of elimination. Its action is prolonged in patients who carry the atypical plasma cholinesterase gene: mildly in heterozygotes and markedly in homozygotes (see "Atypical Plasma Cholinesterase" below). Because the enzyme is synthesized in the liver, its action is also prolonged in patients in hepatic failure.

Reversing a Nondepolarizing Block

Neuromuscular function following administration of a nondepolarizing muscle relaxant will recover with time. The time course of recovery depends on redistribution of these agents in body water and their eventual elimination by metabolism and excretion. Because most of the muscle relaxant molecules are electrically charged at physiologic pH, tissue uptake is slow and duration of action is governed chiefly by the pathways of elimination.

At the end of a surgical procedure, recovery of neuromuscular transmission following administration of a nondepolarizing muscle relaxant is usually not complete. Therefore, it is necessary to terminate the action of the nondepolarizing muscle relaxant with an anticholinesterase—neostigmine, pyridostigmine, or edrophonium. However, the antagonistic action of an anticholinesterase against the neuromuscular blocking action of a nondepolarizing muscle relaxant may not be adequate in the presence of a profound block. It is recommended that the anticholinesterase be given only after some spontaneous return of neuromuscular function.

Because anticholinesterases work at both the neuromuscular junction and muscarinic sites (chiefly organs innervated by the vagus nerve), muscarinic side effects of these agents should be blocked with the administration of a vagolytic agent (atropine or glycopyrrolate) at the same time.

Neostigmine and Atropine

A combination of neostigmine, 2.5–5 mg, and atropine, 1.2–2.4 mg, is the preparation most commonly used to reverse the action of a nondepolarizing muscle relaxant. Both drugs are usually mixed in the same syringe and administered intravenously as a bolus. The action of atropine at muscarinic sites always precedes that of neostigmine, and gross disturbance of cardiac rate and rhythm following the administration of this mixture is uncommon. Reversal of neuromuscular blockade is usually seen within 5 minutes. In order to ensure that normal neuromuscular function has returned, the patient should be observed closely during this period (see "Monitoring Neuromuscular Function" in Chapter 14).

Pyridostigmine

Pyridostigmine is an analogue of neostigmine. A dose of 10–20 mg is required for counteracting the effect of a nondepolarizing muscle relaxant in most adults. Its onset of action is somewhat delayed and may take 15 minutes. It has a longer duration of action than neostigmine and produces milder muscarinic side effects. It should be given with 0.6–1.2 mg of atropine.

Edrophonium

In small doses, the effect of edrophonium in reversing the action of nondepolarizing muscle relaxants is transient. However, this effect is sustained if the dose is increased to 1 mg/kg. Compared with neostigmine, edrophonium has a quicker onset of action and milder muscarinic side effects.

Glycopyrrolate

Glycopyrrolate is a potent antisialagogue with no action on the central nervous system and minimal effects on the cardiovascular system. Its duration of action is longer lasting than that of atropine. In order to block the muscarinic effects of neostigmine effectively, it should be given in the ratio of one part by weight of glycopyrrolate to five parts of neostigmine.

Factors Affecting Action

The potency, duration of action, and ease of reversal of nondepolarizing muscle relaxants are known to be affected by many physiologic and pharmacologic factors. They include priming, age, hypothermia, acid-base homeostasis, electrolyte imbalance, renal failure, myasthenia gravis, the Eaton-Lambert syndrome, and drug interactions.

Priming

All nondepolarizing muscle relaxants require a latency of at least 2−3 minutes for peak action to develop. A subparalyzing dose of these agents given before the loading dose can decrease the latency and increase the potency of their action. Herein lies the principle of priming. In practice, 10% of the calculated loading dose is given 3−4 minutes before the full dose. However, this technique does not work consistently in all patients, and sensitive patients may develop significant paralysis following the calculated priming dose.

Age

The development of the neuromuscular junction is incomplete in premature infants and neonates. Many clinicians have found that this group of patients is more sensitive to nondepolarizing muscle relaxants. In addition, geriatric patients have decreased muscle bulk and are more sensitive to the effects of nondepolarizing muscle relaxants than are young adults. Because the rate of elimination of nondepolarizing muscle relaxants (particularly those dependent on renal excretion) is slower in the elderly, generally the duration of action is longer as well.

Hypothermia

Hypothermic patients are said to be relatively resistant to the neuromuscular blocking action of nondepolarizing muscle relaxants. However, the rate of elimination of these agents by the kidneys and liver is also slowed. Therefore, duration of action is prolonged under hypothermic conditions.

Acid-Base Homeostasis

The mechanism of interaction between hydrogen ions and nondepolarizing muscle relaxants is unknown, but it is difficult to reverse the block of nondepolarizing muscle relaxants when the P_aCO_2 is more than 50 mm Hg. That is, respiratory acidosis potentiates the actions of nondepolarizing relaxants. Metabolic alkalosis may potentiate the blockade of nondepolarizing agents also, but metabolic acidosis does not seem to pose the same problem.

Electrolyte Imbalance

Hypokalemia, particularly that of acute onset, potentiates the neuromuscular blockade of nondepolarizing muscle relaxants and diminishes the ability of anticholinesterases to reverse a nondepolarizing neuromuscular block. This enhancement is related to changes in the resting membrane potentials of excitable tissues (muscle and nerves) in the presence of hypokalemia.

Renal Failure

Gallamine, metocurine, and alcuronium are eliminated from the body by renal excretion. Renal failure prolongs the duration of their action, and the standard practice of re-establishing neuromuscular transmission with an anticholinesterase is inadequate. In the absence of renal function, recovery of neuromuscular function is totally dependent on the redistribution of these drugs within the body. Because tissue uptake of these highly charged molecules is slow, recovery from a normal dose can be prolonged indeed. These comments also apply to the long-acting nondepolarizing muscle relaxants pipecuronium and doxacurium.

d-Tubocurarine, pancuronium, and rocuronium are eliminated via both the kidneys and the liver, but pancuronium is slightly more dependent on renal excretion than the others. In the presence of renal failure, clearance by the kidneys is diminished, but hepatic clearance continues unabated and may even be enhanced. Reversal of the effects of these agents with an anticholinesterase is usually successful, even in anephric patients. Because the renal excretion of all anticholinesterases is also diminished in renal failure, there is no danger that the effects of the relaxants will outlast those of the anticholinesterases, unless the patient has been given an overdose.

Vecuronium is broken down in the liver, and 3-deacetylated vercuronium, a major metabolite almost as active as the parent compound, is excreted in urine. Prolonged action of vecuronium following continuous infusion in critically ill patients in the intensive care unit has been reported. Mivacurium, in contrast, is hydrolyzed by plasma cholinesterase. Because plasma cholinesterase activity is decreased in renal failure, the duration of action of mivacurium can be expected to be prolonged by 50%.

Myasthenia Gravis

Patients with myasthenia gravis have a block at the neuromuscular junction similar to that seen following curare administration. This block can be successfully reversed with anticholinesterases. These patients are extremely sensitive to the effects of nondepolarizing muscle relaxants and are resistant to the Phase I block of depolarizing muscle relaxants. Adequate muscle relaxation can usually be obtained in these patients without the use of a muscle relaxant, provided their medication (usually pyridostigmine) is omitted on the day of the operation. The degree of relaxation can be increased even further by using inhalation agents with good muscle-relaxant properties (e.g., isoflurane). If use of a nondepolarizing muscle relaxant is absolutely essential, only a small dose (1/30th to 1/10th the normal dose) should be given. Use of a peripheral nerve stimulator to follow the time course of neuromuscular blockade in this instance is mandatory.

Eaton-Lambert Syndrome

In the Eaton-Lambert (myasthenic) syndrome, originally described in patients with oat cell carcinomas, release of acetylcholine at motor nerve endings is impaired. Affected patients are sensitive to the effects of both nondepolarizing and depolarizing muscle relaxants.

Drug Interaction

All volatile anesthetic agents can potentiate the action of nondepolarizing muscle relaxants, but isoflurane, enflurane, desflurane, and sevoflurane are more potent than halothane in this respect. The mechanism of interaction is probably related to

1. A decline in efferent impulses in motor nerves as a result of depression of the central nervous system
2. An increase in delivery of relaxant molecules to skeletal muscles as a result of increased muscle blood flow

3. Stabilization of muscle cell membrane by the anesthetic agent

Succinylcholine, a depolarizing muscle relaxant usually given to facilitate tracheal intubation, can increase the block of a subsequent dose of nondepolarizing agents by 10–20%. Nondepolarizing muscle relaxants should be given only after the patient has shown signs of recovery from succinylcholine, and the dose should be modified accordingly.

Magnesium antagonizes the action of calcium at motor nerve endings and inhibits the calcium-mediated release of acetylcholine. Magnesium sulfate, an agent used in the treatment of seizures associated with toxemia of pregnancy, enhances the neuromuscular blockade of nondepolarizing muscle relaxants. Similarly, calcium channel blockers (e.g., verapamil) can potentiate the action of these agents.

Aminoglycosides exert an action similar to that of magnesium on prejunctional motor nerve endings and enhance the action of nondepolarizing muscle relaxants. Other antibiotics, by acting on the postjunctional membrane, have a similar effect. Antibiotic agents that have been reported to potentiate nondepolarizing blockade include clindamycin, colistin, gentamicin, kanamycin, lincomycin, neomycin, paromomycin, polymyxin A and B, streptomycin, tetracycline, and viomycin.

In contrast to the drugs mentioned above, anticonvulsants (phenytoin and carbamazepine) can cause resistance to the action of nondepolarizing muscle relaxants.

▮ Pharmacology of Succinylcholine

There are only two useful depolarizing muscle relaxants, but succinylcholine has been used largely to the exclusion of decamethonium. It is composed of two molecules of acetylcholine joined end to end and has a rapid onset of action that is obvious within one vein-to-muscle circulation time. It is most commonly used during induction of anesthesia to facilitate tracheal intubation. The normal intubating dose is 1 mg/kg.

The ester bond of succinylcholine is hydrolyzed rapidly by plasma cholinesterase (pseudocholinesterase). Therefore, succinylcholine is a short-acting agent. Following an intravenous injection, neuromuscular function returns in 3–5 minutes unless paralysis is maintained with an intravenous infusion of appropriate dilution (usually 500 mg in 500 ml of 5% dextrose solution). Phase II block is always a possible complication during prolonged infusion. In order to reduce the incidence of this complication, the total dose of succinylcholine should be limited to 500 mg and the duration of infusion to 60 minutes.

Side Effects

Succinylcholine has several well-known side effects. They include cardiac arrhythmias, salivation, muscle pain, and increases in intragastric pressure, intracranial pressure, intraocular pressure, and serum potassium concentration. Bradycardia and salivation are muscarinic side effects and can be prevented or treated with a parasympatholytic agent. The rest are attenuated by precurarization. In addition, succinylcholine can cause masseter spasm and allergy reaction in some patients.

Cardiac Arrhythmias

Although succinylcholine mimics the action of acetylcholine, sinus bradycardia following its administration is common only in children. Following an intubation dose, heart rate usually increases in adults, but bradycardia and transient asystole have been reported when administration is repeated within 10 minutes. This complication can be prevented by atropine, given either in the premedication or intravenously during induction of anesthesia. Ventricular premature beats have also been reported following administration of succinylcholine, but there are usually other precipitating factors (e.g., hypoxemia, hypercapnia, the administration of exogenous catecholamine, and inadequate depth of anesthesia).

Salivation

Owing to its muscarinic effect on the salivary glands, succinylcholine is a potent sialagogue. The secretion is usually watery and presents little problem. If it is deemed necessary, this side effect can be blocked by the administration of atropine or glycopyrrolate.

Muscle Pain

The incidence of postoperative myalgia following a paralyzing dose of succinylcholine is as high as 90%. Pain is particularly severe in ambulatory and muscular patients. Damage to muscle fibers during fasciculation has been suggested to be the cause of this unpleasant side effect, and myoglobinemia and myoglobinuria have been observed in some patients.

Masseter Spasm

Incidents of jaw muscle spasm following succinylcholine have been reported in young patients, particularly in children between 8 and 12 years of age and following the induction of anesthesia with halothane. The spasm lasts 2−3 minutes, is not relieved by a repeat dose of succinylcholine, and can be overcome by persistent effort. Contrary to previous belief, masseter spasm without rigidity is not a sign of malignant hyperthermia (see "Malignant Hyperthermia" in Chapter 16). Nevertheless, increased vigilance for other signs of malignant hyperthermia should be instituted during the course of anesthesia in these patients.

Increase in Intragastric Pressure

Succinylcholine can cause a rise in intragastric pressure. The magnitude of this increase varies from patient to patient, and pressures large enough to cause regurgitation of stomach contents have been reported. Presumably the increase in pressure is related to fasciculation of the abdominal musculature.

Increase in Intracranial Pressure

During light anesthesia, succinylcholine may cause an increase in intracranial pressure in patients with decreased intracranial compliance. This is likely due to a combination of afferent cerebral stimulation via the muscle spindles and increased carbon dioxide production. Pretreatment with a small subparalytic dose of a nondepolarizing agent or concurrent administration of deep anesthesia will prevent a rise in intracranial pressure.

Increase in Intraocular Pressure

Concurrent with the onset of fasciculation, intraocular pressure increases following administration of succinylcholine. This side effect lasts for only 5 minutes and is due both to fasciculation of extraocular muscles and dilation of choroidal blood vessels. Although this rise in intraocular pressure is of little significance in most patients, it can cause extrusion of intraocular contents (e.g., vitreous) in patients with an open wound of the eye.

Increase in Serum Potassium Concentration

In most surgical patients there is a small rise in serum potassium concentration (approximately 0.5 mEq/L) following administration of succinylcholine. This increase is attributed to the flux of potassium ions escaping from skeletal muscle cells during fasciculation. However, a much larger rise in potassium concentration is seen in certain patients. Hyperkalemic cardiac arrest following the administration of succinylcholine has occurred in severely burned or injured patients, particularly within 1 week to 2 months after the initial trauma. Similarly, cardiac arrest has occurred in patients with neuromedical and neurosurgical disorders, usually in the first 6 months following onset of hemiplegia or paraplegia. A large rise in serum potassium concentration may be found also in uremic patients, patients with severe intra-abdominal sepsis, and patients suffering from peripheral vascular disease complicated by muscle wasting. More recently, attention was drawn to the occurrence of severe hyperkalemia, intractable cardiac arrest, and rhabdomyolysis in apparently healthy children who were subsequently proved to have skeletal muscle myopathies, including Duchenne's muscular dystrophy. These reports prompted the manufacturers of succinylcholine to warn against the use of succinylcholine in children, except in emergencies when immediate tracheal intubation is indicated.

Allergic Reactions

Hypersensitivity reactions to succinylcholine have been reported sporadically in the northern hemisphere but are prevalent in Australia and New Zealand. The reason for this regional difference in prevalence is unclear.

Factors Affecting Action

Many factors can affect the action, potency, and duration of action of succinylcholine. They include precurarization, self-taming, myotonia, myasthenia gravis, and atypical plasma cholinesterase.

Precurarization

Pretreatment of the patient with a subparalyzing dose of nondepolarizing muscle relaxant (e.g., 3 mg of d-tubocurarine, 20 mg of gallamine, or 1 mg of pancuronium) can attenuate but not abolish many of the unwanted side effects of succinylcholine mentioned above. This technique is known as precurarization. Precurarization will certainly attenuate the severity of fasciculation and muscle pain as well as the rise in intragastric, intracranial, and intraocular pressures. However, the effectiveness of precurarization in preventing hyperkalemia is questionable; at best it offers susceptible patients only partial protection against this potentially fatal complication. Precurarization also decreases the potency of succinylcholine and delays the onset of paralysis. In order to overcome these disadvantages of precurarization, the dose of succinylcholine should be increased to 1.5–2 mg/kg.

Self-Taming

Administration of 0.1 mg/kg of succinylcholine before the full intubating dose can attenuate muscle fasciculations seen with this agent. This technique is called self-taming. It is not as effective as precurarization and does not diminish the incidence of succinylcholine-induced myalgia. Nor is there evidence to suggest that self-taming will attenuate the other unwanted side effects associated with succinylcholine.

Myotonia

Myotonia is an inability to relax a muscle after its contraction. It is seen in patients suffering from myotonia dystrophica (myotonia atrophica) and myotonia congenita. The former is the most common form of muscular dystrophy, whereas the latter is rare. Myotonic muscles are not relaxed by succinylcholine. Instead they go into sustained contraction (contracture). Therefore, succinylcholine is contraindicated in myotonic patients.

Myasthenia Gravis

Myasthenic patients are somewhat resistant to Phase I block and are more prone to develop Phase II block. In practice, however, little difficulty is encountered in the use of a single dose of succinylcholine for tracheal intubation in these patients.

Atypical Plasma Cholinesterase

Plasma cholinesterase is a glycoprotein synthesized in the liver. At least five genetic variants determined by genes at two different loci have been identified: the usual, the atypical, the fluoride-resistant, the silent, and the C_5 variants.

The *usual variant* (cholinesterase$_{\text{1st locus}}^{\text{usual}}$ or E_1^u) has a strong cholinesterase activity and is the most common. In persons homozygous for this variant ($E_1^u E_1^u$), hydrolysis of succinylcholine is rapid and its duration of action is limited to 5 minutes. As much as 80% of the enzyme activity of these normal persons is inhibited by dibucaine. This percentage of inhibition is called the *Dibucaine Number*. That is, plasma from homozygotes with the usual enzyme has a Dibucaine Number of 80.

The *atypical variant* (E_1^a) has a weak cholinesterase activity. Succinylcholine is hydrolyzed very slowly in persons homozygous for this variant ($E_1^a E_1^a$), and a single intubating dose produces prolonged paralysis in these patients. Approximately 1 in 2000 patients is homozygous for the atypical enzyme. Paradoxically, only 20% of the intrinsic activity of the atypical enzyme is inhibited by dibucaine; that is, plasma from homozygotes with the atypical enzyme has a Dibucaine Number of 20. A significant number of patients are heterozygotes $(E_1^u E_1^a)$ with both usual and atypical enzymes. The Dibucaine Number of the plasma of such persons ranges from 30 to 70. The duration of action of succinylcholine in these heterozygotes is only moderately prolonged (increased to 10–20 minutes) and is of little clinical significance.

Whereas the *fluoride-resistant variant* (E_1^f) has a moderately reduced cholinesterase activity that is resistant to inhibition by fluoride ions, the *silent variant* (E_1^s) has extremely weak cholinesterase activity. Homozygotes with the fluoride-resistant enzyme $(E_1^f E_1^f)$ are only moderately sensitive to succinylcholine, but those with the silent enzyme $(E_1^s E_1^s)$ are extremely sensitive. Both variants are rare.

The C_5 *variant* is determined by a gene in the second locus (cholinesterase$_{2nd\ locus}$ or E_2). Being 30% more potent than the usual enzyme, it is of little clinical significance.

Other Factors

Many other factors have been observed to be associated with a reduction in plasma cholinesterase activity. They include advanced liver disease, hemodialysis, pregnancy, and the use of oral contraceptive agents, echothiophate (an anticholinesterase eye drop used in the treatment of glaucoma), neostigmine, and cytotoxic agents (e.g., cyclophosphamide). Although the reduction in enzyme activity can be marked, prolonged apnea is rare except in patients who are being treated with echothiophate, neostigmine, or cytotoxic agents.

Local Anesthetics

6

Local anesthetics are drugs that block impulse conduction in nerve fibers. Many substances have local anesthetic properties, but only those that produce a transient and completely reversible inhibition of impulse propagation are clinically useful.

Cocaine, the first local anesthetic discovered, is an alkaloid extracted from the leaves of *Erythroxylon coca*, a shrub that grows in the highlands of Peru and Bolivia. Although its numbing action was described earlier by von Anrep, it was used for the first time as a local anesthetic in 1884 by the Austrian ophthalmic surgeon Karl Koller, who used it topically by instilling it into the conjunctival sac.

Cocaine is toxic and addictive. In many ways its undesirable properties have been an impediment to the development of regional anesthesia, except for experiments with spinal anesthesia. A safer substitute came in the form of procaine in 1905. Lidocaine, the most popular agent in use today, was introduced in 1948.

Anatomy of Peripheral Nerves

The cellular unit of the peripheral nerve is the neuron (Fig. 6–1*A*). It has a cell body and a long process called the axon (also called a "nerve fiber"). All nerve fibers are ensheathed by Schwann cells (Schwann cell sheath or neurolemma). In unmyelinated nerves, approximately 5–20 of these nerve fibers are embedded in the cytoplasm of a single Schwann cell (Fig. 6–1*B*). In myelinated nerves, a substantial layer of myelin (transformed Schwann cell membrane) lies between the nerve fiber and the Schwann cell cytoplasm (Fig. 6–1*C*). This myelin sheath is not continuous along the entire length of the myelinated fiber; it is interrupted periodically at the nodes of Ranvier.

All large peripheral nerves have mixed sensory, motor, and autonomic functions. In a typical peripheral nerve, the fibers are bundled together to form fascicles, which in turn are bundled together to form the nerve trunk. The nerve trunk, the fascicles, and the nerve fibers are supported extensively by con-

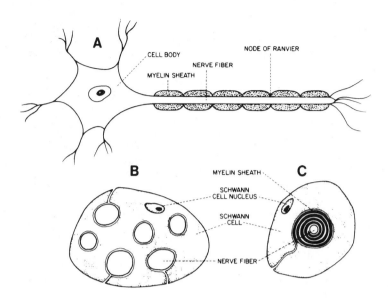

FIGURE 6–1. Anatomy of the peripheral nerve. *A*, A typical neuron. *B*, Cross section of unmyelinated fibers. *C*, Cross section of a myelinated fiber. (Refer to text for details.)

nective tissues known, respectively, as epineurium, perineurium, and endoneurium. Thus there are multiple barriers through which local anesthetics must travel to reach the neuronal membrane, the site of action.

Physiology of Impulse Conduction

The neuronal membrane is a bimolecular layer of phospholipids interspersed with voltage-gated sodium and potassium channels formed by globular protein molecule subunits. Normally this membrane is selectively permeable to positively charged potassium ions, relatively impermeable to positively charged sodium ions, and totally impermeable to negatively charged intracellular protein molecules. Within the membrane, there is also an energy-dependent membrane transport system that actively extrudes intracellular sodium in exchange for extracellular potassium. When the cell is at rest, the ratio of intracellular to extracellular potassium is 30:1 (150 mEq/L inside the cell and 5 mEq/L in the extracellular fluid). This excess of intracellular potassium is counterbalanced by a similar excess of extracellular sodium ions. However, the electronegativity of intracellular protein molecules remains unchecked, and the nerve fiber has a normal resting membrane potential of -70 mV (negative on the internal surface in relation to the external surface).

In the resting state, the sodium-potassium pump in the neuronal membrane is active and the sodium and potassium channels are in the *closed state* (Fig. 6−2*Aa*). When the nerve fiber is depolarized by an excitatory stimulus (e.g., pinprick), the transmembrane potential becomes less negative. When the transmembrane potential reaches -50 mV (the threshold potential), the sodium-potassium transport system is paralyzed and the voltage-gated sodium and potassium channels change to the *open state* and become freely permeable to their respective ion species. Because the sodium channels open faster, influx of positively charged sodium ions according to their electrical and concentration gradients generates an inward current to depolarize that region of the cell membrane even further to $+30$ mV (Fig. 6−2*Ab*). With time, the potassium channels are fully open and efflux of positively charged potassium ions according to their electrochemical gradient generates an outward

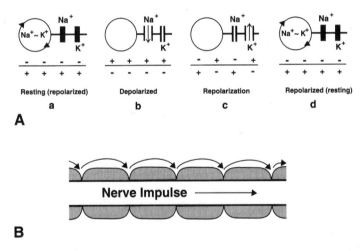

FIGURE 6−2. *A*, The sequence of events during depolarization and repolarization of nerve cell membrane. *a*, When in the resting state, the sodium-potassium pump is active and the sodium and potassium channels are in the closed state. *b*, During depolarization, the pump is paralyzed and sodium channels open before potassium channels. *c*, During repolarization, the pump is still paralyzed and the potassium channels are fully open while the sodium channels are in an inactive state. *d*, Following repolarization, the sodium-potassium pump is again active and the sodium and potassium channels return to the closed state. *B*, A diagram illustrating saltatory conduction in a myelinated fiber.

current and the cell membrane repolarizes (Fig. 6−2*Ac*). During repolarization (when the cell membrane is still "partially de-polarized"), the sodium channels settle into an *inactive state*. The changes in electrical potential during the course of depo-larization and repolarization are called the action potential. Following full repolarization, the resting membrane potential is again `−70 mV, the sodium and potassium channels return to the closed state, and the regional imbalance in sodium and po-tassium ion concentrations resulting from sodium influx and potassium efflux is restored by the sodium-potassium pump (Fig. 6−2*Ad*). This wave of depolarization and repolarization is transferred sequentially to adjacent regions of the cell mem-brane on an unmyelinated nerve fiber, and the impulse passes down its entire length. In myelinated fibers, the wave of exci-tation progresses rapidly through the insulated portion of the nerve fiber, moving from one node of Ranvier to the next (Fig. 6−2*B*), a phenomenon called saltatory conduction. Therefore, impulse propagation in myelinated fibers is much faster than that in unmyelinated fibers.

■ Mechanism of Local Anesthetic Action

Local anesthetics are lipophilic and weakly basic compounds available most commonly as water-soluble hydrochloride salts (XHCl). Except for benzocaine, they dissociate in aqueous so-lution to form the respective base (X) and its acid (XH$^+$) ac-cording to the formulas

$$XHCl \rightleftharpoons XH^+ + CL^-$$
(hydrochloride salt)

$$XH^+ \rightleftharpoons X + H^+$$
(ionized acid)   (nonionized base)

The base (X), being uncharged, diffuses through tissue barriers readily, but it combines with a proton (H$^+$) to become the active acid (XH$^+$) on reaching the axoplasm. Because the pK$_a$ of most local anesthetics lies between 7.5 and 9, the concentration of the ionized acid exceeds that of the nonionized base at tissue pH. If tissue pH becomes more acidic, the concentration of the charged acid form will increase even further.

Several hypotheses have been postulated to explain the ac-tion of local anesthetics that can exist in charged and un-charged forms. They are the membrane receptor hypothesis, the membrane expansion hypothesis, and the surface charge hypothesis.

Membrane Receptor Hypothesis

Local anesthetic molecules in their uncharged base form cross-tissue barriers, including the neuronal membrane, to their site of action. Once inside the axoplasm, they become charged by acquiring a proton and occupy receptor sites on the channel protein subunits of sodium channels. Binding of these receptor sites causes conformational changes in these channel protein subunits, thus blocking the influx of sodium ions and preventing depolarization and impulse propagation. Probably there are multiple receptor sites within the sodium channels, but evidence suggests that all clinically useful agents act on a site located close to the inside surface of the neuronal membrane.

Membrane Expansion Hypothesis

Although the receptor hypothesis explains the action of local anesthetics that can exist in the charged acid form (XH^+), it fails to explain the action of benzocaine, a local anesthetic that exists in the uncharged form only. The membrane expansion hypothesis postulates that uncharged benzocaine molecules "dissolved" in the lipid matrix of the neuronal membrane interfere with bonding of these lipid molecules and allow the membrane to expand. Expansion of the lipid matrix compresses sodium channels, blocks passage of sodium ions, and prevents depolarization and impulse propagation. In this hypothesis, the uncharged base form (X) of other local anesthetics can also act in a similar manner. This hypothesis is an extension of the lipid solubility hypothesis of inhalation anesthetics and implies a single mode of action for both local and general anesthetics (see "Lipid Solubility Hypothesis" in Chapter 1).

Surface Charge Hypothesis

The action of the ionized species of local anesthetic molecules on electric charges on the external and internal surfaces of nerve cell membrane has been proposed in separate hypotheses to explain the action of local anesthetics. In the first hypothesis, it is proposed that positively charged acid forms bound to the external surface of nerve cell membrane make the external surface more positive in relation to the internal surface. (This is equivalent to making the internal surface relatively more negative.) Thus, by hyperpolarizing the nerve cell membrane, positively charged acid forms increase the threshold required to generate an action potential.

In the second hypothesis, it is proposed that positively charged acid forms bound to the internal surface make the internal surface less negative. That is, they cause a "partial depolarization" of the membrane and leave the sodium channels in the inactive state (see "Physiology of Impulse Conduction" above), thus decreasing the excitability of the nerve fiber and blocking impulse propagation.

▒ Systemic Effects of Local Anesthetics

The molecule of a typical local anesthetic has an aromatic (benzene) ring joined to a tertiary amine. If it is formed between an aromatic acid and an amino alcohol, the compound is an aminoester; if it is formed between an aromatic amine and an amino acid, the compound is an aminoamide. Despite these differences, both ester and amide compounds have similar pharmacologic actions and systemic side effects.

Nerve Conduction

Nerve fibers have been classified into three groups according to their function and the degree of myelination: the A fibers of myelinated somatic nerves, the B fibers of myelinated preganglionic autonomic nerves, and the C fibers of nonmyelinated nerves. Furthermore, the A fibers are subdivided into α, β, γ, and δ subgroups, according to their diameter: the largest are α fibers and the smallest are δ fibers. Transmission of pain and temperature is subserved by both Aδ fibers and C fibers.

In general, small and unmyelinated fibers are more sensitive to the action of local anesthetics, but there are exceptions. Whereas the larger myelinated Aδ fibers and the small unmyelinated C fibers are equally sensitive, the myelinated B fibers are even more sensitive to the action of local anesthetic agents. Owing to the sensitivity of these autonomic fibers, sympathetic blockade following spinal or epidural anesthesia is more extensive than sensory blockade. This feature is responsible for the fall in blood pressure associated with these techniques.

When a local anesthetic is deposited around a nerve, it diffuses from the surface toward the core of the nerve trunk. Therefore, conduction in mantle fibers (those on the surface) is blocked before that in core fibers. Because proximal parts of a limb are supplied by mantle fibers while distal parts are supplied by core fibers, it should not be surprising to find that anesthesia first develops proximally during a major nerve block (e.g., brachial plexus block).

Central Nervous System

Local anesthetics are used therapeutically for regional neural blackade. A generalized central nervous system effect is a toxic reaction. Fortunately, central effects are seen only when plasma concentration has exceeded toxic levels, following an overdose or inadvertent intravenous injection. Because impulse transmission in inhibitory pathways is depressed before that in facilitatory pathways, the initial clinical manifestation of central nervous system toxicity is a release phenomenon: excitation and convulsion. With even higher doses, all pathways are depressed, coma ensues, and death is usually due to respiratory arrest (see "Treatment of Systemic Toxicity" in Chapter 17). The propensity for local anesthetics to produce central nervous system toxicity is potentiated by both respiratory and metabolic acidosis.

Cardiovascular System

Most local anesthetics cause some degree of arteriolar dilation. In addition, all of them have direct effects on the myocardium. The myocardial effects of local anesthetics are best exemplified by those of lidocaine.

At therapeutic concentrations, lidocaine decreases the automaticity of Purkinje fibers exposed to a variety of arrhythmogenic stimuli. In this respect, lidocaine (1 mg/kg given as a bolus intravenously or 30 μg/kg/min given as an infusion) is useful in the treatment of ventricular arrhythmias. At toxic concentrations, however, it causes depression of myocardial excitability, conductivity, and contractility, all of which can lead to cardiovascular collapse and death. At equipotent anesthetic doses, bupivacaine and etiodocaine are more cardiotoxic than lidocaine. Cardiotoxicity is increased by hypoxemia, hypercapnia, acidosis, and hyperkalemia and during pregnancy.

Tachyphylaxis

Tachyphylaxis refers to the reduced potency of a local anesthetic agent when it is administered in repeated doses, as in continuous epidural anesthesia. This phenomenon is partly explained by an observed increase in hydrogen ion concentration locally after repeated administration of the acid salt. As tissue acidity increases, availability of the uncharged base form decreases (see "Mechanism of Local Anesthetic Action" above). Because only the uncharged base form can readily diffuse through tissue barriers, a decline in its concentration is seen clinically as reduced potency.

Hypersensitivity

Allergic reactions to local anesthetics, including dermatitis, bronchospasm, and anaphylaxis, have been reported from time to time. Most reports incriminate the ester-type agents. True hypersensitivity to local anesthetic agents may be extremely rare. Bacteriostatic additives may be responsible for some of the reported reactions. Epinephrine added to some preparations can cause tachycardia, diaphoresis, pallor, anxiety, and changes in mental perception, which are often mistakenly regarded as signs and symptoms of an allergic reaction. Skin testing may be helpful in diagnosing true allergy, but its result is not always specific or reliable.

Absorption and Elimination

Systemic absorption of local anesthetic agents is determined by the site of injection, size of the dose, degree of tissue binding, and pharmacologic characteristics of the agent. In general, rate of absorption is faster and peak plasma concentration higher if the site of injection is vascular, the size of the dose is large, the degree of tissue binding is small, and the agent has direct vasodilating property. However, these factors can interact to make prediction difficult. For example, bupivacaine is a more potent vasodilator than lidocaine. Yet the peak concentration of lidocaine is higher than the peak concentration of bupivacaine after injection of equivalent doses of these agents into similar sites. This is because the strong tissue-binding property of bupivacaine retards absorption, although its vasodilating property favors absorption. In addition to the above factors, concomitant use of a vasoconstrictor (usually epinephrine 1:100,000 or less) retards systemic absorption of local anesthetics. As a result, local absorption is delayed, duration of action prolonged, peak concentration lower, incidence of systemic toxicity reduced, and range of safe dose increased.

After absorption, local anesthetics are distributed first by venous blood to the lungs, where they are taken up avidly during this first pass through the pulmonary circulation. Pulmonary uptake reduces the amount reaching the systemic circulation and protects the patient against systemic toxicity. On reaching the systemic circulation, local anesthetics are distributed according to regional blood flow to the vessel-rich viscera and redistributed to lean body mass and vessel-poor tissues in a manner similar to what has been described for intravenous anesthetics (see "Tissue Blood Flow and Tissue Mass" in Chapter 2). Ultimately they are eliminated from the body by metabolic degradation. Urinary excretion of unchanged drugs is relatively insignificant.

Ester-type compounds are hydrolyzed by esterase in the liver and by cholinesterase in plasma. The degree and rate of hydrolysis by plasma cholinesterase vary according to the agent, being most marked for chloroprocaine, less for procaine, and least for tetracaine. It has been suggested that the rate of elimination of these agents may be prolonged in patients with atypical plasma cholinesterase. It is also suggested that procaine, by competing for plasma cholinesterase, can prolong the action of succinylcholine and mivacurium in normal persons.

Unlike ester-type compounds, amide-type agents are detoxified in the liver. The rate of clearance, in decreasing order, is prilocaine > etidocaine > lidocaine > mepivacaine and ropivacaine > bupivacaine. (Prilocaine has extrahepatic sites of metabolism.)

■ The Aminoesters

Cocaine

Cocaine, an ester, is active topically and has the ability to cause vasoconstriction by blocking reuptake of norepinephrine at sympathetic nerve endings. Its use is limited to anesthetizing the mucous membrane of the upper airway by topical application.

Procaine

Procaine is also an ester. Hydrolysis of procaine in the body yields *para*-aminobenzoic acid, which is known to interfere with the bacteriostatic action of sulfonamides. The agent is not active topically. A 0.25% or 0.5% solution is adequate for local infiltration or extensive field blocks, but a 1% or 2% solution is required for nerve blocks. Depending on the concentration used, its duration of action is anywhere from 30 minutes to 1 hour. It is a relatively safe agent; as much as 15 mg/kg can be given without signs of systemic toxicity.

Chloroprocaine

Chloroprocaine is a chlorinated derivative of procaine. The agents have similar properties, but chloroprocaine is more potent. It is also more rapidly hydrolyzed and has a shorter duration of action than the parent compound. The maximum safe dose is 15 mg/kg. There have been reports of neurotoxicity following intrathecal injection of chloroprocaine. Although toxicity may have been due to the presence of sodium bisulfite preservative and the low pH of the solution and not to the drug itself, chloroprocaine is not recommended for spinal anesthesia. A new formulation of chloroprocaine containing ethylene-diaminetetra-acetic acid (EDTA) but not bisulfite is now available. Spasm of back muscles has been reported following epidural injection of this new preparation, probably resulting from chelation of calcium ions in the erector muscles of the spine.

Tetracaine

Tetracaine, another ester, is 10 times as potent as procaine. A dose of over 1.5 mg/kg is toxic. This agent is used almost exclusively for spinal anesthesia. A 1% solution is usually mixed with an equal volume of 10% dextrose to make a 0.5% hyperbaric solution (a solution with specific gravity higher than that of cerebrospinal fluid). Because tetracaine is hydrolyzed four times more slowly than procaine, its duration of action is up to 3 hours; this can be increased even further with the addition of a vasoconstrictor.

▓▓▓ The Aminoamides

Lidocaine

Lidocaine, an amide, is by far a better agent than procaine. The advantages are rapid onset, more intense anesthesia, and a longer duration of action. Onset of action can be hastened and intensity of anesthesia increased even further by the use of carbonated lidocaine in place of lidocaine hydrochloride. Unlike procaine, lidocaine is also active topically. Normally a 0.5%

solution is used for local infiltration, a 1% or 2% solution for nerve blocks, a 1.5% or 2% solution for epidural anesthesia, and a hyperbaric 5% solution in 7.5% dextrose for spinal anesthesia. Epinephrine may be added to increase its duration of action. In addition, 2% and 4% syrups are available for use as a mouthwash or gargle, 4% solution and 10% aerosol for topical anesthesia of the trachea, and 2% jelly and 5% ointment for lubrication of endotracheal tubes. A 1:1 lidocaine-prilocaine preparation in an oil and water emulsion (EMLA cream or patch) is also available for transdermal application. It is suitable for providing anesthesia for needle insertion or other minor surgical procedures. Each gram of the emulsion contains 25 mg each of lidocaine and prilocaine. A generous layer should be applied to the intended area and covered with an occlusive dressing for 30 minutes to 1 hour.

Lidocaine is a safe and effective local anesthetic. It is the most popular agent in current practice. In order to avoid systemic toxicity, its dose should be limited to 7 mg/kg with epinephrine or 5 mg/kg without.

> **Note:** Bilateral posterior leg pain without neurologic deficit that lasts for up to 1 week has been reported after intrathecal injection of hyperbaric 5% lidocaine. The clinical significance of this transient radicular-like pain is unclear. It may be related to a high concentration of lidocaine near the site of injection. The current recommendation is to dilute the 5% solution with an equal volume of cerebrospinal fluid or normal saline before subarachnoid injection.

Dibucaine

Dibucaine, also an amide, is a potent but toxic agent. Its action is slow in onset but lasts 2–3 hours. Prepared as a 0.5% solution, it is used almost exclusively for spinal anesthesia. Systemic toxicity is seen when the dose exceeds 1.5 mg/kg.

Prilocaine

The action of prilocaine, another amide, is somewhat similar to that of lidocaine, but it is less toxic. As much as 9 mg/kg with epinephrine or 6 mg/kg without epinephrine is tolerated by most patients. However, prilocaine can cause the formation of methemoglobin, a product of oxidation of the ferrous iron of normal hemoglobin to the ferric state by toluidine, a metabolite of prilocaine. Methemoglobin does not have the ability to carry oxygen, and signs of severe methemoglobinemia are those of hypoxemia. A patient who develops clinical signs related to methemoglobinemia should be treated with oxygen by mask, and methylene blue, 1–2 mg/kg, should be given intravenously. Methylene blue is a reducing agent capable of converting methemoglobin to normal hemoglobin.

Mepivacaine

Pharmacologically, mepivacaine, also an amide, resembles lidocaine except that its duration of action is somewhat longer. A 1% solution is suitable for local infiltration, but a 1.5% solution is required for major nerve blocks and a 1.5% or 2% solution for epidural anesthesia. A dose of over 5 mg/kg, with or without epinephrine, is toxic.

Bupivacaine

Bupivacaine is structurally very similar to mepivacaine, but it is more potent and has a much longer duration of action (2–5 hours, depending on the site). Onset of action and uptake into the bloodstream are equally slow. Addition of epinephrine does little to increase its duration of action. The 0.25% solution is suitable for local infiltration and epidural analgesia; the 0.5% solution should be used for major nerve blocks and epidural anesthesia. For spinal anesthesia, the hyperbaric 0.75% solution in 8.25% dextrose in water should be used. Bupivacaine is more cardiotoxic than equipotent doses of other agents. The total dose should be limited to 2 mg/kg, with or without epinephrine. Cardiotoxicity of bupivacaine is increased in parturients and can be refractory to treatment. The 0.75% solution for epidural anesthesia (not the hyperbaric solution for spinal anesthesia) has been withdrawn from the market.

Etidocaine

Although etidocaine is related to lidocaine structurally, it is similar to bupivacaine in pharmacologic action but is less toxic. A dose of 6 mg/kg with epinephrine or 4 mg/kg without is tolerated well.

Ropivacaine

Ropivacaine was developed to supplant the cardiotoxic bupivacaine. Structurally it is related both to bupivacaine and mepivacaine; pharmacologically it is slightly less potent than bupivacaine and slightly shorter acting. At equipotent doses it is less cardiotoxic than bupivacaine, and its toxicity does not increase with pregnancy. Furthermore, cardiac arrest produced by ropivacaine is amenable to routine resuscitative measures, whereas that by bupivacaine may be refractory to treatment. However, clinical experience with this new agent is still limited.

7

The Anesthetic Machine and Accessories

The function of the anesthetic machine (also called the gas machine) is to deliver a safe anesthetic mixture to the anesthetic circuit, from which it can be inhaled by the patient. All modern machines have evolved from the continuous-flow Boyle's apparatus. In newer models, mechanical ventilators and monitors are integrated with the basic unit. This chapter is dedicated to a description of the basic components and built-in safety features of the standard gas machine. Discussions of anesthetic circuits, ventilators, and monitors are presented in Chapter 8, 9, and 14, respectively.

Basic Components

Taken in the direction of gas flow, the basic components of an anesthetic machine are arranged in the following sequence (Fig. 7–1):

1. Source of oxygen, nitrous oxide, and other gases (e.g., air)
2. Pressure gauges
3. Pressure regulators (pressure-reducing valves)
4. Flowmeters
5. One or more vaporizers for volatile agents
6. Common gas outlet
7. Oxygen flush control

The assembly of gas lines and their accessories, from the gas supplies to the flowmeter controls, is often referred to as the high-pressure circuit portion of the anesthetic machine; that beyond the flowmeter controls is the low-pressure circuit of the machine.

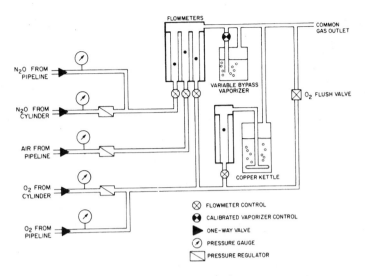

FIGURE 7–1. Basic components of the anesthetic machine. (Refer to text for details.)

Source of Anesthetic Gases

All anesthetic machines have duplicate supplies of both oxygen and nitrous oxide: either two cylinders of each gas or a supply of oxygen and nitrous oxide by pipelines and a spare supply of oxygen and nitrous oxide by cylinder. The duplicate supply of oxygen is mandatory; the duplicate supply of nitrous oxide can be optional. These gas supplies are harnessed to the gas inlets of the machine by noninterchangeable safety systems so that a gas supply cannot be mistakenly connected to the wrong inlet (see "Safety Features" below). Within these inlets are one-way valves to prevent leakage of gases through an open inlet. Some machines are also equipped with noninterchangeable safety harnesses for the supply of air and other gases.

Pressure Gauges

Built into the anesthetic machine are pressure gauges for monitoring the pressure of gas supplies. Oxygen and nitrous oxide are supplied through pipelines at a constant pressure of 50 psi, but oxygen, nitrous oxide, and other gases are also supplied in cylinders at much higher pressures.

Oxygen is compressed to approximately 2000 psi in a full cylinder. At this pressure and at room temperature, compressed oxygen remains in the gaseous state. As the cylinder empties, pressure within it falls progressively, and the pressure registered is directly proportional to the amount of oxygen remaining in the cylinder. For example, a pressure of 1000 psi indicates that the cylinder is half full.

Nitrous oxide, in contrast, is compressed to only about 750 psi in a full cylinder. At this pressure and at room temperature, compressed nitrous oxide is in the liquid state. The pressure registered on the pressure gauge in this instance is the vapor pressure of nitrous oxide at room temperature. As nitrous oxide vapor leaves the cylinder, more liquefied nitrous oxide evaporates to take its place; thus the vapor pressure does not fall as long as there is liquid nitrous oxide in the cylinder. When all the liquid nitrous oxide has evaporated, pressure in the cylinder falls rapidly as it empties. Therefore, pressure in the nitrous oxide cylinder bears no relationship to the amount of liquid nitrous oxide in the cylinder. This is also true for carbon dioxide, which is normally compressed to 840 psi. The only method of determining the quantity of nitrous oxide or carbon dioxide remaining in a cylinder is to compare its weight with that of a full tank.

Pressure Regulators

The pressure of oxygen and nitrous oxide supplied by cylinders must be reduced to a lower and constant working pressure suitable for use in the anesthetic machine (40−50 psi). This is accomplished by means of pressure regulators (pressure-reducing valves). A pressure regulator is also necessary for air and carbon dioxide. Pressure regulators work on the simple principle that high pressure applied to a small area can be balanced by low pressure applied to a large area. In this manner, a high-pressure inflow is transformed to a low-pressure outflow. In some anesthetic machines, the 50-psi pressure of oxygen and nitrous oxide from pipelines and the reduced pressure (40−50 psi) of oxygen and nitrous oxide from cylinders are further reduced to 16 psi by a second-stage pressure regulator before these gases are directed to the flowmeters.

Flowmeters

Flowmeters are tapered glass tubes (Thorpe tubes) calibrated individually for oxygen, nitrous oxide, and other gases. These tubes are mounted vertically and in parallel in a protective casing. The inflow into the flowmeters is regulated by flow-control valves situated at the lower end of the flowmeter assembly, and

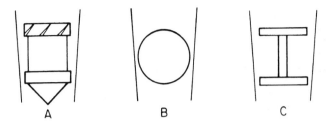

FIGURE 7–2. Types of flowmeter floats. Gas flow should be read from the upper edge of elongated floats (*A* and *C*) and from the equator of a spherical float (*B*).

gas flows are indicated by floats in the centers of these tubes. When the controls are shut off, the floats settle to the lower and narrower ends of the flowmeter tubes. When the control valves are turned on, the floats rise in the tubes according to the magnitude of the gas flows. Gas flows should be read from the upper edge of elongated floats and from the equator of spherical floats (Fig. 7–2). After passing through their respective flowmeters, anesthetic gases mix to form the fresh gas mixture before flowing downstream.

Vaporizers

Vaporizers are devices designed to dispense a measured amount of volatile agent (e.g., halothane, isoflurane, desflurane) into the fresh gas mixture. Almost all of those in use today are concentration-calibrated, variable-bypass vaporizers using a flow-over method for vaporization. However, measured-flow vaporizers illustrate the function of anesthetic vaporizers more vividly and are described first.

The copper kettle is a prototypic *measured-flow device*; the Verni-Trol is another example. They are supplied with their own measured flow of oxygen (Fig. 7–3*A*). As oxygen flows through the vaporizer, it becomes fully saturated with the vapor of the volatile anesthetic. When this vapor-laden oxygen joins the fresh gas mixture, the concentration of anesthetic vapor in the mixture can be expressed as

$$\text{Concentration of vapor in anesthetic mixture} = \frac{\text{Volume of vapor}}{\text{Total volume of mixture}}$$

Because the volume of vapor is directly related to the flow of oxygen through the vaporizer, anesthetic concentration changes according to this flow.

In addition to the flow of oxygen through the vaporizer, there is one other factor that affects the vapor output of the vaporizer:

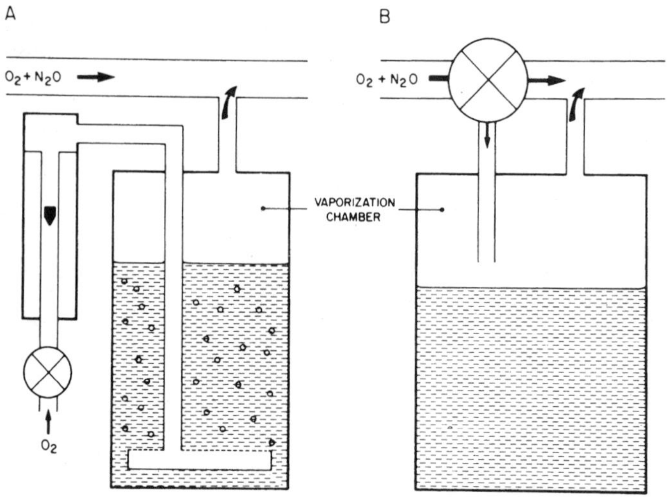

FIGURE 7–3. Types of vaporizers. *A*, A measured-flow vaporizer (e.g., the copper kettle) with its own oxygen supply dispensed from a flowmeter. *B*, A variable-bypass vaporizer (e.g., the Tec 5 and the Vapor 19.1), in which the concentration control dial diverts a fraction of the fresh gas mixture through the vaporization chamber (Refer to text for details.)

cooling through loss of latent heat of vaporization. (Latent heat of vaporization may be defined as the amount of energy removed by molecules on leaving the liquid phase to enter the gaseous phase.) Although heat is absorbed from its surroundings, the temperature of the liquid anesthetic falls with time as it evaporates. Because vaporization is less vigorous when the liquid is cold, the volume of vapor carried by a constant flow of oxygen through the vaporizer is smaller at lower temperatures. That is, concentration of vapor in the anesthetic mixture falls as the liquid anesthetic cools. Therefore, it is necessary to increase continually the flow of oxygen through the copper kettle or the Verni-Trol vaporizer in order to maintain a constant anesthetic vapor concentration as the liquid anesthetic cools.

The *variable-bypass vaporizer* does not have its own oxygen supply (see Fig. 7–3*B*). When such a device is switched on, a fraction of the fresh gas mixture is diverted through the vaporization chamber and flows over the liquid anesthetic to become saturated with vapor. Subsequently this fraction rejoins the main flow downstream to yield the anesthetic mixture. The anesthetic concentration in this mixture can be calculated as for a measured-flow vaporizer and is calibrated directly on the control dial. A variable-bypass vaporizer is equipped with a temperature-sensitive mechanism that increases automatically the fraction of gas flow through the vaporization chamber as the temperature of the liquid anesthetic falls. Thus the output of anesthetic vapor remains constant, despite cooling of the vaporizer and its content. These vaporizers are calibrated individually for specific volatile agents. Filling a vaporizer with the wrong agent can cause serious overdose. The following vaporizers are variable-bypass flow-over devices: the Tec 3, Tec 4, Tec 5, and Ohio calibrated vaporizers by Ohmeda; the Vapor 19.1 vaporizers by North American Dräger; and the PPV Sigma vaporizers by Penlon.

Desflurane has a boiling point around room temperature (23.5° C) and a vapor pressure close to that of the atmosphere (664 mm Hg) at 20° C. This agent requires an injection-type vaporizer (the Tec 6 vaporizer by Ohmeda) heated to 39° C to deliver pure vapor under pressure. Through an electronic servo-controller, metered amounts of desflurane vapor are injected into the fresh gas according both to the concentration dial setting and the fresh gas flow.

Common Gas Outlet

Beyond the vaporizer, the anesthetic mixture is directed by internal circuits to leave the anesthetic machine at the common gas outlet. This fresh gas outlet has a standard 22-mm outer diameter and a 15-mm inner diameter. From this common gas outlet, the anesthetic mixture flows to the anesthetic circuit.

Oxygen Flush Control

All anesthetic machines are equipped with an emergency oxygen flush valve. The control of this valve is usually situated close to the common gas outlet. Irrespective of flowmeter and vaporizer settings, activation of this demand valve will deliver pure oxygen at a flow of 35–75 L/min directly to the common gas outlet, bypassing the flowmeters and vaporizers. In older models, this control can be locked in the "On" position. Using this locking feature is inadvisable because it runs the risk of allowing high pressures to build up in the anesthetic circuit and in the patient's airway. The oxygen flush valve in all modern machines can be activated only on demand.

▨ Safety Features

In order to ensure that a safe anesthetic mixture is delivered to the patient and to avoid abuse, standards organizations, government agencies, and the industry have established safety specifications for the design of anesthetic machines and their accessories. Because there are national, regional, and institutional differences in these standards, the student is advised to become familiar with local practice. These safeguards are by no means foolproof, but in general the following features are recommended:

1. Color codes for all equipment containing or delivering medical gases and volatile anesthetics.
2. Medical gas cylinders built and tested to specifications and equipped with the pin-index safety system and a safety pressure-relief valve.
3. Noninterchangeable safety systems to connect medical gas pipelines to the anesthetic machine.
4. A downstream position for the oxygen flowmeter in the flowmeter assembly and a unique oxygen flowmeter control.
5. A safety system to fill agent-specific vaporizers.
6. Mutually exclusive vaporizer controls.
7. A back-pressure check valve, oxygen failure safety valve, oxygen failure alarm, minimum oxygen–nitrous oxide flow-ratio controller, and oxygen analyzer with alarm.

Color Codes

Color codes for equipment containing or delivering medical gases are designed to minimize accidental confusion sometimes encountered in the use of such equipment. In all English-speaking countries except the United States, the international code is used: white for oxygen, blue for nitrous oxide, white and black for air, gray for carbon dioxide, black for nitrogen, and brown for helium. In the United States, green replaces white for oxygen and yellow replaces white and black for air; otherwise the code is the same for the other gases mentioned. All pipelines, gas cylinders, pressure gauges, and flowmeters and their controls should be appropriately color coded.

Volatile agents are coded according to one universally accepted standard: red for halothane, orange for enflurane, purple for isoflurane, blue for desflurane, and yellow for sevoflurane. This code should be used to differentiate the containers of these agents and agent-specific vaporizers.

Medical Gas Cylinders

The oxygen and nitrous oxide cylinders most commonly mounted on anesthetic machines are size E cylinders made of steel or its chromium-molybdenum alloy. All cylinders in use are tested every 5–10 years; they should withstand a pressure two-thirds higher than the maximum allowable working pressure. However, the pressure in a full cylinder containing liquefied or flammable gases should not exceed the working pressure at room temperature, and the pressure in a full cylinder containing nonliquefied and nonflammable gases should not exceed the working pressure by more than 10%. All information concerning the manufacturing and testing of such a cylinder is engraved on its shoulder (Fig. 7–4A, B). A large label bearing the chemical or common name of its contents is affixed to its body, and a tag indicating whether the cylinder is full or empty is attached to its neck (Fig. 7–4C). When the cylinder is in use, the FULL section of the tag should be removed; when the cylinder is empty, the IN USE section should be removed.

At the upper end of the cylinder, there is an elongated block in which resides the cylinder valve (Fig. 7–5). Gas flow through the outlet port of this valve is controlled by turning the valve stem counterclockwise with a wrench. Two safety features are

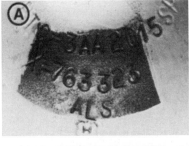
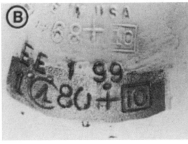
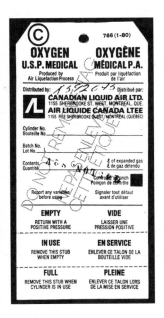

FIGURE 7–4. Markings and label on medical gas cylinders. A, The specification number of the cylinder is *3AA, 2015* is the service pressure in psi, *X-763323* is the serial number, and *ALS* identifies the owner. B, The marking *EE19.9* is the elastic expansion in millimeters at 3360 psi, *1-80* is the retest date, the symbol between *1* and *80* identifies the testing facility, and *+10* indicates that 10% overfill is allowable. C, The label attached to the neck of the cylinder.

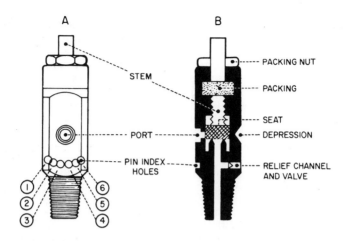

FIGURE 7–5. The cylinder valve. *A*, Frontal view illustrating the loci of the pin-index holes. *B*, Cross section illustrating the valve mechanism and the safety pressure-relief valve. (Refer to text for details.)

built into this valve block: the pin-index safety system and the safety pressure-relief valve.

Pin-Index Safety System

Gas cylinders are secured to the anesthetic machine by yokes. The pin-index safety system is designed to prevent the attachment of a cylinder to the wrong inlet on the anesthetic machine (e.g., a nitrous oxide cylinder to the oxygen inlet). This is achieved by the presence of two holes just below the exit port of the valve block. These holes are matched by two corresponding pins on the yoke. Each of these holes, with the corresponding pin, occupies one of six loci describing an arc (see Fig. 7–5*A*). Two exclusive loci of holes and pins have been assigned to each gas. If a cylinder is attached to the wrong yoke, the unmatched position of pins and holes will prevent proper alignment of the outlet port of the cylinder and the inlet port of the anesthetic machine. The loci allocated for oxygen are 2 and 5; those for nitrous oxide are 3 and 5; those for air are 1 and 5.

Safety Pressure-Relief Valve

The safety pressure-relief valve (see Fig. 7–5*B*) is designed to prevent rupture of the cylinder should the pressure within rise rapidly above working pressure (e.g., during a fire). Usually one of three valve mechanisms is employed: a metal disk that ruptures at high pressure, an alloy that has a relatively low melting point (e.g., Wood's metal), or a spring-loaded one-way valve that yields to high pressure.

Noninterchangeable Pipeline Connections

Pipelines delivering compressed gas are also attached to the anesthetic machine by noninterchangeable connections. Two such systems exist: the diameter-index safety system and the quick-mount system.

The *diameter-index safety system* is illustrated in Figure 7–6A. It consists of a female component having two concentric bores (M and N) that will mate with a corresponding male component having two concentric diameters (M' and N'). The diameters of M and N and those of M' and N' are specific for each gas. As diameters M and M' increase, those of N and N' decrease. In this manner, the female component designed for a specific gas is absolutely incompatible with the male component of all other gases.

The *quick-mount system* allows rapid connection and disconnection without special tools. There is more than one type of quick-mount system. Figure 7–6B illustrates one type in which the index skirt of the male component must fit the index groove of the female counterpart. The two components are held

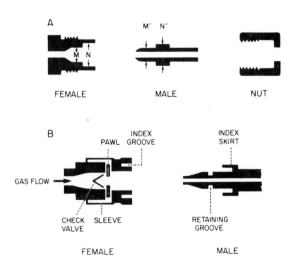

FIGURE 7–6. Noninterchangeable pipeline connections. *A*, The diameter-index safety system. *B*, One type of quick-mount system. (Refer to text for details.)

together by a spring-loaded catch (the pawl) engaging the retaining groove. Turning the sleeve clockwise will release this catch and allow rapid disconnection. In another type, the female component has concentric bores that match the concentric diameters of the corresponding male component. Noninterchangeability is ensured in a manner similar to that of the diameter-index safety system. These two components are held together by plunging the male element into the female element and locking them together with a counterclockwise twist.

Oxygen Flowmeter and Its Control

In order to minimize the possibility of delivering a hypoxic gas mixture as a result of leaks, all anesthetic machines manufactured in North America since 1974 have their oxygen flowmeter located downstream of all other flowmeters in the flowmeter assembly. If oxygen flowmeter were mounted in the upstream position, oxygen could escape through cracks in all flowmeters (see Fig. 7–7A). This can result in the delivery of a hypoxic gas mixture if nitrous oxide is also turned on. With the oxygen flowmeter mounted downstream, oxygen is lost only if there is a leak in its own flowmeter tube (Fig. 7–7B), so the chance of a hypoxic mixture being delivered is reduced.

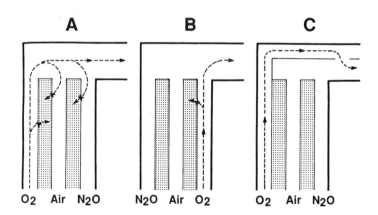

FIGURE 7–7. Position of oxygen flowmeter. *A*, If it is mounted upstream, a leak in any of the flowmeters can result in the delivery of a hypoxic gas mixture. *B*, If it is mounted downstream, a hypoxic gas mixture is delivered only when the leak is in the oxygen flowmeter itself. *C*, If the oxygen flowmeter is upstream but oxygen is allowed to flow in its own conduit to a point distal to all other flowmeters, the risk of oxygen leak is the same as that in *B*.

In English-speaking countries other than the United States and Canada, the oxygen flowmeter is left in the upstream position but oxygen flows in its own conduit to enter the mainstream at a point distal to all other flowmeters (Fig. 7–7C). This arrangement has the same margin of safety as that used in North America.

Much effort has also been put into the design of the oxygen flowmeter control. To allow it to be distinguishable from others under all lighting conditions, certain features are recommended: it should be coded by color, have the chemical formula O_2 affixed to its face, have a fluted profile unique to sight and to touch, and be the largest and most accessible of all the flowmeter controls.

Agent-Specific Filling System for Vaporizers

All modern variable-bypass vaporizers are agent specific. Accidental filling of a vaporizer with the wrong agent not only can cause serious misunderstandings but also can lead to fatal overdose. The agent-specific filling system for vaporizers is designed to avoid such accidents.

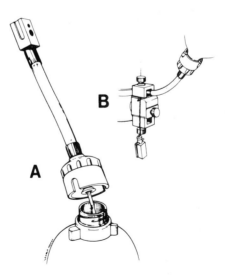

FIGURE 7–8. Filling spout used in agent-specific filling system for vaporizers. *A*, The index groove at the tip and the index notches in the cap of the spout allow filling of an agent-specific vaporizer from a bottle containing liquid of that agent only. *B*, A drawing showing how the spout fits the filling port of the agent-specific vaporizer.

The filling port of a vaporizer without this system is simply a funnel, but that of a vaporizer with this system is housed in a block that will accept only the tip of a spout with an index groove carved into its side (Fig. 7–8). At the other end of the spout, the bottle cap also has grooves at its side so that it will fit only containers that have a collar with matching ridges. The vaporizer, the spout, and the bottle are also color coded for the agent.

With a boiling point around room temperature, desflurane vaporizers cannot be filled by a simple funnel system. The Tec 6 vaporizer has a unique filler port that will accept only the adaptor that comes mounted on the desflurane bottle.

Exclusive Vaporizer Control

In order to prevent more than one vaporizer from being switched on simultaneously, vaporizer controls should be exclusive. In older models, the intended agent must be selected on a separate control first. Only then can the control of the vaporizer containing that agent be switched on. No amount of tampering will allow the control of a second vaporizer to be turned on simultaneously. In current models, the controls of these vaporizers are mutually exclusive. That is, once the control of one vaporizer is switched on, the controls of the others are automatically locked in the "Off" position.

Back-Pressure Check Valve

During positive-pressure ventilation of the patient, intermittent positive pressure applied to the anesthetic circuit will travel in both anterograde and retrograde directions. Therefore back-pressure is transmitted to the vaporization chamber of the vaporizer that is in use. At the commencement of expiration, the rapid fall in back-pressure will cause a simple vaporizer (e.g., the Boyle's bottle) to discharge at both its inlet and its outlet (Fig. 7–9), thereby increasing the anesthetic output of the vaporizer. A second problem related to back-pressure is bouncing movements of flowmeter floats: a fall in the levels of the floats when positive pressure is applied and a rise to normal levels when positive pressure is removed. Interposition of a one-way check valve between the distal vaporizer and the common gas outlet eliminates these problems. (Back-pressure has no effect on the vapor output of a modern vaporizer.)

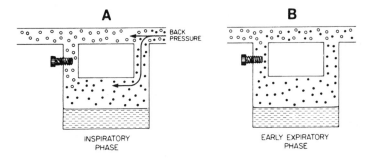

FIGURE 7–9. The effect of back-pressure on a simple variable-by-pass vaporizer. *A*, During the inspiratory phase of controlled ventilation, back-pressure from the ventilator will pressurize the vaporization chamber. *B*, During the early expiratory phase, dissipation of this back-pressure will cause the discharge of vapor at both the inlet and the outlet of the vaporizer. (The fresh gas is represented by open dots and the vapor-laden mixture by solid dots.)

Oxygen Failure Safety Valve

The oxygen failure safety valve is a mechanical device designed to interrupt the flows of nitrous oxide and other inert gases to their respective flowmeters if oxygen supply pressure has fallen to 25 psi. (Oxygen supply pressure is the pressure of oxygen in the pipeline or of oxygen from the cylinder after it has gone through the first-stage pressure regulator: 40–50 psi.) This interruption of inert gas flow is achieved by shutting off the supply of all gases before they reach the flowmeters. It must be stressed that this safety valve ensures only that no hypoxic gas mixture is delivered to the anesthetic circuit when oxygen supply fails. It does not protect against failure in oxygen supply, nor does it prevent the delivery of a hypoxic gas mixture as a result of leaks in the flowmeter assembly or at a point distal to this assembly. Unless the machine is also equipped with a minimum oxygen–nitrous oxide flow-ratio controller (see below), it is still possible to turn on the flow of nitrous oxide without switching on the oxygen flow, if oxygen supply pressure is normal.

Oxygen Failure Alarm

The oxygen failure alarm is an adjunct to the oxygen failure safety valve. As oxygen supply fails, the alarm will sound a high-pitched warning for at least 7 seconds. In some of these devices, the failing source of oxygen is used to sound the alarm, which will stop when the supply of oxygen is depleted. Stoppage of the audio signal in this instance should not be regarded as correction of the problem. In another type, the audio alarm is powered by nitrous oxide. However, if nitrous oxide is not in use, the alarm will fail to function. A third type powered by battery is also available, but will not function if the battery becomes exhausted. Therefore these devices should not be regarded as foolproof.

Minimum Oxygen–Nitrous Oxide Flow-Ratio Controller

This controller is a mechanical link between the oxygen and nitrous oxide flowmeter controls. Its function is twofold: to provide a minimal flow of oxygen at 200 ml/min and to maintain oxygen flow above 25% of total flow at all times. When both oxygen and nitrous oxide are in use (e.g., 2 L/min flow each), nothing will happen to nitrous oxide flow if oxygen flow is increased beyond 2 L/min. Nothing will happen to nitrous oxide flow either if oxygen flow is reduced to less than 2 L/min, as long as oxygen flow remains above 25% of total flow. However, if oxygen flow is reduced to below 667 ml/min (less than 25% of total flow), then nitrous oxide flow will decrease pro rata automatically to maintain oxygen flow at 25% of total flow. When oxygen flow falls to 200 ml/min, nitrous oxide flow shuts off automatically. In the same example, oxygen flow will rise pro rata automatically if nitrous oxide flow is increased beyond 6 L/min so that oxygen flow is maintained at not less than 25% of total flow; or, depending on the device, it would not be possible to increase the nitrous oxide flow beyond 6 L/min.

Introduction of this oxygen–nitrous oxide flow-ratio controller represents another step to prevent dispensing hypoxic mixtures from the anesthetic machine. Again this effort is not foolproof. Because this controller links the oxygen and nitrous oxide flowmeter controls only, addition of a second inert gas can result in the delivery of hypoxic mixtures.

Oxygen Analyzer with Alarm

Besides prevention, it is equally important to be warned of the danger when a hypoxic gas mixture is being delivered. Addition of an oxygen analyzer with an alarm is a step in this direction. This device is an add-on feature in older machines but a built-in component of newer models. It emits an audible alarm and a visual signal when oxygen concentration of the gas mixture falls below 21%. If the alarm does go off, the sole means of resetting it is by increasing oxygen concentration to 21% or more.

An add-on oxygen analyzer used for this purpose has a slow response time and becomes inaccurate if moisture condenses on the surface of its electrode (see "Galvanic Fuel Cell and Polarographic Oxygen Analyzers" in Chapter 14). Therefore, locating the analyzer electrode in the expiratory limb of any anesthetic circuit is undesirable. It should be incorporated into the inspiratory limb of the circle system and be positioned at the common gas outlet when other circuits are used.

■ Checking the Anesthetic Machine

Equipment failure, including machine failure, is a major cause of anesthesia morbidity and mortality. Therefore, it is mandatory that the operator should check out the anesthesia machine before use at the start of a working day. The checkout should begin with going over the manual of an unfamiliar machine to make sure that it is equipped to meet current standards. Having ascertained that it is, the user should proceed to check the machine in the following sequence:

1. Inspect the machine and its accessories visually for damage.

2. Check that the vaporizers are properly filled and tighten their filler caps.

3. Verify that the flowmeter controls and the vaporizer control dials are off. With the master switch still turned off, attach a suction bulb to the common gas outlet and squeeze it repeatedly until it is fully collapsed. (If the bulb will not remain collapsed for at least 10 seconds, a leak exists in the low-pressure system between the flowmeter controls and the fresh gas outlet.) Complete the checkout of the low-pressure system by repeating the above maneuver with the vaporizer control dials switched on one at a time to check for leaks in the vaporizers.

4. Confirm that the pipeline connections are secure. The pipeline pressure gauges should register 50 psi.

5. Verify that the gas cylinders are properly seated and are turned off. Turn on the oxygen cylinder and check its pressure gauge. It should register at least 500 psi, indicating that the cylinder is at least a quarter full. ***Turn off the oxygen cylinder again after this maneuver***. (Cylinder oxygen is used only as a backup to pipeline supply. If it is not turned off, the oxygen flowmeter will draw on this supply first until the cylinder pressure falls to equal the pipeline pressure of 50 psi. At this pressure, the cylinder is practically empty and would be useless as a backup.)

6. Turn on the master switch of the anesthesia machine and check the range of flow of the individual gases by adjusting the flowmeter controls.

7. Set both the oxygen and nitrous oxide flows at 3 L/min each and check the function of the oxygen–nitrous oxide flow-ratio controller by turning down the oxygen flow slowly to below 1 L/min. If this device is functioning properly, the nitrous oxide flow will fall pro rata to maintain an oxygen–nitrous oxide flow ratio of 1:3 (25% oxygen).

8. Set both the oxygen and nitrous oxide flows at 3 L/min again and check the function of the oxygen failure safety valve and oxygen failure alarm by disconnecting the pipeline supply of oxygen. If these devices are functioning properly, the nitrous oxide flow will be shut off as the oxygen flow fails and a high-pitched alarm will sound for at least 7 seconds. *Reconnect the anesthesia machine to the oxygen pipeline after this maneuver.*

9. Calibrate the oxygen analyzer, if it is part of the anesthesia machine, and check its reading against the known composition of oxygen in the fresh gas flow.

> **Note:** The maneuvers enumerated above are generic methods of checking out an anesthesia machine. They represent the minimum one should do to prepare the machine for service. Special conditions may demand more vigorous checkout procedures. The user should check the manuals of brand-name machines for special checkout procedures that may be required. Checkout of the anesthetic circuit and its accessories is reviewed in Chapter 8.

Anesthetic Circuits 8

The anesthetic circuit or anesthetic system delivers the anesthetic mixture from the machine to the patient's upper airway. Common to all anesthetic circuits are the tubings, adjustable pressure-limiting valve, reservoir bag, and pressure gauge. Because the lungs can be injured by high pressures built up accidentally in the circuit, a safety device that limits this pressure to around 50 cm H_2O also should be incorporated into the system. This safety feature can be in the form of a special blow-off valve (e.g., the Norry valve) interposed between the circuit mount and the anesthetic circuit or in the form of a specially constructed reservoir bag (see "Reservoir Bag" below).

Circuit Components

Anesthetic Tubings

Corrugated anesthetic tubings are made of antistatic black rubber or lightweight plastic. The corrugations are for strength, flexibility, and kink resistance. These tubings form a low-resistance conduit through which the anesthetic mixture is delivered to the patient's upper airway, and they act as a reservoir in which fresh anesthetic mixture is stored during expiration. Tubing for adult circuits has a 22-mm inner diameter and that for pediatric circuits a 15-mm inner diameter.

Adjustable Pressure-Limiting Valve

In current anesthetic practice, the rate at which fresh gas is added to the circuit is higher than the rate of uptake by the patient. Therefore, it is necessary to include an adjustable pressure-limiting (APL) valve (also called a relief valve, expiratory valve, or pop-off valve) in the circuit to vent excess gas to the atmosphere or to a scavenging system. A prototype APL valve is illustrated in Figure 8–1A. The valve is shut by turning the control clockwise; it is opened by turning the control in the

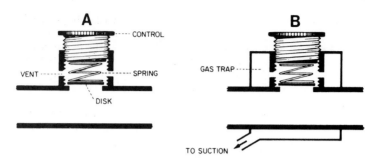

FIGURE 8–1. Illustration of an adjustable pressure-limiting (APL) valve. *A*, A simple APL valve. *B*, An APL valve with a gas trap for scavenging. (Refer to text for details.)

other direction. When the valve is shut, compression of the spring pushes the valve disk tight against its seat, so that no gas can escape. When the valve is open, the spring is only lightly compressed; excess gas escapes through the vent by unseating the valve disk with a pressure of less than 1 cm H_2O. Some APL valves are built within a gas trap (see Fig. 8–1*B*) from which the overflow is directed to the outflow of a central evacuation system. These are called scavenging devices; they are designed to reduce pollution of the operating room atmosphere.

The setting of the APL valve varies according to the mode of ventilation. During spontaneous ventilation, the valve should be set fully open so that excess gas can vent at a low pressure during expiration. During manual ventilation, the valve should be set partially closed so that pressure applied to the reservoir bag and transmitted to the circuit can inflate the patient's lungs until the opening pressure of the valve is reached, when some of the gas mixture is vented. During mechanical ventilation, the valve should be shut and excess gas should be allowed to overflow through the ventilator. The APL valve should never be completely shut except during mechanical ventilation.

Reservoir Bag

Most reservoir bags are made of latex rubber, although bags made of plastic are also available for special use. As an integral component of the patient's breathing circuit, the reservoir bag has four major functions:

1. It is a reservoir for the anesthetic mixture. This is necessary because inspiratory flow varies during inspiration. It is zero at the beginning of inspiration, it rises to approximately

30 L/min at its peak, and it settles back to zero at the end of inspiration. Fresh gas flow from the anesthetic machine, in contrast, is constant and is not set nearly as high as peak inspiratory flow. Therefore, there are moments during inspiration when a large discrepancy between fresh gas flow and inspiratory flow exists. This shortfall is drawn from the reservoir bag as required.

2. It serves as a monitor of the patient's ventilatory pattern during spontaneous ventilation. Excursion of the bag is a reflection of the patient's tidal volume; frequency of this excursion is equal to the patient's respiratory rate.

3. It provides a means by which the patient's lungs can be ventilated manually.

4. It acts as a safety device, protecting the patient's airway and lungs from exposure to pressure greater than 50–60 cm H_2O, which can cause barotrauma. This function exploits the characteristic compliance (pressure-volume relationship) of these bags mandated by the American Society for Testing and Materials and other institutions overseeing standards and quality. For bags that have a nominal volume of 1.5 liters or smaller, the internal pressure should remain within the range of 30–50 cm H_2O when they are inflated up to four times nominal volume. For bags larger than 1.5 liters nominal volume, the pressure should remain between 35 and 60 cm H_2O when they are inflated up to four times nominal volume. Thus the airway is protected from exposure to pressure higher than 50–60 cm H_2O in an accident (e.g., when the APL valve is inadvertently left in the shut position during spontaneous ventilation).

Pressure Gauge

A gauge of aneroid type is usually built into the circuit mount to measure pressure that is transmitted to the airway from the anesthetic circuit. The importance of monitoring this pressure is discussed under "Airway Pressure" in Chapter 14.

Type of Circuits

In the past it has been popular to classify anesthetic circuits (also called anesthetic systems) into open, semiopen, semiclosed, and closed systems, and the respective terms were used ambiguously. Classifying circuits as rebreathing and nonrebreathing systems is equally unsatisfactory because some degree of rebreathing occurs with all commonly used circuits. In this chapter, circuits are identified by their common names. The most popular circuits in current use are the anesthetic circle, the Magill circuit, the modified T-piece, and the Bain circuit. For completeness, the Waters to-and-fro system and circuits employing nonrebreathing valves are also mentioned.

The Circle System

The anesthetic circle is the most popular circuit in use in North America. When the fresh gas flow added to the circle is low, rebreathing of expired gas is marked, but carbon dioxide in the expired gas is removed by a soda lime or Baralyme canister incorporated into the circuit.

Soda lime comes in 4- to 8-mesh granules hardened with a small amount of silicates. (A 4-mesh strainer has 16 quarter-inch square openings per square inch; an 8-mesh strainer has 64 eighth-inch square openings per square inch. Four- to 8-mesh granules will pass through a 4-mesh strainer but be retained by an 8-mesh strainer.) The granules are composed of 4% sodium hydroxide, 1% potassium hydroxide, 76–81% calcium hydroxide, 14–19% moisture, and a dye indicator. The reactions involved in carbon dioxide absorption are as follows:

$$CO_2 + H_2O \rightarrow H_2CO_3$$

$$2NaOH + H_2CO_3 \rightarrow Na_2CO_3 + 2H_2O$$

$$Ca(OH)_2 + H_2CO_3 \rightarrow CaCO_3 + 2H_2O$$

These reactions generate heat. Although water is also generated, the presence of moisture is essential to initiate these reactions. A change in the color of the pH-sensitive dye indicator is a sign of exhaustion of the absorbent. The exact color change varies with the brand.

Baralyme is a mixture of 20% barium hydroxide octahydrate and 80% calcium hydroxide. (The water content, which is incorporated into barium hydroxide as octahydrate, equals 13% of the mixture by weight.) It also comes in 4-mesh to 8-mesh granules. Carbon dioxide reacts with barium hydroxide octahydrate directly according to the equation

$$Ba(OH)_2 \cdot 8H_2O + CO_2 \rightarrow BaCO_3 + 9H_2O$$

The new inhalation anesthetic sevoflurane can react with soda lime and Baralyme to produce compound A, a nephrotoxin in laboratory rats (see "Sevoflurane" in Chapter 3). However, no such toxicity has been reported in humans. In addition, there have been sporadic reports of mild to moderately severe carbon monoxide poisoning in anesthetized patients in whom the carbon dioxide absorption circle system was used. Available evidence points to the reaction of halogenated inhalation anesthetics with carbon dioxide absorbents (soda lime or Baralyme) that has remained dormant and unused in the circle system for some time as the source of carbon monoxide. Under artificial laboratory conditions, soda lime with a critical water content of less than 4.8% and Baralyme with a critical water content of less than 9.5% can react with desflurane, enflurane, and isoflurane (but not halothane or sevoflurane) to produce toxic or near-toxic levels of carbon monoxide. Under similar conditions, desflurane produces much more carbon monoxide than an equipotent concentration of enflurane or isoflurane, and reaction with Baralyme produces more carbon monoxide than with soda lime. It is still unclear how or whether these laboratory conditions are achieved in the clinical situation. Further study is required to clarify the issue. Until more information becomes available, it may be prudent to change soda lime or Baralyme canister that has been lying dormant in carbon dioxide absorption anesthetic circuits regularly and to flush the anesthetic circuit and canister with 100% oxygen for at least 1 minute before the first case of the day.

The most popular arrangement of the circle is illustrated in Figure 8–2. There are two APL valves in the circle: one near the patient on the Y-piece and one close to the reservoir bag. In spontaneous ventilation, overflow occurs during the second half of expiration. This should be allowed to take place at the APL valve near the patient to vent expired gas. In manual ventilation, overflow occurs during inspiration. To minimize escape of fresh gas through the valve near the patient, this valve should be shut and overflow allowed to take place at the one

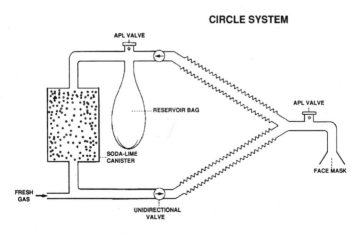

FIGURE 8–2. The circle system

close to the reservoir bag. The circle system has these advantages over other circuits:

1. Economy of lower fresh gas flow
2. Partial warming and humidification of the inspired mixture because reaction of carbon dioxide with alkaline absorbents generates heat and water
3. Smaller overflow of excess gas and less pollution of the operating room atmosphere
4. Reduced fire hazard when flammable agents are used

A major disadvantage of the system is its high resistance, which is less than ideal for small children. Resistance can be reduced by removing the unidirectional valves and using a circulator instead to direct gas flow.

Most anesthesiologists using the circle system choose a fresh gas flow of 2–3 L/min. With this magnitude of fresh gas flow, rebreathing is only partial. The technique is safe so long as the fresh gas mixture contains at least 25% oxygen. Yet to maximize the advantages of the anesthetic circle requires reduction of fresh gas flow to around 200–300 ml/min of 100% oxygen, just enough to meet the basal metabolic rate for oxygen. At this very low flow, rebreathing is maximal. This closed-circuit technique carries certain risks. Owing to dilution of fresh gas by exhaled gases, there is always a huge discrepancy between oxygen concentration of the fresh gas (which is 100%) and that of the mixture in the inspiratory limb of the circle. Large changes in vaporizer settings are required to bring about small changes in anesthetic concentration of the inspired mixture, and minor incompetence of unidirectional valves can cause dangerous accumulation of carbon dioxide in the circuit. Oxygen concentration and carbon dioxide tension of inspired and expired gases should be monitored at the airway when low-flow technique is practiced.

Magill Ciruit

The arrangement of the Magill circuit (also called the Mapleson A circuit) is illustrated in Figure 8–3. Because carbon dioxide absorption is not employed, adequate flow of fresh gas is required to purge the circuit of expired gas. In order to minimize rebreathing, fresh gas flow equal to the patient's minute ventilatory volume (approximately 100 ml/kg body weight) is sufficient during spontaneous ventilation. However, a very high gas flow is required to minimize rebreathing during controlled ventilation, a feature that makes this circuit impractical for this purpose.

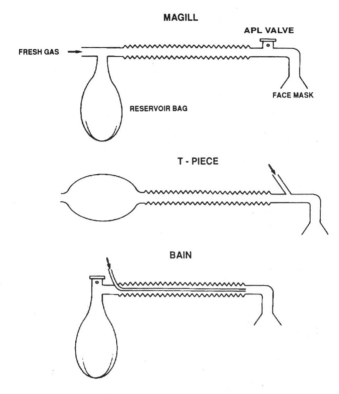

FIGURE 8–3. The Magill circuit, the T-piece, and the Bain circuit.

Ayre's T-Piece

There are many modifications of the original Ayre's T-piece; the most popular is the Jackson-Rees version (see Fig. 8–3). (This circuit is called the Mapleson E circuit if the reservoir bag is omitted.) Being valveless, it offers little resistance to gas flow; this feature makes it a popular pediatric circuit. During spontaneous ventilation, overflow from the system is allowed to escape through the open end of the reservoir bag; during manual ventilation, the open end of the reservoir bag is occluded as the bag is compressed; and during mechanical ventilation, this bag is replaced by the bellows of the mechanical ventilator. The modified T-piece is not as efficient as the Magill circuit in eliminating expired gas during spontaneous ventilation: A fresh gas flow 2.5–3 times the patient's minute volume is required to prevent rebreathing. However, it is more efficient than the Magill circuit during controlled ventilation; fresh gas flows required to maintain normocapnia in the patient are

1. For patients weighing 10–30 kg: 100 ml/kg body weight plus 1000 ml
2. For patients weighing more than 30 kg: 50 ml/kg body weight plus 2000 ml

Bain Circuit

The Bain circuit (see Fig. 8–3) is made of lightweight plastic and is a modification of the Mapleson D circuit. It has a coaxial design and its extra length allows the anesthetic machine to be positioned well away from the field of operation, which has made it popular in anesthesia for head and neck surgery. During spontaneous ventilation, a fresh gas flow of 100–150 ml/kg body weight is required to minimize rebreathing. Unlike the Magill circuit, the Bain circuit is more efficient during controlled than during spontaneous ventilation. A fresh gas flow of 70 ml/kg body weight is sufficient to maintain normocapnia.

Waters To-and-Fro Circuit

The Waters to-and-fro circuit (Fig. 8–4) is a carbon dioxide absorption system that offers low resistance to gas flow yet has all the advantages of the circle system. Being located close to the patient's head, the Waters canister is cumbersome and can shed irritant alkaline dust into the airway. Its popularity is waning.

Circuit with Nonrebreathing Valves

A nonrebreathing valve (e.g., Ambu, Fink, Reuben, Stephen-Slater) is one that directs fresh gas mixture to the patient during inspiration and expired mixture to the atmosphere during expiration. A prototype circuit is illustrated in Figure 8–4. During spontaneous ventilation, fresh gas flow should be adjusted so that the reservoir bag is around three-fourths full at the end of expiration and at least one-fourth full at the end of inspiration. During controlled ventilation, fresh gas flow should equal the patient's minute volume. Unfortunately, many of these valves have a significant apparatus dead space, some can become incompetent with use, others can stick when wet, and all are difficult to clean and sterilize. These circuits are not popular except as a backup to conventional anesthetic circuits or in cardiopulmonary resuscitation.

WATERS TO-AND-FRO

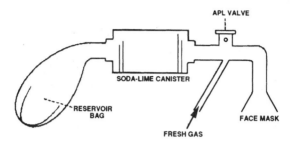

NON-REBREATHING

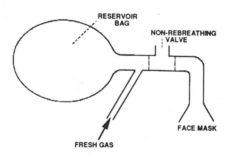

FIGURE 8-4. The Waters to-and-fro circuit and a circuit with non-rebreathing valve.

■ Checking the Anesthetic Circuit

The anesthetic machine should be checked at the beginning of a workday, but the anesthetic circuit should be checked before the start of each case. The checkout procedure should include the following steps:

1. Verify the calibration of the oxygen analyzer. (This device may be an add-on accessory to the anesthetic circuit or it may be built into the monitor modules of the anesthetic machine. This procedure has been described in "Checking the Anesthetic Machine" in Chapter 7.)

2. Inspect the circuit for damage. If it is the Bain or a similar coaxial circuit, pay special attention to the integrity of the inner tube.

3. Turn off the flowmeters and switch the anesthetic machine to the "Manual" mode (as opposed to the "Ventilator" mode)

and check for leaks in the anesthetic circuit by closing the APL valve and blocking the patient's end of the anesthetic circuit. Using the oxygen flush control on the anesthetic machine, fill the reservoir bag until the pressure in the circuit registers 30 cm H_2O or more on the pressure gauge. The pressure in the circuit should remain unchanged for at least 10 seconds.

4. Check the safety device that limits the maximum pressure in the circuit as in Step 3 but keep activating the oxygen flush control to increase the pressure within the circuit. If the device is a Norry valve, it will blow off when the circuit pressure reaches 40 cm H_2O. If the device is the reservoir bag, the inflation pressure will not exceed 50 cm H_2O for a bag that has a nominal volume of 1.5 liters or smaller and will not exceed 60 cm H_2O for a bag that has a nominal volume larger than 1.5 liter. (Do not overinflate the reservoir bag.)

5. Open the APL valve fully and check the low-pressure venting function of the valve by occluding the patient's end of the anesthetic circuit and activating the oxygen flush control at the same time. When the reservoir bag is inflated to its full nominal capacity, excess gas should vent with hardly any pressure registered on the pressure gauge of the circuit.

6. Check the scavenging device and the integrity of its connection to the vacuum outlet.

7. If the circuit is the circle system, make sure that the anesthetic machine has not been lying dormant. Consider changing the carbon dioxide absorbent if it has. Otherwise, inspect the carbon absorption canister and make sure that it is properly filled with active absorbent. (Exhaustion of the absorbent is indicated by a color change unique to the brand of the absorbent.)

Mechanical Ventilators

Mechanical ventilators are devices that generate positive pressure rhythmically to inflate the lungs during artificial ventilation. Advances in electronics have changed the crude pneumatically driven ventilator into a sophisticated machine that can deliver pressure and flow in complicated waveforms and control inspiration and expiration with precision. This chapter deals with the basic principles behind mechanical ventilators and mechanical ventilation rather than the mechanics and electronics of brand-name ventilators.

All ventilators have the following functions: (1) to inflate the lungs during inspiration, (2) to change over from inspiration to expiration, (3) to allow the lungs to deflate during expiration, and (4) to change over from expiration to inspiration. In order to ensure safe mechanical function, all modern ventilators are equipped with a pressure gauge to monitor pressure in the circuit, a pressure-limiting device to protect the lungs from barotrauma, high- and low-pressure alarms, and a spirometer to measure ventilatory volumes.

▨ Phases of Ventilation

Inspiratory Phase

All mechanical ventilators are driven either by compressed gas or by an electric motor. When the generated pressure is applied to the upper airway, flow of air into the lungs and the volume of inflation are determined by the following equations:

$$\text{Flow} = \frac{\text{Airway-alveolar pressure gradient}}{\text{Airway resistance}}$$

$$\text{Volume} = \text{Increase in alveolar pressure} \times \text{Compliance}$$

The magnitude of positive pressure a ventilator generates can be low or very high. When it is low but constant, the *pressure* transmitted to the upper airway is *constant* throughout inspiration (see Fig. 9–1A). Flow into the lungs is high initially but falls exponentially to zero at the end of inspiration (see Fig. 9–1B). A ventilator producing this type of pressure is called a *constant-pressure generator*.

When the generated pressure is very high, this pressure is usually applied to the airway gradually so that airway pressure increases through inspiration (see Fig. 9–1C). *Flow* into the lungs, however, is *constant* (see Fig. 9–1D). A ventilator producing this type of air flow is called a *constant-flow generator*.

Changes in compliance or airway resistance of the lungs will affect the performance of these ventilators in different ways. A constant-pressure generator delivering a set volume to normal lungs will have difficulty delivering this same volume when compliance falls, airway resistance increases, or both happen simultaneously. A constant-flow generator, in comparison, is a powerful machine. It delivers the same volume at the expense of higher airway pressure, even when compliance and airway resistance deteriorate.

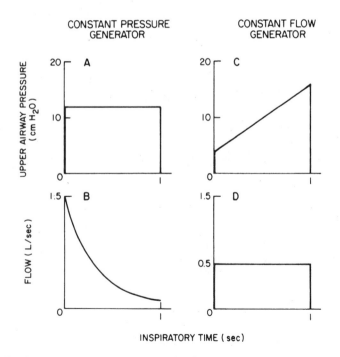

FIGURE 9–1. The pressure and flow waveforms of a constant-pressure generator and a constant-flow generator. (Refer to text for details.)

When volume delivered is the sole criterion, performance of a constant-pressure generator is affected by changes in lung characteristics, whereas that of a constant-flow generator is not. The right type of ventilator should be chosen to match the patient's lung characteristics. In the operating room, use of a constant-pressure generator is not unreasonable because most anesthetized patients have stable lung characteristics. In critically ill patients whose pulmonary compliance and airway resistance can change from moment to moment, only a constant-flow generator can deliver a constant volume of ventilation.

Changeover from Inspiration to Expiration

For a ventilator to function effectively, it must stop inflation periodically to allow the lungs to deflate. There are four types of changeover mechanism: volume cycling, time cycling, pressure cycling, and flow cycling.

In *volume cycling*, changeover occurs after the ventilator has delivered a preset volume. Owing to the presence of small leaks, the compression of gases, and the distention of delivery tubings, this cycling volume is always larger than the actual volume received by the patient. Nevertheless, volume cycling is a common design used in many ventilators.

Time cycling is equally popular, and changeover occurs after a preset inspiratory time. When time cycling is used in a constant-flow generator, changeover occurs only after a preset volume has been delivered (volume is the product of flow and time).

In *pressure cycling*, changeover occurs when pressure at the upper airway has reached a preset value. When a ventilator is pressure cycled, the volume it delivers varies according to the changing characteristics of the lungs. That is, a pressure-cycled constant-flow generator behaves like a constant-pressure generator.

In *flow cycling*, changeover occurs when inspiratory flow has fallen to a preset value. This mechanism is used only in low-pressure generators.

Expiratory Phase

During the expiratory phase, the lungs are allowed to deflate, usually against atmospheric pressure but in some cases against a positive end-expiratory pressure (PEEP). Use of negative pressure in the expiratory phase is now out of favor.

Changeover from Expiration to Inspiration

Ability of the ventilator to change over from expiration to inspiration is as important as that from inspiration to expiration. Although the same four changeover mechanisms can be defined, only changeover after a preset expiratory time (i.e., time cycling) is practical.

▨ Safety Features

Mechanical ventilation is indispensable in a modern operating room, and safeguards should be in place to monitor its function. Some of these devices are built into the ventilator and some are add-on components. When the mechanical ventilator is an integral part of the modern anesthetic machine, these devices are integrated into the array of monitors of the machine.

Bellows Design

When the anesthetic machine is set to the "Ventilator" mode (as opposed to the "Manual" mode), the ventilator bellows housed in a transparent rigid casing replaces the reservoir bag of the anesthetic circuit. During expiration, the bellows is filled by the fresh gas mixture from the anesthetic machine and exhaled gases from the patient. During inspiration, a driving gas (either compressed air or oxygen) cycled into the rigid casing empties the contents of the bellows into the patient's lungs. Tidal volume is determined by a control dial that limits bellows excursion.

Two types of bellows design are used. In older machines, the bellows descends as it fills during expiration. This descending (hanging) bellows design is relatively unsafe. In the presence of a disconnection in the anesthetic circuit, the bellows will continue to fill by sucking in air from the atmosphere and will empty its contents into the atmosphere, giving the illusion that the ventilator is ventilating the patient. In newer models, the bellows ascends as it is filled by the fresh gas mixture and the patient's exhaled gases during expiration. In the presence of a disconnection, the ascending (standing) bellows will collapse completely, giving warning of the disconnection.

Pressure Monitor

Pressure in the anesthetic circuit during mechanical ventilation is monitored by either an aneroid pressure gauge or an electronic pressure transducer (see "Airway Pressure" in Chapter 14) in all modern ventilators. Normally this pressure is near zero during end expiration (unless PEEP is applied) and does not exceed 30 cm H_2O at peak inspiration. A subatmospheric pressure usually means the patient is breathing spontaneously against the ventilator. A large increase in pressure during inspiration could mean an increase in airway resistance (e.g., bronchospasm or kinked endotracheal tube); a decrease in chest wall or pulmonary compliance (e.g., recovery from muscle relaxant, pneumothorax, or pulmonary congestion); or, rarely, mechanical failure of the ventilator (e.g., blocked expiratory vent). A large fall in pressure during positive-pressure ventilation always means a major leak in the anesthetic circuit or even total disconnection.

Pressure Alarms

Disconnection in the anesthetic or ventilator circuit is a critical incident. All modern ventilations have a low-pressure alarm to warn the user of this danger. It is activated if a preselected threshold pressure less than the patient's peak inspiratory inflation pressure is not sensed after a preset delay of around 15 seconds. In order to protect against barotrauma to the airway, a high-pressure alarm is activated by pressures above an upper limit (usually 60 cm H_2O). In addition to these basic alarms, some brand-name anesthetic ventilators are equipped with pressure alarms to warn against subatmospheric pressures of less than -10 cm H_2O and continuously elevated pressure of more than 15 cm H_2O.

Pressure-Limiting Device

Excess pressure generated by mechanical ventilators (particularly by constant-flow generators) can cause barotrauma to the airway and lungs (e.g., pneumothorax). Therefore, the high-pressure alarm described above is an integral component in ventilator design. Most ventilators also have a pop-off valve in the internal circuit to limit the pressure that can be delivered to the bellows housing. The pressure at which it pops off is preset by the manufacturer. It is around 60 to 100 cm H_2O.

Spirometer

The bellows of the ventilator is usually calibrated to indicate the volume of gas mixture it delivers with each breath. Owing to compression of the gas mixture, distention of anesthetic tubing, and minor leaks, the tidal volume received by the patient is always less than what is registered by the bellows. A spirometer mounted on the expiratory limb of the anesthetic circuit can give independent verification of tidal and minute volumes. Changes in ventilatory volume can raise a warning of changes in lung characteristics and disconnections (see "Ventilatory Volumes" in Chapter 14).

Other Monitors and Alarms

Advances in electronics have greatly improved the self-monitoring and alarm functions of modern mechanical ventilators. In some brand-name models these additional monitors and alarms are available: electric power failure alarm, ventilator failure alarm, low driving gas supply pressure alarm, excessive PEEP alarm, and alarms to indicate ventilator settings beyond the capability of the machine. The user should check with the operating manuals of brand-name models to benefit from the full capability of these alarms.

■ Checking the Ventilator

Like the anesthetic circuit, function of the mechanical ventilator should be checked before the start of each case. The following maneuvers are recommended:

1. Use a reservoir bag as the model lung and attach it to the patient's end of the anesthetic circuit. Select the "Ventilator" setting (as opposed to "Manual") on the circuit mount and close the APL valve if required. (In most setups, selection of the "Ventilator" setting will automatically exclude the APL valve from the anesthetic circuit.)

2. Set the oxygen flow to 200–300 ml/min.

3. Select a ventilator setting with respect to tidal volume, respiratory rate, and inspiration-expiration ratio appropriate for the patient (see "A Practical Guide to Mechanical Ventilation" below).

4. Switch on the ventilator and use the oxygen flush control to fill the bellows and reservoir bag (model lung) to capacity.

5. Observe the excursion of the bellows during inspiration. It should deliver the selected tidal volume at the selected rate. Observe the excursion of the bellows during expiration. An ascending bellows should return to the top of its casing unless there is a leak. (A descending bellows will fill to capacity in the presence of a leak. To check for leaks in these models re-

quires obstruction of the patient's end of the anesthetic circuit. No leak is present if the high-pressure alarm is activated with minimal upward excursion of the bellows during the inspiratory phase.)

6. Check the reading on the pressure monitor of the ventilator during the inspiratory phase. It should register a peak pressure of 20–30 cm H_2O when inflating the reservoir bag used as the model lung. Failure to inflate the reservoir bag is another indication of leaks, whether the bellows is ascending or descending.

7. If the anesthetic circuit is the circle system, check the excursions of the unidirection valves (see Fig. 8–2) during the respiratory cycle. These valves are positioned in the inspiratory and expiratory limbs of the circle and should open in phase with inspiration and expiration.

■ A Practical Guide to Mechanical Ventilation

Pulmonary capillary blood absorbs oxygen from and excretes carbon dioxide into the alveoli. The purpose of pulmonary ventilation is to bring oxygen into and remove carbon dioxide from the alveoli. When this is done properly, not only is an adequate volume of air moving in and out of the lungs, but also the distribution of this volume to the alveoli matches their perfusion (see Chapter 10). Therefore, choice of tidal volume, respiratory rate, and inspiration-expiration ratio (or inspiratory and expiratory times) is important. In addition, the positive intrathoracic pressure during mechanical inflation of the lungs can impede venous return to the heart. In order to minimize this undesirable side effect of positive-pressure ventilation, proper selection of inspiration-expiration ratio again is important.

Tidal Volume

Tidal volume delivered by mechanical ventilators can be set by adjusting the volume control or by adjusting both the inspiratory flow and inspiratory time controls. (Volume is the product of flow and time.) The tidal volume of a normal person in the awake state is approximately 7 ml/kg body weight. For reasons stated in Chapter 10, the tidal volume of normal anesthetized persons should be increased by 50% during mechanical ventilation to reduce ventilation-perfusion inequalities.

Respiratory Rate and Inspiration-Expiration Ratio

The respiratory rate on a mechanical ventilator can be set by the rate control alone or by adjusting both the inspiratory and expiratory time controls. The rate should be set at a normal level of 10–15 breaths per minute. In order not to impede venous return, the inspiratory phase should be as short as is practical. However, delivering a set tidal volume in a short time encourages maldistribution of inspired gas and ventilation-perfusion inequalities. Experience has shown that an inspiration-expiration ratio between 1:2 and 1:1 is acceptable in normal persons. In patients who are hypovolemic, a smaller ratio of 1:3 or 1:4 may be indicated to promote venous return.

Hypocapnia is a common complication when the carbon dioxide absorption circle system is used. The magnitude of hypocapnia can be decreased by lowering the fresh gas flow and respiratory rate.

Inspiratory Flow

Like short inspiratory time, a fast inspiratory flow encourages ventilation-perfusion inequalities. Therefore, inspiratory flow should be slow. Obviously it should not be so slow that the selected tidal volume cannot be delivered in the chosen inspiratory time.

Summary

Effective pulmonary ventilation can be achieved in patients who have normal lungs with the following ventilator settings: tidal volume, 10 ml/kg; rate, 12 breaths per minute (8 per minute when the anesthetic circuit is the circle system); inspiration-expiration ratio, 1:2; and inspiratory flow, relatively slow. Capnography is a useful aid in the fine adjustment of fresh gas flow, tidal volume, and respiratory rate and to keep end-tidal carbon dioxide tension between 35 and 40 mm Hg (see "Capnographs" in Chapter 14).

Effect of Anesthesia on Respiratory Function

10

Of the many systemic side effects of anesthetic drugs (see Chapters 2 through 6), none is more serious than those that affect the respiratory system. Depression of ventilation and maldistribution of pulmonary ventilation and blood flow are part and parcel of general anesthesia. Both can cause hypercapnia and hypoxemia. In addition, airway resistance and pulmonary compliance are also affected. In this chapter, these important complications of anesthesia are described, and their effects on elimination of carbon dioxide and oxygenation are reviewed.

■ Alveolar Ventilation

Normally a 70-kg human breathes 10–15 times each minute and has a tidal volume of 500 ml per breath (7 ml/kg body weight per breath). However, only 70% of each tidal breath is distributed to the alveoli; the other 30% is wasted in ventilation of the conducting airways. Gas in these anatomic airways does not take part in gas exchange, and the space it occupies is called the *anatomic dead space*. In addition, there is no gas exchange in alveoli that are ventilated but not perfused; this space constitutes the *alveolar dead space*. The sum of anatomic dead space and alveolar dead space is called *physiologic dead space*. The relationship between alveolar ventilation per minute ($\dot{V}_A$) and tidal volume (V_T), physiologic dead space (V_D), and respiratory rate (RR) is represented by the following equation:

$$\dot{V}_A = (V_T - V_D) \times RR$$

A fall in tidal volume or respiratory rate or an increase in physiologic dead space will decrease "effective" alveolar ventilation.

Under the influence of inhalation anesthetics, tidal volume is smaller than normal. Usually there is also an increase in respiratory rate, which is most pronounced with halothane but less so with the other agents. This pattern of shallow breathing is much less efficient than normal breathing. As the difference between tidal volume and physiologic dead space narrows, "effective" alveolar ventilation falls, despite an increase in respiratory rate.

Under the influence of narcotic analgesics, in contrast, respiratory rate is reduced but tidal volume remains unchanged. This pattern of breathing is also inefficient, and "effective" alveolar ventilation falls in proportion to the decrease in respiratory rate.

During anesthesia, alveolar ventilation is also reduced by an increase in physiologic dead space. Protruding the jaw and extending the neck will double the anatomic dead space, and decrease in pulmonary perfusion as a result of hypotension will increase alveolar dead space. This increase is further exaggerated by instrument dead space in face masks, connectors, and rebreathing circuits. Although tracheal intubation halves the anatomic dead space, this decrease may not be enough to offset other added instrument dead space.

In summary, "effective" alveolar ventilation is less than normal in anesthetized patients who are breathing spontaneously. Its effect on elimination of carbon dioxide and oxygenation is discussed in later sections.

■ Control of Breathing

Breathing is under the control of the respiratory center at the brain stem, respiratory muscles being its effectors. To meet widely different ventilatory demands imposed by activities of the body, the respiratory center receives many sensory inputs. They include impulses from central and peripheral chemoreceptors and those from receptors in the lungs and airways, in muscles and joints, and in systemic and pulmonary vasculature. This center is also under the direct influence of higher centers and the cerebral cortex.

The central chemoreceptors are located on the ventral surface of the medulla and are anatomically distinguishable from the respiratory center itself. They are sensitive to changes in the hydrogen ion concentration of cerebrospinal fluid. An increase in hydrogen ion concentration stimulates breathing, and a decrease inhibits it.

When P_aCO_2 rises above normal, carbon dioxide crosses the blood-brain barrier and reacts with cerebrospinal fluid to yield hydrogen ions:

$$CO_2 + H_2O \rightleftharpoons H_2CO_3 \rightleftharpoons H^+ + HCO_3^-$$

The action of these hydrogen ions on the central chemoreceptors stimulates breathing. Because carbon dioxide excretion is increased during hyperventilation, stimulation of breathing will return both the carbon dioxide level of arterial blood and the hydrogen ion concentration of cerebrospinal fluid toward normal; that is, P_aCO_2 regulates breathing by its effect on hydrogen ion concentration of cerebrospinal fluid. It is the most important factor in the control of normal ventilation.

Less important are the peripheral chemoreceptors located at the bifurcation of the common carotid arteries and at the aortic arch. Breathing is stimulated via this route by hypoxemia, but this mechanism does not operate until P_aO_2 has fallen to less than 60 mm Hg. Although these receptors are stimulated also by hypercapnia, they account for less than 20% of the normal ventilatory response to carbon dioxide. Receptors in the carotid bodies, but not those in the aortic bodies, are stimulated also by acidemia.

All anesthetics depress the sensitivity of the central and peripheral chemoreceptor reflex. That is, normal increases in ventilation in response to hypercapnia or hypoxemia are either depressed or abolished by these agents. Whereas anesthetic levels of thiopental and inhalation agents depress the ventilatory response to both hypercapnia and hypoxemia, subanesthetic levels of inhalation agents (consistent with those found in patients in the postanesthesia care unit) are enough to abolish the ventilatory response to hypoxemia. Ventilatory depressant effects of anesthetic agents are dose related and additive. Among the inhalation agents, nitrous oxide has the least depressant effect. If it is used as part of the anesthetic gas mixture, the concentration of volatile agents can be reduced, thus sparing the more potent depressant effects of volatile agents.

In short, anesthetized patients are ill-equipped to cope with hypercapnia and/or hypoxemia resulting from depression of the normal ventilatory control mechanism. developing hypercapnia or hypoxemia may go unnoticed if only ventilatory volumes are monitored.

Ventilation-Perfusion Inequalities

Ideally all alveoli should receive an equal share of inspired gas and cardiac output, but in reality some mismatch of ventilation and perfusion exists in normal persons. Regardless of whether the individual is erect, supine, or in the lateral decubitus position, pulmonary blood flow gravitates to dependent zones of the lungs. At the same time, alveolar ventilation is better in dependent zones. However, in terms of blood flow, dependent zones of the lungs are relatively underventilated and nondependent zones overventilated. In other words, dependent zones of the lungs have a low ventilation-perfusion ratio, and nondependent zones have a high ventilation-perfusion ratio. This ratio is commonly expressed as $\dot{V}/\dot{Q}$.

Blood perfusing areas of the lungs with a low $\dot{V}/\dot{Q}$ ratio does not become fully saturated with oxygen; these areas act as right-to-left shunts to cause desaturation of arterial blood. Ventilation of areas of the lungs with a high $\dot{V}/\dot{Q}$ ratio is more than what is necessary to oxygenate the small amount of blood perfusing these areas. Much of the tidal exchange to these areas is wasted (like dead space gas). The volume of this wasted ventilation constitutes the *alveolar dead space*.

Factors that decrease the $\dot{V}/\dot{Q}$ ratio of dependent zones increase arterial desaturation, and factors that increase the $\dot{V}/\dot{Q}$ ratio of nondependent zones increase alveolar dead space and decrease "effective" alveolar ventilation. Three such factors are important in the conscious state: airway closure, functional residual capacity (FRC), and hypoxic pulmonary vasoconstriction. Two others are important in anesthetized patients: the effect of anesthesia itself and that of mechanical ventilation.

Airway Closure and Functional Residual Capacity

The membranous respiratory bronchioles are compressible. When their intraluminal pressure is less than pleural pressure, these microscopic airways collapse. Consequently, their alveoli are isolated and cannot take part in tidal exchange. This phenomenon is called *airway closure*. The lung volume at which airway closure commences is called *closing capacity*. (The term *closing volume* is also used. It is the difference between closing capacity and residual volume.) Airway closure takes place only in dependent zones. In young healthy adults, closing capacity is well below *FRC*, which is the lung volume at the end of a normal expiration; therefore, no airway closure occurs during normal tidal breathing.

Functional residual capacity can fall (e.g., in obese or pregnant patients), and closing capacity can increase above normal (e.g., in smokers and geriatric patients). When FRC is below closing capacity, small airways in dependent zones of the lungs close prematurely during normal tidal exchange. When these airways are closed, their alveoli cannot receive a full share of the tidal volume, so the $\dot{V}/\dot{Q}$ ratio of these dependent zones falls.

Hypoxic Pulmonary Vasoconstriction

Pulmonary vessels in regions where the alveoli are underventilated and low in oxygen content tend to constrict. As a result, blood is directed to well-ventilated alveoli. Although residual perfusion of those areas with a low $\dot{V}/\dot{Q}$ ratio persists, hypoxic pulmonary vasoconstriction is a functional protective mechanism that reduces ventilation-perfusion mismatch in both dependent and nondependent zones of the lungs.

Effects of Anesthesia

If distribution of ventilation and perfusion is not perfectly balanced in the conscious state, it is even worse during anesthesia. Following induction of anesthesia, the $\dot{V}/\dot{Q}$ ratio falls in dependent zones and increases in nondependent zones. This deterioration is qualitatively similar in all anesthetized patients, whether they are breathing spontaneously or are mechanically ventilated. Although the mechanism has not been fully explained, anesthesia is known to produce certain effects on factors that affect the distribution of ventilation and perfusion:

1. A 15–20% fall in FRC is a consistent feature following induction of anesthesia. Functional residual capacity may even fall below closing capacity in some anesthetized patients. When this happens, the $\dot{V}\dot{Q}$ ratio of dependent zones falls below normal.

2. Hypoxic pulmonary vasoconstriction, a protective mechanism that reduces ventilation-perfusion inequalities, may be inhibited by inhalation anesthetics. In its absence, mismatch of ventilation and perfusion in both dependent and nondependent zones of the lungs will increase. (The magnitude of inhibition of hypoxic pulmonary vasoconstriction by inhalation anesthetics is being debated. Clinical studies in patients undergoing single-lung anesthesia have demonstrated only minimal inhibition.)

3. Blood flow to nondependent zones of the lungs is impeded by gravitational force. If pulmonary hypotension is a complication following induction of anesthesia, blood flow to nondependent regions will likely decrease, and consequently the $\dot{V}/\dot{Q}$ ratio in these regions will be higher than normal.

Effect of Mechanical Ventilation

In the supine position, abdominal contents act as a column of fluid, and the pressure against the diaphragm is highest in dependent zones. Following induction of anesthesia, there is cephalad displacement of the end-tidal position of the diaphragm; this displacement is most pronounced in these dependent regions. Whereas most of the diaphragmatic movement occurs in these dependent regions during spontaneous breathing, diaphragmatic movement takes place mainly in nondependent regions during mechanical ventilation (Fig. 10–1). Therefore, the effect of mechanical ventilation is an increase in the $\dot{V}/\dot{Q}$ ratio of nondependent zones at the expense of a fall in the $\dot{V}/\dot{Q}$ ratio of dependent zones. However, the low $\dot{V}/\dot{Q}$ ratio of dependent zones during mechanical ventilation can be reversed partially by delivering a larger-than-normal tidal breath. During a large tidal exchange, a larger share of the tidal volume is delivered to dependent zones when alveoli in nondependent zones have reached the limit of their distensibility.

In addition, a longer inspiratory phase (i.e., a larger inspiration-expiration ratio) improves intrapulmonary distribution of gases and oxygenation. This is of special importance in patients with significant lung disease. However, a prolonged inspiratory phase during positive-pressure ventilation can impede venous return, decrease cardiac output, and impair oxygenation (see "Oxygenation" below). In some critically ill patients, it may be necessary to monitor cardiac output while adjusting ventilatory parameters so as to obtain the best degree of oxygenation.

In summary, induction of anesthesia is accompanied by an increase in shunt-like effects as a result of falls in the $\dot{V}/\dot{Q}$ ratio in dependent zones of the lungs. Similarly, there is an increase in alveolar dead space as a result of increases in the $\dot{V}/\dot{Q}$ ratio in nondependent zones.

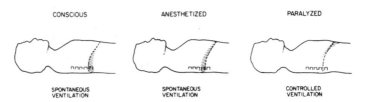

FIGURE 10–1. Excursion of the diaphragm, indicated by shaded areas, in conscious and anesthetized persons breathing spontaneously and in the paralyzed person ventilated mechanically. The dotted line marks the position of the diaphragm at the end of a normal expiration (i.e., at FRC) in a conscious person breathing spontaneously. (Refer to text for details.)

Airway Resistance and Pulmonary Compliance

Airway resistance (not including that caused by the anesthesia apparatus) can double during an uncomplicated anesthetic procedure. Increases in airway resistance can occur at both the upper and lower airways. At the upper airway, it is mainly due to the tongue falling back to lie against the posterior pharyngeal wall, causing obstruction to air flow. This obstruction can be corrected by lifting the jaw forward and inserting a pharyngeal or laryngeal mask airway or an endotracheal tube. Increase in resistance of the lower airway, in comparison, is the result of a reduction in the caliber of small airways following a fall in FRC. Airway resistance can increase even further in the presence of anesthetic complications: laryngospasm will increase resistance of the upper airway and bronchospasm will increase that of the lower airway. In addition, pulmonary compliance has been observed to decrease during anesthesia, but the magnitude of this change is small and its significance is not clear.

Carbon Dioxide Elimination

Arterial carbon dioxide tension in healthy, conscious subjects lies between 36 and 40 mm Hg, but values approaching 70 mm Hg have been reported in anesthetized persons breathing spontaneously. This increase in P_aCO_2 is a reflection of impairment of carbon dioxide elimination, even when the anesthetic is simple and uncomplicated.

Carbon dioxide elimination is directly proportional to alveolar ventilation. When alveolar ventilation falls, P_aCO_2 rises. During anesthesia, not only is ventilation depressed (see "Alveolar Ventilation" above), but also "effective" alveolar ventilation is decreased (see "Ventilation-Perfusion Inequalities" above). In addition, ventilatory response to an increase in P_aCO_2 is depressed by anesthetic agents (see "Control of Breathing" above). All of these factors contribute to carbon dioxide retention during anesthesia. Because carbon dioxide excretion can be increased by increasing ventilation, carbon dioxide retention can be rectified easily with larger tidal volumes delivered by either assisted or mechanical ventilation.

Oxygenation

The oxygen tension of arterial blood is 5–10 mm Hg below that of alveolar gas in healthy adults breathing room air. This alveolar-arterial oxygen tension difference is due to the presence of

1. An *anatomic shunt*, which is the venous return of bronchial and coronary circulations. It drains directly into the left heart and accounts for 2% of cardiac output.

2. *Venous admixture*, which is blood flowing through areas of the lungs with a low $\dot{V}/\dot{Q}$ ratio. This accounts for approximately 3% of normal cardiac output.

It is well known that arterial oxygenation is impaired during anesthesia. This is reflected in the desaturation of arterial blood and in a larger-than-normal alveolar-arterial oxygen tension difference. The major cause of arterial desaturation during anesthesia is an increase in shunt-like effects of blood flowing through areas of the lungs with a low $\dot{V}/\dot{Q}$ ratio (see "Ventilation-Perfusion Inequalities" above).

Falls in cardiac output that are often seen during anesthesia also can contribute to impairment of arterial oxygenation. Figure 10−2 illustrates the mechanism of this impairment. A hypothetical patient "A" consumes oxygen at the rate of 200 ml/min and has a cardiac output of 5 L/min, of which 20%, or 1 L/min, is shunt. From each 100 ml of cardiac output, 4 ml of oxygen must be extracted; the oxygen content of mixed venous blood is 15 ml O_2/100 ml blood. Blood going through the lungs is fully oxygenated and has an oxygen content of 20 ml/100 ml blood, but blood in the shunt has an oxygen content equal only to that of mixed venous blood. Therefore, the arterial oxygen content is 19 ml O_2/100 ml blood.

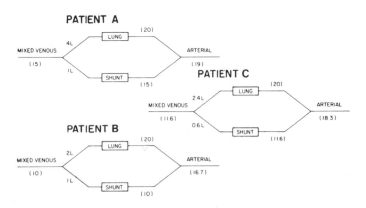

FIGURE 10−2. Effects of a fall in cardiac output on arterial oxygenation on hypothetical patients *A*, *B*, and *C* (refer to text for details). The oxygen content of blood (ml/100 ml blood or volume percent) along each route is shown in parentheses.

In patient "B" cardiac output has fallen to 3 L/min but the shunt has remained fixed at 1 L/min. Because almost 6.7 ml of oxygen must be extracted from each 100 ml of cardiac output to satisfy the same oxygen consumption of 200 ml/min, mixed venous oxygen content has fallen to 10 ml O_2/100 ml blood. The outcome is a lower arterial oxygen content of 16.7 ml O_2/ 100 ml blood. Similar desaturation of arterial blood would have occurred even if the shunt fraction had remained at 20% of cardiac output. this is illustrated by patient "C," whose cardiac output has fallen to 3 L/min but the shunt has fallen proportionately to 0.6 L/min. To satisfy oxygen demand, 6.7 ml of oxygen must be extracted from each 100 ml of arterial blood. As a result, mixed venous oxygen content has fallen to 11.6 ml O_2/100 ml blood and arterial oxygen content to 18.3 ml O_2/100 ml blood.

It is clear that desaturation of mixed venous blood is the underlying cause of impaired arterial oxygenation following a fall in cardiac output. This desaturation is also seen when the hemoglobin concentration is low or when there is a shift of the oxygen-hemoglobin dissociation curve to the left. These factors too may contribute to arterial hypoxemia in patients undergoing surgery.

Alveolar hypoventilation is another factor that can cause arterial desaturation in patients under anesthesia. This is because alveolar oxygen tension (P_AO_2) is determined not only by the oxygen tension of inspired gas (P_IO_2) but also by the carbon dioxide tension of alveolar gas (P_ACO_2). If the respiratory quotient is R, the relationship among these three variables can be expressed as

$$P_AO_2 = P_IO_2 - \frac{P_ACO_2}{R}$$

From this relationship, it can be seen that an extremely high P_ACO_2 as a result of ventilatory depression can result in a low P_AO_2 and arterial hypoxemia.

■ Practical Guidelines

In addition to depression of ventilation, depression of ventilatory control, and increase in ventilation-perfusion inequalities following induction of anesthesia, cardiac output may fall under certain conditions. Although these changes are tolerated well by healthy young adults, they can cause serious hypercapnia and hypoxemia in ill patients. When hypercapnia is a complication of ventilatory depression, ventilation should be assisted or controlled. When hypoxemia is a complication of ventilation-perfusion mismatch, attention should be directed to improving the abnormal distribution of ventilation and perfusion. In general, some or all of the following maneuvers can be tried:

1. Oxygenation of blood perfusing areas where the alveoli have a low $\dot{V}/\dot{Q}$ ratio can be improved by increasing the inspired oxygen fraction.

2. Ventilation to richly perfused dependent zones can be improved by minimizing forces that restrict the expansion of these regions (e.g., reducing the Trendelenburg tilt and removing unnecessary surgical packings).

3. During artificial respiration, ventilation of dependent zones can be improved with a larger-than-normal tidal breath. Mechanical dead space can be added to reduce the tendency to hypocapnia during large-tidal-volume ventilation when necessary.

4. Application of PEEP to increase FRC can improve the $\dot{V}/\dot{Q}$ ratio of dependent zones and improve arterial oxygenation. However, PEEP can cause a fall in cardiac output by impeding venous return. Because a large drop in cardiac output can itself cause impairment of arterial oxygenation, the magnitude of PEEP should be appropriate in order to obtain a salutary effect.

5. During thoracotomy in the decubitus position, ventilation and perfusion of the dependent lung can be improved by collapsing and packing the nondependent lung so that it is neither ventilated nor perfused.

Even if these measures fail, oxygen delivery can be improved by increasing cardiac output or the hemoglobin content of blood. When oxygen delivery to tissues is improved by either method, mixed venous blood will become less desaturated and arterial oxygenation will improve.

Anesthesia and Systemic Illness

11

The responsibility of the anesthesiologist would be simple indeed if all surgical patients were healthy. Unfortunately, many have other illnesses that can complicate the course of anesthesia and subsequent recovery. Certain considerations are reason for concern:

1. Patients whose homeostatic mechanisms are ravaged by disease are very sensitive to the systemic side effects of anesthesia.

2. Systemic illness can alter uptake, distribution, and elimination of anesthetic drugs.

3. Drugs used in the treatment of systemic illness can interact adversely with anesthetic agents.

4. Systemic illness can interfere with the execution of anesthetic procedures.

Therefore, it is mandatory that all patients be carefully assessed and prepared before surgery. In general, no elective operation should be scheduled unless the patient is in the best possible state of health that is consistent with his or her organic illness. There is nearly always sufficient time for treatment to be instituted and take effect, even when an operation is urgent. In the following sections, risks associated with anesthesia in patients with some common illnesses are reviewed.

Ischemic Heart Disease

Approximately 5% of the population in North America and western Europe has chronic myocardial ischemia. Affected patients are prone to have catastrophic cardiac complications during surgery and in the postoperative period, particularly if they have uncontrolled hypertension, congestive heart failure, major arrhythmias, respiratory failure, and hepatic or renal dysfunction. These abnormalities should be brought under control before the scheduled operation. Patients with a history of myocardial infarction also deserve special attention, because they

137

are at risk of having another infarction following surgery. According to the classic study reported by Tarhan and his colleagues in 1972, this risk is highest (36%) in patients whose previous infarction occurred 3 months or less before the operation; it is lower (16%) when the previous infarction occurred 4–6 months before the operation; and it is stable at 5% if the previous infarction occurred more than 6 months before the operation. Moreover, the mortality rate is over 50% among patients who suffer recurrence of myocardial infarction in the perioperative period. Although a follow-up study reported in 1978 by the same group of authors showed essentially the same risks, Rao and associates showed in 1985 that outcome can be improved dramatically if invasive hemodynamic monitoring and aggressive treatment of hypertension and tachycardia (factors that can precipitate myocardial ischemia) are practiced. They reported a reinfarction rate of only 5.7% in patients who have a history of myocardial infarction within the last 3 months and a rate of 2.3% in those whose previous infarction occurred within the last 4–6 months. Therefore, patients should not be exposed to the stress of anesthesia and surgery within 6 months of myocardial infarction if the operation is elective in nature. If the operation is urgent but not life threatening, a delay of 3 months is advisable. Only the life-threatening nature of a surgical illness justifies earlier operation. When early surgery is planned, aggressive measures to balance myocardial oxygen supply and demand are indicated.

If ischemic heart disease increases the anesthetic and surgical risk of these patients, drugs used in its treatment also give reason for concern. Cardiac glycosides used in the treatment of congestive heart failure or tachyarrhythmias are potentially toxic. During surgery and in the postoperative period, many factors, including fluid and electrolyte shifts, acid-base abnormalities, hypoxemia, and abnormal renal and hepatic function can precipitate life-threatening complications. Therefore, it is important to maintain normal oxygenation, normocapnia, and normal fluid, electrolyte, and acid-base balance in patients being treated with digitalis.

Diuretics used in the treatment of hypertension or fluid retention can cause hypokalemia by increasing urinary excretion of potassium. As a result, action of nondepolarizing muscle relaxants is prolonged, toxic side effects of digitalis are increased, and the heart is more irritable. Serum potassium concentrations below 3 mmol/L should be corrected before the scheduled operation in these patients.

In contrast, beta-adrenergic antagonists as well as calcium-channel blockers used in the treatment of arrhythmias, hypertension, or myocardial ischemia are myocardial depressants. Interaction between these agents and anesthetic drugs can cause bradycardia, hypotension, and congestive heart failure. However, experience has shown that the myocardial depressant effects of these drugs and anesthetic agents are simply additive and predictable. Abrupt withdrawal of these drugs can precipitate an acute attack of coronary insufficiency and is contraindicated. Therefore, maintenance therapy with beta-adrenergic antagonists or calcium-channel blockers should be continued right up to the time of surgery, unless there are signs of overdose.

The heart is an aerobic organ and relies entirely on oxidative metabolism to do work. During surgery in patients with ischemic heart disease, it is important to avoid complications that can increase myocardial work (e.g., tachycardia, hypertension, left ventricular failure, myocardial stimulation) or those that can decrease myocardial oxygen supply (e.g., hypotension, anemia, hypoxemia). Manipulation of circulatory dynamics and myocardial mechanics may be necessary to maintain a balance between myocardial oxygen demand and supply. In these situations, invasive monitoring is indicated (see "Invasive Hemodynamic Monitoring" in Chapter 14).

Essential Hypertension

Arterial hypertension is a manifestation of many organic disorders: renal failure, endocrine disorders (e.g., pheochromocytoma, Cushing's syndrome, primary aldosteronism), coarctation of the aorta, and toxemia of pregnancy. However, in approximately 80% of patients affected by hypertension no cause can be established. These patients are said to have primary essential hypertension. Many develop end-organ dysfunction (e.g., encephalopathy, nephropathy, heart failure) if the hypertension is not brought under control.

Many agents—diuretics, sympatholytic agents, calcium-channel blockers, direct-acting vasodilators, rauwolfia alkaloids—are used to treat hypertension. Management of affected patients has been influenced in the past by reports of severe hypotension and bradycardia during anesthesia. These complications were attributed to interactions between antihypertensive drugs and anesthetic agents. Therefore, past practice was to stop all antihypertensive drugs for 1–2 weeks before the scheduled operation.

Current experience has shown that the danger of uncontrolled hypertension is worse than that of drug interaction. With careful titration of anesthetic drugs, circulatory complications are now rare in hypertensive patients even if their medications are continued right up to the time of operation. While these patients are being prepared for anesthesia and surgery, end-organ complications should be brought under control, hypokalemia caused by diuretics should be corrected, and the dose of sympatholytic agents, calcium-channel blockers, or vasodilators should be reviewed if disabling orthostatic hypotension or bradycardia (signs of an excessive dose) develops. If control of blood pressure is optimal, the treatment regimen should continue.

▪ Common Cold

The common cold is a viral infection of the upper respiratory tract. Those who are afflicted have an irritable airway and so are more prone to develop bronchospasm and laryngospasm in response to instrumentation in the pharynx and larynx. Although no serious consequence has been observed following operations on the extremities, this is not true for abdominal procedures, even when they are minor (e.g., inguinal hernia repair). Guarding of the painful abdominal wound will decrease respiratory excursion, impair clearing of secretions, and increase the risk of respiratory complications; constant coughing in the early postoperative period, conversely, can disrupt the suture line. Common sense dictates that patients at the extremes of age and those who are afflicted with chronic illness should not be exposed to anesthesia and surgery when they are debilitated by viral infection. When incessant cough is accompanied by high fever, leukocytosis, and severe systemic manifestations, other infectious disease should be ruled out. In general, a patient should recover completely from the acute phase of a common cold before elective surgery is undertaken.

▪ Chronic Obstructive Lung Disease

Approximately 20% of adult males and 5% of adult females in North America and Western Europe have chronic generalized small airway disease, although most are not disabled. Cigarette smoking is without doubt a major cause of chronic airflow obstruction, and workers in polluted atmospheres (e.g., coal mines, farms, cotton mills) also have an obstructive component in their occupational lung disease. Afflicted patients have impaired pulmonary function that may be further compromised by ventilatory depression and deterioration of ventilation-perfusion inequalities under anesthesia. In the postoperative period, hypoventilation caused by residual effects of anesthesia, guarding of painful surgical wounds, and recumbency can cause retention of secretion, atelectasis, and other pulmonary complications. These patients would benefit from careful preoperative evaluation and preparation.

Patients who are severely disabled should be attended to well in advance of the scheduled operation. All symptoms, signs, and progress of the disease should be documented, and a chest film should be ordered to exclude unsuspected active lesions. Other recommended laboratory investigations include arterial blood gas measurement and pulmonary function studies. Whereas arterial blood gas measurement will yield useful information on overall respiratory function, pulmonary function tests can define the nature of abnormal function (restrictive versus obstructive) and delineate reversible components of abnormal function. Because it has no side effects on respiratory function, regional anesthesia (if practical) is a real alternative to general anesthesia. The advantages and disadvantages of these techniques should be discussed with the patient.

To prepare these patients for surgery, regardless of whether regional or general anesthesia is planned, an active program aimed at improving respiratory function should be instituted. Breathing exercise, postural drainage, inhalation therapy with a mucolytic agent or bronchodilator, and incentive spirometry are helpful measures. All smokers have an irritable airway and a propensity to cough or develop bronchospasm and bronchorrhea following tracheal intubation or extubation. Refraining from smoking at this point is unlikely to eliminate this irritability, but it can reduce the amount of carbon-monoxyhemoglobin in the blood and improve oxygenation. (Carbon-monoxyhemoglobin concentration can be as high as 10% in heavy smokers.) Patients who are receiving bronchodilators should be allowed to continue their medication right up to the time of surgery, but the use of prophylactic antibiotics is not warranted.

▨ Liver Disease

The liver is a major depot from which drugs are eliminated. Intravenous anesthetics and narcotic analgesics are largely detoxified by hepatocytes; succinylcholine is broken down by plasma cholinesterase synthesized in the liver; and d-tubocurarine, pancuronium, vecuronium, and rocuronium depend in part on hepatic clearance. Fortunately, detoxification or excretion of these agents in most patients with liver disease is adequate unless hepatic damage is severe. A fall in serum albumin concentration and reversal of the albumin-globulin ratio are important indicators of altered drug sensitivity in liver disease. Requirements for drugs bound to albumin (e.g., thiopental) will be decreased, and requirements for drugs bound to globulin (e.g., d-tubocurarine) will be increased. Therefore, it is important to titrate the dose of a drug against its effect in this group of patients. Furthermore, attention should be directed to correction of biochemical and hematologic abnormalities and to avoidance of hepatotoxic agents.

Biochemical Abnormalities

Hyperbilirubinemia, hypoalbuminemia, and elevated levels of liver enzymes and ammonia are typical findings in patients with liver disease. Dilutional hyponatremia is frequently observed in patients with ascites and edema, although total body sodium may be above normal. Hypokalemia from excessive urinary loss is usually a sign of secondary aldosteronism. The glycogen store in the livers of patients suffering from fulminating hepatocellular damage is depleted; these patients can pass quickly into hypoglycemic coma. Yet many patients with chronic liver disease cannot cope with a carbohydrate load and have a glucose tolerance curve indistinguishable from that of diabetics. The need to maintain normoglycemia and fluid, electrolyte, and acid-base homeostasis in patients with liver disease is obvious.

Hematologic Abnormalities

Anemia resulting from hemolysis or chronic blood loss from esophageal varices is a common feature in patients with liver cirrhosis. Because these patients already have a hyperdynamic circulation, they tolerate blood loss poorly.

Coagulopathy is also a common complication of liver disease. Thrombocytopenia is the result of hypersplenism secondary to portal hypertension, and low titers of soluble factors II (prothrombin), V, VII, IX, and X the result of decreased hepatic synthesis. Synthesis of factors II, VII, IX, and X is vitamin K dependent. These factors are deficient not only in hepatocellular disease but also in obstructive jaundice because absorption of fat-soluble vitamin K is impaired. Treatment of coagulopathy should be directed to replenishing these clotting factors. Platelet transfusion is indicated when the platelet count falls below 50,000/mm^3 (50 × 10^9/liter). Transfusion of fresh frozen plasma is indicated if prothrombin time is prolonged. Prolonged prothrombin time in patients with obstructive jaundice can be corrected with parenteral injection of vitamin K, but the salutary effect is not seen for 6–8 hours and can take 3 days.

Hepatotoxicity of Anesthetic Agents

There are clear indications that hepatic function is disturbed by both general and spinal anesthesia. Not only is hepatic blood flow depressed in the intraoperative period, but bromsulphalein (sodium sulfobromophthalein) clearance is decreased and liver enzyme levels are elevated in the postoperative period. However, intra-abdominal procedures can also cause reduction in liver blood flow, retention of bromsulphalein, and elevation of liver enzyme levels. Therefore, the precise effect of anesthesia alone on liver function remains unclear. Halothane is the only agent that has clearly been identified as a potential hepatotoxin. Elevation of liver enzyme levels is increased both in frequency and in severity after repeated exposure to halothane, and cases of postoperative jaundice after halothane anesthesia have been reported. It is therefore only prudent to refrain from using halothane in patients with severe liver disease.

Chronic Renal Insufficiency

Systemic complications are unavoidable in chronic renal insufficiency. With the advent of dialysis, uremic complications have become relics of the past. However, when patients with chronic renal failure require surgery, risks associated with hypertension, severe anemia, and fluid and electrolyte abnormalities cannot be ignored. Moreover, some anesthetics are nephrotoxic and others are eliminated only by the kidneys. Therefore, choice of agents should be appropriate.

Hypertension

Not all patients with chronic renal failure are hypertensive, but when hypertension occurs it is mediated by overactivity of the angiotensin-renin system and exacerbated by hypervolemia. Elevated blood pressure may be difficult to control, and damage to end-organs (cardiomyopathy, encephalopathy, retinopathy) is a potential complication. Hemodynamic monitoring and aggressive treatment are indicated for these seriously ill patients.

Anemia in Chronic Renal Failure

Anemia of renal origin is resistant to conventional treatment, and repeated transfusion is neither practical nor advisable. Fortunately, many affected patients have a normal cardiovascular and respiratory system and tolerate chronic anemia relatively well. Chronic anemia is not a contraindication to anesthesia and surgery unless there are other associated disabilities (see "Anemia" below).

Fluid and Electrolyte Abnormalities

Patients with abnormal renal function have difficulty excreting a fluid or electrolyte load. Although periodic dialysis can remove excess fluid and electrolytes, between dialyses these patients are vulnerable to the threat of hyperkalemia, hypernatremia, acidemia, and hypervolemia. Overzealous dialysis, in contrast, can cause electrolyte and volume depletion. Therefore, the records of dialysis should be reviewed so that abnormalities can be corrected.

In the presence of hyperkalemia, a further increase in serum potassium concentration following administration of succinylcholine can cause cardiac standstill (see "Increase in Serum Potassium Concentration" in Chapter 5). If there is not enough time for dialysis, as in an emergency, sodium bicarbonate to correct acidemia and cationic exchange resin, with or without glucose and insulin intravenously, to lower serum potassium concentration to normal values should be given. Precurarization before the administration of succinylcholine also is helpful, but it does not eliminate altogether the possibility of a large rise in serum potassium concentration (see "Precurarization" in Chapter 5).

Nephrotoxicity of Anesthetic Agents

The kidney is another organ that is especially susceptible to the toxic effects of anesthetics and other drugs. Polyuric renal failure has been well documented in patients following methoxyflurane anesthesia. Nephrotoxicity is due to a high plasma concentration of fluoride ions produced by metabolism of methoxyflurane. This agent is absolutely contraindicated in patients with chronic renal insufficiency and has been removed from anesthesia practice. Enflurane, another fluorinated agent, has also been identified as potentially toxic to failing kidneys; however, this has been difficult to substantiate. Sevoflurane, the newest inhalation agent, is associated with plasma fluoride concentrations as high as that seen following methoxyflurane anesthesia. Yet no clinical or subclinical nephrotoxicity has been reported, probably because of its rapid elimination from the body (see "Sevoflurane" in Chapter 3).

Renal Excretion of Muscle Relaxants

Like the liver, the kidneys play a major role in elimination of drugs. Because gallamine, metocurine, alcuronium, pipecuronium, doxacurium, and decamethonium rely heavily on the kidneys for elimination, these agents' duration of action is related to the degree of the patient's renal impairment. They are absolutely contraindicated in functionally anephric patients, and they are relatively contraindicated in patients who have biochemical evidence of renal insufficiency.

▨ Diabetes Mellitus

Diabetes mellitus affects close to 2% of the general population. Not only can its systemic manifestations (generalized atherosclerosis, nephropathy, neuropathy, retinopathy) complicate anesthesia, but anesthesia and the consequence of surgery also can complicate the treatment of the underlying metabolic disorder. There are two diametrically opposing factors that can influence the control of carbohydrate metabolism in diabetic patients undergoing surgery. The natural response to the stress of surgery is an increase in blood sugar by glycogenolysis and gluconeogenesis, but at the same time the reduced caloric intake of surgical patients in the perioperative periods tends to lower blood sugar. Because anesthesia can mask the signs of hypoglycemia, it is important to monitor blood sugar regularly.

Proper anesthetic and surgical management of diabetic patients depends on the treatment they receive. Patients with mature-onset diabetes that is treated by diet alone rarely require other than routine management. Those treated with oral hypoglycemic agents deserve more attention. In general, oral hypoglycemic agents should be discontinued on the day of the operation and for as long as caloric intake is reduced. (Note that the action of chlorpropamide can last well into the next day; patients on a reduced-calorie intake can become hypoglycemic up to 36 hours after receiving the last dose of this drug.) Fasting blood sugar concentration should be checked daily, and urine reaction should be checked every 4 hours during waking hours. Occasionally, administration of insulin in the perioperative period is necessary to obtain control, but this is uncommon.

Management of diabetics treated with insulin requires careful monitoring. Insulin-dependent diabetics are very sensitive to the reduction of caloric intake in the perioperative period and to the metabolic response to surgery. Ideally, elective operations for these patients should be scheduled in the morning. Like other patients scheduled for surgery, they are allowed nonfatty food intake until 5 hours and unlimited clear fluid intake until 3 hours before surgery. On the morning of surgery, the fasting blood sugar concentration should be checked, an intravenous infusion started, 5% dextrose in 0.45% saline infused at a rate of 100 ml/hr, and half the morning dose of insulin given sub-cutaneously. In the operating room, a 5% dextrose solution should be continued for maintenance, at a rate of 100 ml/hr, but third-space and other losses should be replaced with dex-trose-free salt solutions (see also Chapter 21). During the op-eration and in the postoperative period, blood sugar concentra-tion should be checked and regular insulin given according to the result or to urine reaction (the sliding-scale method). De-pending on the surgical operation, the daily insulin require-ment may have to be adjusted even after caloric intake has re-turned to normal.

Severe hyperglycemia can cause impairment of leukocyte function and wound healing. Some anesthesiologists advocate tighter control of blood sugar level in insulin-dependent dia-betics during the perioperative period; the aim is to maintain the blood glucose level between 100 and 150 mg/100 ml (5.5–8.25 mmol/L). Many regimens have been proposed. A typical protocol follows:

1. Allow the patient to have nonfatty food intake until 5 hours before the operation as described earlier.

2. Check fasting blood sugar concentration and start an in-travenous infusion on the morning of the operation. Infuse 5% dextrose in 0.45% saline at the rate of 100 ml/hr.

3. Infuse regular insulin at a rate of 1 unit/hr simultaneously with the help of a constant infusion pump.

4. Repeat the measurement of blood sugar at 1–2 hour in-tervals and adjust the insulin infusion accordingly.

5. Replace other fluid loss with dextrose-free saline and add potassium chloride to the infusion as required.

▓▓▓ Adrenocortical Insufficiency

Functional suppression of the adrenal cortex by chronic ster-oid therapy, rather than organic disease, is the most common cause of adrenocortical insufficiency. The normal adrenal cor-tex secretes 20 mg of cortisol per day, and the plasma level is approximately 14 μg/100 ml (0.38 μmol/L). Both this daily out-put and the plasma level of cortisol increase in response to the stress of surgery. They rise to around 200 mg/day and 30 μg/ 100 ml (0.8 μmol/L), respectively, following herniorrhaphy and around 400 mg/day and 50 μg/100 ml (1.35 μmol/L), respec-tively, after abdominal or hip surgery. Unless there are post-operative complications, these levels return to normal by the third postoperative day. It was long believed that the adrenal cortex required at least 2 years to recover its ability to respond to stress after discontinuation of chronic steroid therapy. Cur-rent experience indicates that the adrenal cortex can recover as early as a few weeks after withdrawal of chronic treatment. Steroid supplement is necessary only for patients who are currently on steroid therapy and for those whose therapy was discontinued within the last 6 months.

In these patients, steroid replacement therapy should be instituted during the perioperative period. For those who are currently on steroid (usually prednisone) therapy, hydrocortisone up to 400 mg or a dose equivalent to their daily dose of prednisone, whichever is greater, should be given in four divided doses intramuscularly or intravenously on the day of operation. (The potency of prednisone in relation to hydrocortisone is 4:1.) This should continue for 2 days postoperatively, after which they can return to their oral maintenance dose of prednisone or an equivalent parenteral dose of hydrocortisone if they must abstain from oral intake. For those who have discontinued steroid therapy in the last 6 months, hydrocortisone, 400 mg in divided doses, should be started parenterally on the day of surgery and continued for 2 days postoperatively. If long-term therapy has been discontinued for more than 6 months, only careful observation is necessary. If signs of addisonian crisis become apparent, hydrocortisone should be given intravenously.

There has been inconclusive evidence that steroid coverage in the perioperative period can interfere with wound healing and increase the risk of infection. However, the benefit of appropriate coverage outweighs the risks.

Anemia

Determination of hemoglobin concentration is an accepted routine in preoperative evaluation. A hemoglobin concentration below 10 g/100 ml (100 g/L) or a hematocrit less than 30% was often considered a contraindication to anesthesia and surgery. However, experience has shown that many anemic patients without cardiovascular, respiratory, and other systemic illnesses can tolerate anesthesia and surgery quite well. The reason for postponing an elective operation for an anemic patient is not simply the anemia but the fact that anemia is a common manifestation of other systemic maladies.

When anemia is discovered unexpectedly, the following questions should be answered:

1. Is the anemia acute or chronic?
2. Is the anemia related to the underlying surgical illness (e.g., hypochromic and microcytic anemia from iron deficiency associated with chronic bleeding from the gastrointestinal tract or menorrhagia; normochromic and normocytic anemia caused by hemodilution after fluid resuscitation following hemorrhage)?

3. Is the anemia related to some other systemic illness (e.g., hepatic or renal disease)?

4. Is the anemia causing symptoms (e.g., dyspnea, palpitation, even angina)?

5. Is the operation elective or emergent?

6. Will the patient benefit from therapy with hematinics? (A patient with anemia related to systemic illnesses or heavy chronic blood loss may not benefit from hematinics.)

7. Is the anemia severe enough and the situation urgent enough that the patient should receive homologous blood transfusion?

If the operation is not urgent, the nature and cause of the anemia should be fully investigated and treatment should be instituted before the operation. When the surgical illness is not causing the patient distress and the operation is truly elective, it is not unreasonable to postpone the operation until the patient responds to treatment. However, a hemoglobin concentration of less than 10 g/100 ml (100 g/L) or a hematocrit lower than 30% should not be regarded as an absolute contraindication to surgery. In fact, the surgical illness itself may be the cause of anemia, in which case the operation would be curative (e.g., vagotomy and pyloroplasty for duodenal ulcer; hysterectomy for metromenorrhagia).

With respect to homologous blood transfusion, it should be remembered that donor blood can be a medium for disease transmission (see "Other Complications of Homologous Blood Transfusion" in Chapter 22) and should not be undertaken lightly. Many patients who have a hemoglobin concentration as low as 8 g/100 ml (80 g/L) or a hematocrit as low as 25% can tolerate major surgery without transfusion; the lowest hemoglobin or hemotocrit below which an urgent operation should not be performed without transfusion remains undefined. However, it must be stressed that blood with a low hemoglobin concentration has a poor capacity for carrying oxygen, so cardiac output increases in anemic patients in order to maintain normal oxygen delivery. If it is necessary to proceed with surgery in such a patient, attention should be given to meticulous surgical hemostasis, repletion of circulatory volume, maintenance of normal hemodynamics, and avoidance of arterial oxygen desaturation.

▄▄▄ Obesity

Severe obesity is a common nutritional problem among citizens of affluent countries. All obese patients have a smaller-than-normal FRC; a few also have hypoxemia and are prone to carbon dioxide retention (the pickwickian syndrome). Endocrine abnormalities (e.g., diabetes), hypertension, and heart failure are other associated complications.

Problems associated with anesthesia and surgery in the obese are related to size. Whereas the mildly to moderately obese patient requires minimal additional care, a morbidly obese patient challenges the wits of the operating room personnel. Even a simple procedure (e.g., transporting the patient to the operating room, positioning on the operating table, finding a mask or blood pressure cuff of the right size, or starting an intravenous infusion) can present a nearly insurmountable problem. Intubation of the trachea can be difficult, and surgical access nearly impossible. The obese patient is more likely to have gastric reflux while lying supine and is at increased risk for postoperative respiratory complications, deep vein thrombosis, and pulmonary embolism.

During evaluation, the morbidly obese patient should be checked routinely for pituitary, adrenal, thyroid, and islet cell dysfunction. Arterial blood gas and pulmonary function studies should be part of the preoperative laboratory investigation. A histamine H_2-receptor antagonist (e.g., cimetidine or ranitidine) should be prescribed to reduce the acidity and volume of gastric contents, and low-dose heparin to prevent deep vein thrombosis should be started on the day of operation and continued until the patient is fully ambulatory. During anesthesia and surgery, the airway should be protected with a cuffed endotracheal tube and ventilation should be controlled. Endotracheal intubation should be accomplished either with the patient awake or by rapid-sequence induction technique (see "Rapid-Sequence Induction" in Chapter 15). At the end of the operation, the endotracheal tube should be left in place until protective laryngeal reflexes have returned. In order to promote better ventilatory exchange, the patient should be nursed in Fowler's position if this is permissible. Deep breathing and coughing should be encouraged, and early ambulation is the best safeguard against deep vein thrombosis and pulmonary embolism.

▧ Arthritis

Approximately 3% of the general population are afflicted with arthritis, and more than 1/10th of them are partially or totally disabled. Whereas rheumatoid arthritis is more common among women and usually involves peripheral joints, ankylosing spondylitis is more common among men and involves axial joints. Both are systemic illnesses with other manifestations (e.g., anemia and pulmonary fibrosis in rheumatoid arthritis, aortic regurgitation and conduction abnormalities in ankylosing spondylitis).

Arthritis can be the cause of many difficulties in the operating room. Crippling skeletal deformities can make it difficult to position the patient on the operating table, and stiffness of the temporomandibular joints and the cervical spine can make direct laryngoscopy and tracheal intubation nearly impossible. Involvement of synovial joints of the larynx limits the choice of endotracheal tubes to smaller sizes, and fusion of costovertebral joints may be a cause of respiratory insufficiency under anesthesia. Therefore, all the joints involved should be noted, and a plan should be devised to cope with these difficulties before induction of anesthesia. Obviously, systemic complications also should be investigated and abnormalities should be corrected before the operation. Because many arthritis patients are on long-term steroid treatment, it is important to review their steroid requirement in the perioperative period (see "Adrenocortical Insufficiency" above).

■ Alcohol and Drug Abuse

Alcoholism is more than a social problem. Liver cirrhosis is a common complication in all alcoholics, beriberi heart disease caused by thiamine deficiency is found in the malnourished, and alcoholic cardiomyopathy is an entity found in well-nourished alcoholics. Encephalopathy and poor vasomotor control caused by autonomic dysfunction (a consequence of peripheral neuropathy) are other important complications of chronic alcohol abuse. The patient who is acutely intoxicated tends to have a low gastric pH and a large volume of gastric contents. Because alcohol acts as a diuretic by inhibiting the secretion of ADH, dehydration may be also a problem. In addition, significant hypoglycemia may be present during recovery from inebriation.

Anesthesia requirements vary among alcoholic patients. Because cross-tolerance exists between many central nervous system depressants, chronic alcoholics who are not acutely intoxicated require a larger than normal dose of both intravenous anesthetics for induction and inhalation anesthetics for maintenance. Conversely, the depressant effects of alcohol, anesthetics, and narcotic analgesics are additive. Therefore, anesthesia requirements are lower than normal in acutely intoxicated persons. Alcoholics who have autonomic dysfunction are very sensitive to the circulatory depressant action of anesthetics, whether they are acutely intoxicated or not. A large drop in blood pressure without compensatory tachycardia during positive-pressure ventilation is another feature seen in these patients. If hypotension is severe, expansion of the intravascular volume is indicated, and treatment with an alpha-adrenergic agonist (e.g., phenylephrine) may be necessary.

Besides abuse of alcohol, abuse of drugs is a growing problem in the more tolerant "new society"; a large number of illicit drugs are available. Heroin addiction in particular is a common problem in many large cities. Because all street drugs are of questionable purity, addicts may present with problems other than drug dependency: granulomatous lesions in the lungs, septicemia, and subacute bacterial endocarditis of the triscupid and pulmonic valves. All intravenous drug addicts are at risk for hepatitis B and C infection and acquired immunodeficiency syndrome (AIDS); blood and body fluid precautions should be practiced when anesthetizing these patients.

Although it is not unreasonable to postpone elective operations until successful withdrawal is achieved, emergency operations cannot be delayed and no attempts at withdrawal should be made until recovery from surgery is complete. Heroin addiction is not a contraindication to general anesthesia or to regional techniques. However, opioids having both agonist and antagonist actions should not be used because they can precipitate the withdrawal syndrome. Methadone is the analgesic of choice. It is as potent as heroin and has a duration of action of up to 12 hours. The dose should be large enough to match the quantity of heroin habitually used.

In addition, to their dependency, many addicts have adrenocortical insufficiency. Although prophylactic administration of steroids is not indicated, addisonian crisis may be the cause of unexplained hypotension during an otherwise uneventful anesthesia. Sudden withdrawal is another cause of unexplained hypotension in addicts. Hydrocortisone and methadone should be given intravenously when indicated.

The labile circulatory function of addicts underlines the importance of establishing an intravenous infusion before inducing anesthesia. Owing to absence of suitable superficial veins on the extremities, cannulation of a central vein may be the only recourse.

Cocaine, another street drug that is gaining popularity, is a stimulant. Sudden withdrawal causes paranoid ideation, delirium, insomnia, lassitude, and depression, but it is not life threatening. Cocaine addicts who snort, smoke, or inhale the drug can present with unique airway problems from damage to mucosal linings of the respiratory tract and the lungs caused by intense vasoconstriction. Like heroin addicts, those who inject cocaine intravenously are potential victims of hepatitis B and C infection, AIDS, and septicemia.

Acute cocaine intoxication is characterized by central nervous system irritability (restlessness, delirium, seizures) and increased sympathetic activity (tachycardia, hypertension, mydriasis). The intoxicated may present with tachyarrhythmias and myocardial ischemia, and some develop a hyperpyrexic, hypermetabolic state not unlike that seen in malignant hyperthermia. Because cocaine is broken down in plasma by cholinesterase, patients who have atypical plasma cholinesterase are particularly susceptible to this drug.

Many cocaine addicts are dependent on one or more central nervous system depressants as well in order to alleviate the undesirable side effects of central nervous system stimulation. Such mixed addiction can present the clinician with a therapeutic challenge. It is important to recognize all of a patient's habits before prescribing treatment.

Preoperative Assessment and Preparation of the Patient

12

In anesthesia practice, "preparation" has two different meanings. In one sense, it means evaluation and care of the patient so that he or she is in the best possible state of good health before coming to the operating room; in the other, it means anticipation by the anesthesiologist of any possible complications during the operation or in the postoperative period. Adequate preparation in either sense cannot be achieved without knowledge of the patient's organic illness. Therefore, a careful history should be obtained and the patient should be examined before the scheduled operation, as is described in the following sections.

Preoperative Assessment

The Anesthetic History and Examination

Cases of mistaken identity and misdirected surgery are not just horror stories. They are true! Prevention of these mishaps begins with the preoperative visit. Each patient should be identified by name, date of birth, and hospital number. Information on the identification bracelet worn by the patient should be checked against that on the operating room schedule and the patient's chart. The patient should be questioned about the nature and site of the intended operation. Such confirmation can be obtained unobtrusively during the course of introduction. A tactful approach is the best way to establish rapport with the patient.

During the interview, the patient's medical history and progress in the hospital should be reviewed. Special attention should be given to previous exposure to anesthesia, medication and treatment, allergies and atopy, personal habits, state of dentition, the airway, and concurrent illness.

At the conclusion of the interview, some time should be spent on explaining the potential risks of anesthesia procedures and the patient should be given the opportunity to ask questions. Taking into consideration the patient's wish, an "anesthetic plan" should be formulated with the full understanding of the patient. Many patients express concern or even fear of what is to come, indicating the need for psychological support. Words of reassurance are the best medicine to alleviate anxiety.

Previous Exposure to Anesthesia

A history of previous exposure to anesthesia, with dates and agents used as well as known adverse reactions, should be recorded for the following reasons:

1. Exposure to halothane should not be repeated within 3 months.
2. Agents that have caused problems in the past should be avoided (e.g., succinylcholine causing prolonged apnea).
3. There may be a history of previous difficulties, such as difficult intubation or awareness during anesthesia.

Some patients may describe side effects (e.g., nausea and vomiting or muscle pain) as complications, but obtaining a detailed history of the event will help to make clear the distinction. It is also worthwhile to note adverse reactions to anesthesia among family members because both atypical plasma cholinesterase and malignant hyperthermia are genetically determined (see "Atypical Plasma Cholinesterase" in Chapter 5 and "Malignant Hyperthermia" in Chapter 16).

Medication and Treatment

It is essential to obtain complete information about past and present medication in the medical history. A knowledge of present medication is especially important in order to anticipate interaction with anesthetic agents. It has been the practice in the past to discontinue vasoactive and psychotropic agents before elective operations. Current experience has shown that patients are in a better position to cope if treatment they receive is optimal. These drugs are no longer discontinued before elective operations if their choice and dose are appropriate.

Allergies and Atopy

All pharmaceutical agents are potential allergens. Obtaining a history of known allergies before prescribing a drug is a basic principle that should not be violated. Many patients may refer to a drug's side effect as an allergic reaction (e.g., dyspepsia from salicylate compounds); these patients should be questioned carefully about the details of the event in order to differentiate a true allergic reaction from side effects.

In addition to drugs, many substances that the patient may be exposed to are also potential allergens (e.g., latex rubber). Therefore, history of environmental allergy should also be sought and recorded.

State of Dentition

The upper incisors are vulnerable to damage by instrumentation during anesthesia (e.g., direct laryngoscopy). Documentation of the state of dentition—the presence of chips or cracks on the enamel, loose teeth, dentures, and crowns—can be important for future reference. The possibility of accidental damage to crowns made of porcelain or synthetic material, no matter how remote this possibility may be, should be made clear; patients who are forewarned are more likely to accept the consequence without attributing blame.

The Airway

Although tracheal intubation may not be planned for the anesthetic, the patient should nevertheless be examined for features that can make this procedure difficult because of possible need for emergency laryngoscopy and intubation in case of complications. Many features of the head and neck can make laryngoscopy and intubation difficult. Some of the features that have been examined more closely include *mouth opening, thyromental distance, cervical spine mobility,* and *view of hypopharynx.*

Mouth Opening.   In adults, the distance between the edges of the upper and lower incisors when the mouth is fully open should be at least 4 cm (equivalent to the breadth of two male or three female fingers). Mouth opening short of this will not accomodate a conventional laryngoscope to view the larynx during intubation. Limited mouth opening may be due to degenerative or traumatic disease of the temporomandibular joint; it may also be due to trismus (masseter spasm) as a result of painful conditions affecting the head and neck (e.g., an infective process such as cellulitis). However, it should not be assumed that trismus will disappear following induction of anesthesia. It may not!

Thyromental Distance.   This is the distance from the mental protuberance of the mandible to the thyroid notch. Normally it should be greater than 6.5 cm in adults (equivalent to the breadth of three male or four female fingers). A shorter distance means mandibular hypoplasia (micrognathia) or anterior/superior displacement of the larynx. Both can make direct laryngoscopy and intubation difficult.

Cervical Spine Mobility. The neck should be flexed and the head extended at the atlanto-occipital joint for optimal laryngoscopy and intubation. An inability to assume this position can mean difficulties. When the patient is sitting with the head and neck in the neutral position, the head should be able to extend at the atlanto-occipital joint (i.e., to tilt backward on the neck) for at least 35 degrees. This examination should be done by facing the patient from the side. A reduction in the range of this movement by one third or any limitation in the movement of the neck may make it difficult to align the long axes of the oral cavity, pharynx, and trachea for easy intubation (see "Posture of Head and Neck" in Chapter 13).

View of Hypopharynx. A tongue that is large in comparison to the oral cavity can make visualization of the larynx during laryngoscopy difficult. Mallampati et al. described the relative size of the tongue versus the oral cavity in four views of the hypopharynx when the tongue is maximally protruded (Fig. 12–1). In the Class I view, the soft palate, fauces, tonsillar pillars, and uvula can be seen. In the Class II view, all of the above sturctures except the tonsillar pillars can be seen. In the Class III view, only the base of the uvula can be seen. In the Class IV view, none of the above structures can be seen. Although studies have shown that frequency of difficult intubation increases with the Mallampati class, most of the patients with a Class IV view of the hypopharynx can still be intubated without difficulties.

Other Features. In addition to the above, acromegaly, prominent upper incisors, prognathia, a long and narrowly arched

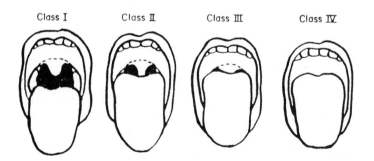

FIGURE 12–1. Classification of views of the pharynx according to Mallampati et al. Class I, the soft palate, fauces, tonsillar pillars, and uvula are seen. Class II, all of the above structures except the tonsillar pillars are visible. Class III, only the base of the uvula is in view. Class IV, none of the above structures is visible (From Samsoon GLT, Young JRB: Difficult tracheal intubation: a retrospective study. Anaesthesia 42: 487, 1987; reprinted with permission.)

palate, a short and thick neck, or the presence of neck masses, disease of the pharynx or larynx, and deviation of the trachea from midline can also make laryngoscopy and intubation difficult. Unfortunately, the power of discrimination of all these features, except mouth opening, are relatively low. Nevertheless, the presence of these features in a patient should heighten the anesthesiologist's anticipation of difficulties. In general, features that can give rise to difficulties in tracheal intubation have the potential to render maintenance of a patent airway by mask difficult.

Concurrent Illness

Many patients have other medical illnesses that can complicate the course of anesthesia and surgery. This subject is reviewed in Chapter 11.

Laboratory Tests

Laboratory tests done routinely have only a small chance of helping to identify unsuspected systemic illness and are not cost effective. Instead, they should be ordered only when indicated by the patient's medical history, physical findings, and intended surgery, to clarify the diagnosis and to follow progress after treatment. Many institutions, however, insist on certain standard laboratory tests on all surgical patients, even when they show no symptoms or signs of systemic illness (e.g., hemoglobin concentration or hematocrit and urinalysis on all patients, 12-lead electrocardiogram on patients older than 50 years). Such practices should be evaluated in view of the economic cost and the minimal benefits of these tests.

Fitness for Anesthesia

Whether the patient is "fit" for anesthesia must be determined at the end of the preanesthetic examination. However, what is "fitness" for anesthesia?

It is known that the systemic side effects of anesthesia can compromise vital functions. It is also known that abnormalities in systemic functions can affect the action and uptake, distribution, and elimination of anesthetic drugs. In short, healthy patients are less likely to have anesthetic complications. In this sense, "fitness" means good health. However, there cannot be a single criterion of fitness; otherwise no surgical patient with concurrent medical illness would ever be able to reap the benefit of an operation. In general, patients are acceptable candidates for anesthesia and surgery if they are in the *best possible state of good health that is consistent with their organic illness.*

Although good health is the criterion of fitness, the nature of the surgical procedure is the overriding factor in determining the timing of an operation. Elective surgery can be postponed indefinitely if time is required to improve the condition of an "unfit" patient. However, if the operation will cure the "unfitness" or if it is urgent, then unnecessary delay should be avoided. For example, a child who is having respiratory difficulty is unfit. However, if distress is due to the presence of a foreign body in the bronchus, then its removal via a bronchoscope is curative; there is no reason for procrastination. Similarly, a patient in congestive heart failure who requires urgent surgery to revascularize an ischemic leg is equally unfit. In this case, however, a little time well spent is necessary to bring heart failure under control. An aggressive approach to treatment can bring remarkable results, even in a short time.

Therefore, fitness is only relative. It is a decision to be made jointly between the anesthesiologist and surgeon. Colleagues in other specialties may have to be consulted, but the anesthesiologist cannot forsake his or her part of the responsibility. In determining fitness, it is helpful to ask the following questions:

1. Does the patient have abnormal systemic function?
2. What is the underlying cause of the abnormality?
3. Can it be improved with treatment?
4. What is the treatment?
5. How much time is available for treatment to take effect?

If the answer to Question 3 is affirmative, then treatment should be initiated immediately to improve the patient's systemic function to an optimum within the time available.

Classification of Physical Status

All patients should be classified according to their physical capacity as part of the preoperative evaluation. The most common classification of physical status in use is that recommended by the American Society of Anesthesiologists:

Class I   A fit and healthy patient
Class II   A patient with mild systemic illness
Class III A patient with severe systemic illness that is not incapacitating
Class IV   A patient with an incapacitating systemic illness that is a constant threat to life
Class V   A moribund patient who is not expected to live for more than 24 hours, with or without surgery

In addition to this rating, the letter "E" should be entered if the operation is an emergency.

This classification of physical status is not a predictor of anesthetic risk because the insult of anesthesia cannot be divorced from that of surgery. However, attempts at arriving at a classification do serve at least two important purposes:

1. They ensure that the attending anesthesiologist has a clear overview of the patient's general state of health, without which an attempt at classification would be impossible.

2. They allow proper selection of patients for outpatient surgery. All Class I and II patients are suitable candidates, but only those in Class III whose systemic illness and its treatment are not complicated by the procedure are acceptable (see also "Selection Criteria for Outpatient Surgery" in Chapter 20).

▇ Preparation of The Patient

Oral Intake before Anesthesia

The protective laryngeal reflex is obtunded during anesthesia. Regurgitation of stomach contents and soiling of the airway are major risks in anesthetized patients. In order to minimize this risk, all patients scheduled for an elective operation should abstain from oral intake for a period of time before induction of anesthesia. However, experience has shown that the previous practice of "nothing by mouth after midnight" was too stringent. The current practice allows nonfatty foot intake until 5 hours and unlimited clear fluid intake until 3 hours before surgery. In addition, oral medication with a small amount of water is allowed up to 1 hour before the operation.

Total reliance on a fixed time interval for gastric emptying can be misleading. Patients who have gastric stasis owing to disorders of the gastrointestinal tract and obstetric patients who are at term can have a large volume of gastric contents even after a prolonged fast. Similarly, the stomach of a trauma patient empties slowly; food ingested before the accident can stay in the stomach for a long time. If incomplete gastric emptying is suspected, other means of protecting the airway should be planned (see "Rapid-Sequence Induction" in Chapter 15).

Premedications

The practice of premedication (preanesthetic medication) is rooted in the era of ether anesthesia. The traditional indications were alleviation of anxiety, facilitation of the induction of anesthesia, reduction of salivary and bronchial secretions, and minimizing anesthetic requirement. Drugs commonly used were sedatives (e.g., barbiturates), antisialagogues (e.g., atropine or hyoscine), and narcotic analgesics (e.g., morphine, meperidine, or pantopon).

With modern anesthetic techniques, however, induction of anesthesia is smooth and pleasant, copious salivary and bronchial secretions are rare, and anesthetic requirements can be adjusted as the needs arise. Times have changed and so have the reasons for premedication. It is still indicated for the relief of anxiety, but some new indications have emerged, including protection against acid aspiration pneumonitis and prophylaxis against other complications.

Relief of Anxiety

Anxiety is a natural reaction when one is faced with uncertainty. There is no better anxiolytic agent than words of understanding, support, and reassurance. This puts emphasis on the importance of establishing rapport with and gaining the confidence of the patient during the preoperative visit. For the patient who needs it, the prescription of a tranquilizer (e.g., 10–15 mg of diazepam orally or 2–4 mg of lorazepam sublingually, given 1–2 hours before the scheduled operation) is more appropriate than a sedative. If anxiety is due to pain, a potent analgesic should be prescribed also.

Protection against Acid Aspiration Pneumonitis

Aspiration of gastric contents during anesthesia is a major cause of morbidity. As little as 25 ml of gastric juice with a pH of 2.5 or less is enough to produce acid pneumonitis. Some patients' basal gastric contents may well exceed these limits despite prolonged fasting; if so, they are at risk of regurgitation and aspiration. Therefore, many methods of modifying this volume and acidity with pharmacologic agents have been proposed (see also "Preoperative Fasting and Premedication" in Chapter 20):

1. Neutralizing gastric juice with antacid before induction of anesthesia (e.g., 30 ml of one-third molar sodium bicitrate within 30 minutes before induction of anesthesia).

2. Giving histamine H_2-receptor antagonist (e.g., 600 mg cimetidine or 150 mg ranitidine) orally 1–2 hours before induction of anesthesia, to reduce both the acidity and volume of gastric contents.

3. Giving 20 mg metoclopramide orally 1–2 hours before induction of anesthesia, to encourage gastric emptying.

It must be stressed that these methods of modifying gastric volume and acidity are only added safety measures. They are not meant to supplant rapid-sequence induction in susceptible patients (see "Rapid-Sequence Induction" in Chapter 15).

Prophylaxis against Other Complications

Some anesthetic side effects or complications can be prevented by other drugs given before induction of anesthesia. These drugs should be included as premedication if indicated. They include antiemetics (e.g., prochlorperazine) for patients prone to nausea and vomiting, antihistamines (e.g., chlorpheniramine) for atopic persons, hydrocortisone for patients on chronic steroid therapy, and dantrolene for suspected victims of malignant hyperthermia. In addition, patients who are receiving antianginal, antihypertensive, and antiarrhythmic drugs or bronchodilators should be allowed to continue with their medications right up to the time of surgery.

Airway Management in Anesthetized Patients

13

When an anesthetized patient is lying supine, the tongue tends to fall backward into the hypopharynx, causing upper airway obstruction. This is the most common correctable respiratory complication of general anesthesia and must be rectified promptly. If indicated, tracheal intubation is a reliable method of relieving this type of airway obstruction (see "Direct Laryngoscopy and Tracheal Intubation" below). However, if tracheal intubation is not planned, and particularly when the procedure is relatively short, other simpler methods can be tried. They include the head tilt–jaw thrust maneuver, insertion of a pharyngeal airway, or insertion of the laryngeal mask airway.

Simple Airway Management Methods

Head Tilt–Jaw Thrust Maneuver

Extending the head on the neck at the atlanto-occipital joint and thrusting the jaw forward by grasping the angle of the patient's mandible on either side and displacing it anteriorly (Fig. 13–1A) can lift the tongue off the posterior pharyngeal wall and relieve the airway obstruction described above. With practice, a mask attached to an anesthetic circuit can be applied to the patient's face at the same time (Fig. 13–1B) and anesthesia maintained with the patient breathing an inhalation agent delivered through the circuit. For this maneuver to work, the patient must have patent nasal passages. If the nasal passages are not patent, a pharyngeal airway should be inserted in addition to the head tilt–jaw thrust maneuver.

162

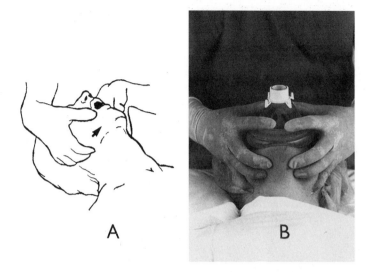

FIGURE 13–1. The head tilt–jaw thrust maneuver. *A*, The head is extended at the atlanto-occipital joint and the jaw lifted forward by grasping the ramus of the mandible bilaterally. *B*, An anesthetic face mask is applied to the patient's face together with the head tilt–jaw thrust maneuver.

Pharyngeal Airway

Pharyngeal airways are molded tubes inserted through the nose or mouth to keep the airway patent. A *nasopharyngeal* airway is made of latex rubber (Fig. 13–2*A*). It is soft and supple and has a flange at the external end to prevent it from disappearing beyond the naris of the nose into the lower airway. It should be well lubricated and inserted with gentle pressure in order to avoid damage to nasal mucosa and nosebleed. An *oropharyngeal* airway is made of plastic (Fig. 13–2*B*). It also has a flange at the external end to prevent it from disappearing beyond the lips. Being rigid in construction, it can also be used as a bite block to prevent semiconscious patients from biting on the laryngeal mask airway or the endotracheal tube, thus occluding the lumens of these conduits. It should be inserted upside down, with its concavity facing cephalad, and then turned 180 degrees when it is well within the oral cavity.

Adult nasopharyngeal airways come in four sizes according to diameter: 28, 30, 32, and 34 French units. (The French scale is a system used to denote the outer dimension of a tubular instrument. When the thickness of the instrument's wall is taken into account, the inner diameter of the airway in millimeters is roughly equivalent to its size in French units divided by 4.) The larger the size, the longer the airway. Adult oropharyngeal airways, in comparison, come in three sizes according to length: 8 cm (size 3), 9 cm (size 4), and 10 cm (size 5). For a nasopharyngeal or oropharyngeal airway to function properly, its tip should be just above the glottic opening, keeping the tongue from lying against the posterior pharyngeal wall.

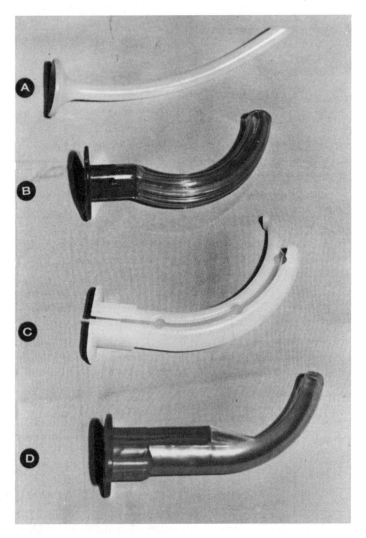

FIGURE 13–2. Pharyngeal airways. *A,* Nasopharyngeal airway. *B,* Oropharyngeal airway. *C,* Berman intubating airway. *D,* Williams intubating airway.

Modified oropharyngeal airways are available also for fiberoptic laryngoscopy and intubation via the orotracheal route (Fig. 13−2*C*, *D*). The Williams intubating airway has a large-bore lumen that can accommodate an endotracheal tube, the Berman airway has a side slit along its entire length so that it can be removed after intubation, and the Ovassapian airway has both a large bore and a side slit. The functions of these special airways are explained under "Flexible Fiberoptic Laryngoscopy and Intubation" below.

Laryngeal Mask Airway

The laryngeal mask airway is a spoon-shaped device (Fig. 13−3) consisting of a wide-bore conduit ending in a mask with an inflatable cuff built into its perimeter. Once the mask is positioned in the larynx, only the tubular conduit protrudes from the mouth, similar to an endotracheal tube—thus providing a secure airway without occupying the user's hands. Unlike the face mask, it allows easy surgical access to the head and neck; unlike the endotracheal tube, it does not evoke the pressor response (tachycardia and hypertension) during its insertion. A properly placed laryngeal mask airway will even allow short-term positive-pressure ventilation of the lungs, so long as the peak airway pressure does not exceed 15−20 cm H_2O. However,

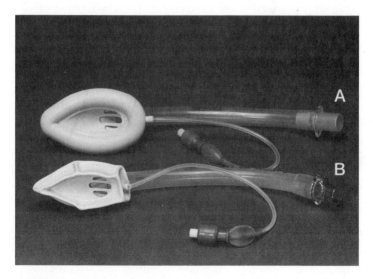

FIGURE 13−3. Laryngeal mask airways. *A*, A size 4 airway with its cuff inflated. *B*, A size 3 airway with its cuff deflated.

inflation of the stomach is always a possibility, and positive-pressure ventilation of the lungs via an endotracheal tube is safer in long procedures. A major disadvantage of the laryngeal mask airway is its inability to protect the airway from soiling by stomach contents. In patients who are at risk of gastric aspiration, tracheal intubation is indicated. Other uses of this specialized airway device include providing an emergency airway in case of a failed tracheal intubation, providing a conduit for blind orotracheal intubation, and providing a conduit for fiberoptic orotracheal intubation.

Positioning the Laryngeal Mask Airway

Laryngeal mask airways come in six sizes, each of which has a cuff that should not be inflated beyond its maximum capacity and each of which has a conduit that can accommodate an endotracheal tube of a finite size or smaller. The guidelines in Table 13–1 are helpful in matching patient to laryngeal mask airway.

Normally the laryngeal mask airway is introduced after induction of general anesthesia using an intravenous or inhalation agent. When the intravenous route is used, propofol is the preferred agent because it is better than thiopental in suppressing airway reflexes. If thiopentone is used, a significant number of patients will develop laryngospasm following insertion of the airway. If it is desirable to use the laryngeal mask airway as a conduit to assist awake fiberoptic orotracheal intubation, it can be positioned under local anesthesia. The method of local anesthesia is similar to that described for awake tracheal intu-

TABLE 13–1. Guidelines for Selection of Laryngeal Mask Airways*

PATIENT'S SIZE	MASK AIRWAY SIZE	MAX. CUFF CAPACITY (ml)	MAX. ENDOTRACHEAL TUBE SIZE (mm)
Neoantes/infants up to 6.5 kg	1	4	3.5 (uncuffed)
Infants/children up to 20 kg	2	10	4.5 (uncuffed)
Children between 20 and 30 kg	2½	14	5.0 (uncuffed)
Children/small adults over 30 kg	3	20	6.0 (cuffed)
Normal/large adults	4	30	6.0 (cuffed)
Large adults	5	40	7.0 (cuffed)

*From Laryngeal mask airway quick reference. Gensia, Inc., San Diego, CA; reprinted with permission.

bation (see "Intubation under Local Anesthesia" below). The proper procedure of positioning the laryngeal mask airway is

1. Choose a laryngeal mask airway appropriate for the patient.
2. Check and deflate the cuff; lubricate the mask generously with water-soluble jelly.

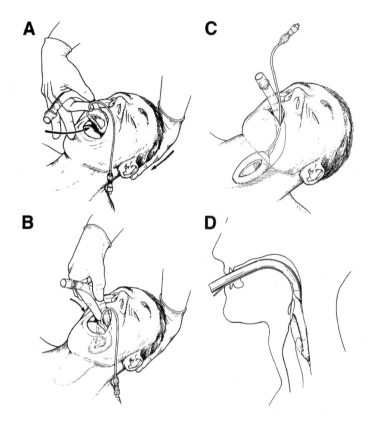

FIGURE 13-4. Positioning the laryngeal mask airway. *A,* Advance the airway with the aperture of the mask facing caudad and the back of the mask pressed against the hard palate. *B,* Allow the mask airway to round the palatopharyngeal angle and slide into the larynx. Occasionally resistance may be met at this point because the tip of the mask is impinging on the posterior pharyngeal wall. This difficulty can be corrected by using a finger in the mouth to guide the mask into the larynx. *C,* Inflate the cuff to no more than its maximum capacity. *D,* In its optimum position, the tip of the laryngeal mask airway is at the level of the upper esophageal sphincter. (From Laryngeal mask airway quick reference. Gensia, Inc., San Diego, CA; and Brain AIJ: The laryngeal mask—a new concept in airway management. Br J Anaesth 55: 801, 1983; reprinted with permission.)

3. Induce general anesthesia or local anesthesia of the airway as indicated.

4. Position the patient supine and the head in the "sniffing" position (neck flexed with head extended at the atlanto-occipital joint).

5. Open the patient's mouth and advance the device with the aperture of the mask facing caudad and the back of the mask pressed against the hard palate until the mask is seated opposite the larynx, as shown in Figure 13–4*A*, *B*, and *C*. (When correctly positioned, the tip of the mask is at the level of the upper esophageal sphincter and the mask envelops the glottis without pushing the epiglottis downward, as shown in Figure 13–4*D*. Occasionally resistance is met before the mask disappears into the larynx, in the position shown in Figure 13–4*B*, because its tip is impinging on the posterior pharyngeal wall. This difficulty can be corrected by using a finger in the mouth to guide the mask into the larynx while constant pressure is applied to advance it.)

6. Let go of the device and inflate the cuff to no more than its maximum capacity (Fig. 13–4*C*). (If the mask airway is correctly positioned, it will slide back out of the mouth for a very short distance at this point.)

7. Connect the laryngeal mask airway to the anesthetic circuit and ventilate the lungs manually by gently squeezing the reservoir bag with the APL valve partially closed. Check the capnograph for CO_2 waveform, auscultate over the apices of the lungs to check for air entry, auscultate over the epigastrium to rule out inflation of the stomach, and auscultate over the larynx to rule out leaks around the cuff. Adjust the position of the device if necessary. (When the laryngeal mask airway is correctly positioned, there should be no inflation of the stomach or leaks around the cuff at a peak inflation pressure of 15–20 cm H_2O or less.)

8. Insert an oropharyngeal airway to prevent the patient from biting on the conduit of the laryngeal mask airway and secure the device in its proper position by using tapes or ties.

Removing the Laryngeal Mask Airway

The laryngeal mask airway is well tolerated by the patient during emergence from anesthesia and can be left in place until the patient is obeying commands or is ready to remove it voluntarily. Just before removal, the oropharynx should be suctioned thoroughly to remove all secretions. Extraction of the device is usually simple following deflation of the cuff. Because the patient has a tendency to bite on the device during the semiconscious state of emergence, the oropharyngeal airway should be left in place as a bite block and removed after the laryngeal mask airway is extracted.

▨ Direct Laryngoscopy and Tracheal Intubation

Tracheal intubation was first described in humans in 1788, when it was recommended for resuscitation of drowning victims, but another century elapsed before the procedure was introduced into anesthesia practice. Tracheal intubation is a safe procedure and has several advantages over the laryngeal mask airway:

1. Control of the airway when the patient must assume an awkward position during the operation.
2. Protection of the airway from contamination by blood, pus, debris, or stomach contents.
3. Long-term positive-pressure ventilation of the lungs, even when the peak airway pressure exceeds 20 cm H_2O.

However, unlike the laryngeal mask airway, tracheal intubation can evoke a pressor response (tachycardia and hypertension) during and immediately following insrumentation.

Depending on the surgical procedure, the face mask—pharyngeal airway combination, the laryngeal mask airway, or tracheal intubation may be used to maintain a patent airway during anesthesia. The choice depends on a combination of characteristics that are unique to each technique (Table 13–2).

TABLE 13–2. Characteristics of Airway Management Techniques

	FACE MASK AND AIRWAY	LARYNGEAL MASK AIRWAY	TRACHEAL INTUBATION
User's attention	One/both hands	Hands free	Hands free
Quality of airway	Very good	Very good/ excellent	Excellent
Skill required	Minimum	Minimum	Easily acquired
Pressor response	No	No	Yes
Access to head and neck	Poor	Excellent	Excellent
Spontaneous ventilation	Short procedure	Long procedure	Long procedure
Controlled ventilation	Very short term	Short term	Long term
Protection of airway	None	Poor	Excellent

Equipment

Laryngoscopes

The laryngoscope is an instrument used for direct inspection of the larynx. Conventional laryngoscopes used by anesthesiologists have two separate components: a handle that provides a housing for the batteries and a detachable and interchangeable blade with a light for illumination. There are two basic designs of laryngoscope blades (Fig. 13–5): curved (e.g., MacIntosh) and straight (e.g., Magill or Miller). All blades are available in different lengths suitable for use in neonates, children, or adults.

A flexible fiberoptic laryngoscope (Fig. 13–6) is available, usually for awake intubation. By manipulating a lever on its handle as well as rotating the scope, the operator can point its tip in all directions so as to obtain a view of the glottic opening otherwise not accessible through a rigid laryngoscope.

In addition, rigid laryngoscopes with fiberoptic viewing designs are available for difficult intubations. Examples are the Bullard and Upsher scopes. The blades of these scopes have a right-angle curve and a fiberoptic bundle for light and viewing. This bundle extends almost to the tip of the blade, and laryngeal structures can be viewed through an eyepiece or on a video monitor via a camera attached to the eyepiece. Current models come with built-in intubating stylets.

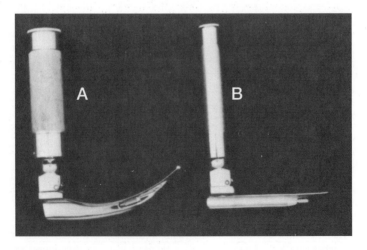

FIGURE 13–5. Laryngoscopes. *A*, A laryngoscope with the MacIntosh blade. *B*, A laryngoscope with a Magill-type blade.

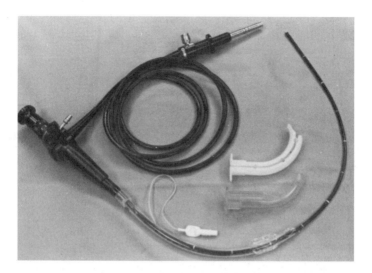

FIGURE 13-6. A flexible fiberoptic bronchoscope shown with two intubating airways.

Endotracheal Tubes

Endotracheal tubes are made of either rubber or plastic (Fig. 13-7). Some are plain and shaped into a curve, some have metallic or nylon coils embedded in their walls to prevent kinking or compression, and some have a slim tracheal portion and a fat laryngeal position so that the "shoulder" at the junction will limit advancement of the tube beyond the larynx and prevent inadvertent bronchial intubation. All tubes should be made of nontoxic and nonirritant material, and they should conform to certain basic designs. Endotracheal tubes that meet these standards bear the codes "IT" and "Z-79."

Most endotracheal tubes have an inflatable cuff near the distal end. Tubes without a cuff are used primarily in pediatric patients. The purpose of the cuff is to provide an airtight seal between the outer wall of the tube and the trachea. By using a syringe, this cuff can be inflated with air via a separate catheter. A pilot balloon is incorporated into this catheter to indicate whether the cuff is inflated or deflated.

Several scales have been used in the past to indicate the physical dimensions of endotracheal tubes (the French, the Davol, and the Magill systems). In current practice, the indicated size is the actual inner diameter in millimeters. In general, adult men require an 8- to 9-mm tube and adult women a 7- to 8-mm tube for orotracheal intubation. For nasotracheal intubation, the size of tubes should be reduced by 1-2 mm. In children, appropriate tube size can be estimated according to

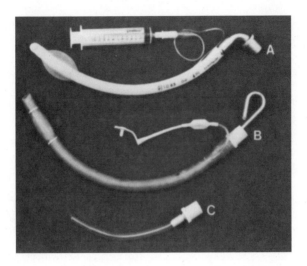

FIGURE 13–7. Endotracheal tubes. *A,* A plastic disposable endotracheal tube with a curved connector. *B,* A reinforced tube with a malleable stylet in its lumen. *C,* A Cole's tube with a straight connector. It has a slim tracheal portion and a fat laryngeal portion.

the formula

$$\text{Tube size} = \frac{\text{Age in years}}{4} + 4.5 \text{ mm}$$

Selecting an endotracheal tube of correct length is as important as selecting one of correct size. There are many ways to estimate the correct length of an endotracheal tube. A popular one based on anatomic landmarks is to measure the distance between the ear lobe and the corner of the mouth on the same side of the face. An orotracheal tube should be cut to twice this length, and a nasotracheal tube to 2 cm longer. The correct length of the selected tube can be confirmed by placing it alongside the patient's face and neck. An endotracheal tube of the correct length should extend from the lower incisor or the nose to a point midway between the cricoid cartilage and Louis's angle (the sternal angle).

Intubating Forceps

During nasotracheal intubation, it is difficult to manipulate the tip of the endotracheal tube. Magill forceps (Fig. 13–8A) are designed specifically for the purpose of guiding the end of the endotracheal tube through the glottic opening. They are also helpful in placing nasogastric tubes under direct vision.

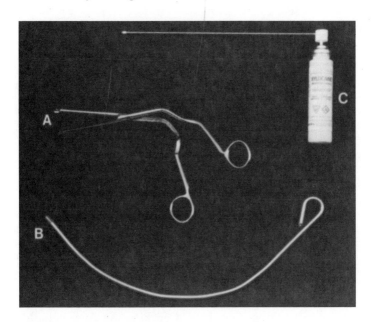

FIGURE 13–8. Endotracheal equipment. *A*, Magill intubating forceps. *B*, A malleable stylet. *C*, A laryngeal spray.

Malleable Stylet

The stylet is a thin piece of metal or plastic that can be threaded through the lumen of an endotracheal tube (Fig. 13–8*B*). It is a useful aid when exposure of the larynx is difficult. Being malleable, it can be used to shape the endotracheal tube into curves that will facilitate intubation. A stylet should be lubricated well so that it can be introduced and withdrawn with ease.

Laryngeal Spray

The laryngeal spray is designed to nebulize a fixed dose of local anesthetic solution (usually lidocaine) and deposit it on the mucosal surface of the larynx and trachea (Fig. 13–8*C*). This method of topical anesthesis is necessary if intubation of a conscious patient is attempted. It is said that topical anesthesia can attenuate reflexes provoked by tracheal intubation (e.g., arrhythmias, hypertension, laryngospasm). Although the issue is controversial, some anesthesiologists routinely spray the cords and trachea with a local anesthestic solution before tracheal intubation, even after general anesthesia has been induced.

Lubricant

Lubrication of orotracheal tubes is optional, but nasotracheal tubes and stylets should always be lubricated with water-soluble jelly or ointment, with or without lidocaine. Products containing oil can cause lipid pneumonia. (Some anesthesiologists believe that use of a local anesthetic lubricant can minimize tissue irritation and the incidence of sore throat.)

Techniques of Intubation

Planning and preparation are vital in all aspects of anesthesia, and tracheal intubation is no exception. During the preoperative visit, the patient should be examined for features that can make tracheal intubation difficult (see "The Airway" in Chapter 12). Before an attempt at intubation is made, the following preparations are mandatory:

1. Verify that the anesthetic machine and the anesthetic circuit are in working order (see "Checking the Anesthetic Machine" in Chapter 7 and "Checking the Anesthetic Circuit" in Chapter 8).

2. Select an endotracheal tube of appropriate size and cut it to the appropriate length. Confirm the integrity of its cuff and make sure that it has the right connector for the anesthetic circuit. (Because size cannot be accurately judged, endotracheal tubes 0.5 mm larger and smaller than the estimated size should also be readily available.)

3. Ascertain that the laryngoscope is in working order.

4. Check that the cuff inflator, intubating forceps, malleable stylet, and laryngeal spray are readily available and easily accessible.

5. Ascertain that a means of pharyngeal suction is available on demand.

6. Have a trained person available to give assistance.

Posture of the Head and Neck

The correct posture of the head and neck for direct laryngoscopy is the same, regardless of the type of laryngoscope blade used or the route of intubation; the position is characterized by flexion of the cervical spine and extension of the head at the atlanto-occipital joint (tip the head backward while it is resting comfortably on a pillow). When the head and neck are correctly positioned, the long axes of the oral cavity, larynx, and trachea lie almost in a straight line (Fig. 13–9A). Incorrect positioning of the head and neck is the most common cause of difficult

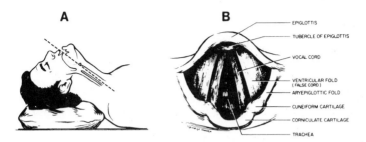

FIGURE 13–9. Technique of tracheal intubation. *A*, Correct posture of the head and neck is flexion of the cervical spine and extension of the head on the neck at the atlanto-occipital joint. In this position, the long axes of the oral cavity, larynx, and trachea lie almost in a straight line. *B*, A view of the glottis through the laryngoscope.

intubation. A mistake made by many beginners is to extend the head and neck fully.

Orotracheal Intubation

Endotracheal intubation, whether by the orotracheal or the nasotracheal route, is a skill that can be acquired only through practice. However, a few words of advice for beginners are helpful. The following steps describe the technique of orotracheal intubation using a curved blade.

1. Position the patient's head correctly on a pillow.
2. Hold the laryngoscope in the palm of the left hand and introduce the blade into the right side of the patient's mouth. Advance the blade posteriorly and toward the midline, sweeping the tongue to the left and holding it away from the visual path with the flange of the blade while doing so. Check that the lower lip is not caught between the lower incisors and the laryngoscope blade.
3. When the epiglottis is in view, advance the tip of the laryngoscope blade into the vallecula formed by the base of the tongue and the epiglottis. Check that the upper lip is not caught between the upper incisors and the laryngoscope blade.
4. Lift the laryngoscope upward and forward, in the direction of the long axis of the handle, to bring the larynx into view. If the epiglottis is seen to overhang the larynx, advance the tip of the blade further into the vallecula. If the esophagus is in sight, withdraw the blade until the larynx falls into view. (A common mistake made by inexperienced operators at this point is to use the upper incisors as a fulcrum for leverage. This not only damages the upper incisors but also pushes the larynx out of sight.)

5. When the larynx is in view (Fig. 13–9B), introduce the endotracheal tube from the right with its concave curve facing downward (caudad) and toward the right side of the patient. Have the assistant retract the angle of the patient's mouth on the right side if room is required to maneuver the endotracheal tube into the larynx. (Another common mistake made by the beginner is to obstruct one's own view by introducing the endotracheal tube centrally, along the curve of the laryngoscope blade.)

6. If only the posterior aspect of the glottis (the arytenoids) is in view, have the assistant apply gentle backward pressure on the thyroid cartilage so that the larynx can be brought into full view. (An alternative is to use the stylet or the intubating forceps to direct the tip of the endotracheal tube into the anterior larynx.)

7. Once the endotracheal tube is in place, apply positive-pressure ventilation to the lungs while the assistant inflates the cuff gradually until an airtight seal is obtained.

8. Continue to ventilate the lungs and rule out esophageal intubation by auscultation over both the chest wall and the epigastrium. (Auscultation over the chest wall alone should not be relied on to verify the position of the endotracheal tube because noise of air moving down the esophagus may not be distinguishable from breath sounds. Air entering the stomach usually but not always gives off a gurgling sound over the epigastrium that is unique. Visually confirming that the endotracheal tube is sitting between the vocal cords is helpful, but the most reliable method to confirm endotracheal intubation is capnography. *Appearance of the expiratory carbon dioxide waveform rules out esophageal intubation.*)

9. Rule out bronchial intubation by checking movement over the apices of the lungs and by auscultation over the apical and axillary regions of the chest wall. (Unequal movement and unequal air entry are signs of bronchial intubation.)

10. Fasten the endotracheal tube securely with adhesive tape or tie after its correct position is confirmed.

The technique of direct laryngoscopy and intubation using a straight laryngoscope blade is essentially similar. The only difference is that the blade should be slipped beneath the epiglottis so that it too is lifted upward and forward. Once the technique of direct laryngoscopy and intubation is mastered, the choice of blades becomes a matter of personal preference. In general, techniques that use curved blades are easier to learn and therefore more popular.

Nasotracheal Intubation

Orotracheal intubation is generally the method of choice in the operating room, but nasotracheal intubation is indicated for operations in the oral cavity. Use of the nasotracheal route for intubation requires some modifications to the technique described before.

1. Topical cocaine, 10%, or phenylephrine, 0.25%, should be applied to the nasal passages to shrink the muscosal lining before nasotracheal intubation is attempted.

2. The nasotracheal tube should be 2 cm longer and 1–2 mm smaller than the orotracheal tube.

3. A curved connector is more convenient than a straight connector.

4. The tube must be lubricated well.

5. The tube should be advanced through the nose directly backward (not cephalad) toward the nasopharynx. When it has been maneuvered into the pharynx, direct laryngoscopy is performed as described, and the nasotracheal tube is guided into the glottis with a pair of intubating forceps.

6. Once the endotracheal tube is in place, the cuff is inflated and esophageal and bronchial intubation is ruled out, as described above.

Intubation under Local Anesthesia

Tracheal intubation for surgical procedures is usually done following induction of anesthesia and administration of a muscle relaxant. In a small number of cases intubation without the benefit of general anesthesia is indicated—specifically in patients in whom induction of anesthesia is considered unsafe unless the airway is secured first:

1. Patients with disease (tumors, trismus, trauma) affecting the patency of the airway.

2. Patients in whom difficult intubation is anticipated.

3. Patients with an unstable cervical spine. (Manipulation of the head and neck in such patients can injure the spinal cord; response to pain in the awake state can warn the anesthesiologist of this trespass.)

"Awake intubation" can be attempted with the help of either conventional laryngoscopes or a fiberoptic scope. In either case, the airway can be anesthetized with lidocaine according to these steps:

1. Have the patient use 5 ml of 4% viscous lidocaine as a mouthwash and gargle to anesthetize the oral cavity and the pharyngeal wall. Repeat this step once with a second 5 ml of 4% viscous lidocaine.

2. Apply 150–200 mg of lidocaine to the larynx and trachea with the aid of the laryngoscope and a laryngeal spray. Pay special attention to the piriform fossa bilaterally, the vocal cords, and the trachea beyond. (The superior laryngeal nerve is submucosal in the piriform fossa and can be anesthetized topi-

cally with anesthetic solution at this site. Blocking the superior laryngeal nerve bilaterally will anesthetize the larynx from the posterior surface of the epiglottis to the upper surface of the vocal cords.)

3. Anesthetize the nasal passage with topical cocaine if the nasal route is used.

Although the above steps will produce adequate anesthesia for cooperative patients, more solid local anesthesia requires the performance of invasive nerve blocks.

1. Anesthetize the oral cavity and pharyngeal wall using 4% viscous lidocaine as described above.

2. Anesthetize the glottid inlet between the posterior surface of the epiglottis and the upper surface of the vocal cords by performing a superior laryngeal nerve block as follows. Palpate for the greater horn of the hyoid bone and deposit 2–3 ml of 1% lidocaine deep to the thyrohyoid membrane but superficial to the laryngeal mucosa using a short 25-gauge needle. (Always aspirate before injection. If the return is blood, adjust the position of the needle. A return of air means the tip of the needle is in the interior of the larynx. In that case, withdraw the needle slowly until air cannot be aspirated and deposit the anesthetic solution in that plane. Perforation of the larynx with a fine needle is of no consequence.) Repeat the block on the opposite side.

3. Anesthetize the trachea below the vocal cord by injecting 5 ml of 2% lidocaine through the cricothyroid membrane as follows. Palpate for the cricoid ring in the midline. Raise a skin wheal and puncture the cricothyroid membrane with a 20-gauge intravenous cannula. Confirm that the tip of the needle is in the tracheal lumen by aspiration for air. Thread the plastic cannula into the tracheal lumen and withdraw the needle. Inject the solution quickly through the plastic cannula during inspiration. (Because of the risk of causing laceration to the trachea when the patient coughs in response to the injected lidocaine solution, use of a plain steel needle for this procedure is not recommended.)

4. Anesthetize the nasal passages when indicated.

"Awake intubation" is unpleasant for the patient. Time must be allowed for the local anesthetic to take effect. Direct laryngoscopy should be done with skill and gentleness. Fentanyl, with or without diazepam, given intravenously for sedation, can be most helpful in securing the cooperation of the patient.

Flexible Fiberoptic Laryngoscopy and Intubation

This technique is particularly useful in difficult intubation or when manipulation of the head and neck is contraindicated (e.g., in fracture of the cervical spine). All practitioners of anesthesia should acquire this skill; use of this technique by the inexperienced in an emergency is seldom successful.

When difficulty in visualizing the glottis with a conventional rigid laryngoscopy is anticipated, fiberoptic laryngoscopy should be the method of choice rather than of last resort. Accumulation of secretions and blood from unsuccessful attempts at rigid laryngoscopy and intubation can make visualization of the larynx with the fiberoptic scope nearly imposible.

Both the nasal and the oral route can be used for this technique. In either case, the airway should be anesthetized topically and by nerve blocks as described earlier. The lubricated endotracheal tube should be threaded onto the lubricated stem of the scope, as illustrated in Figure 13–6, before the procedure. Suction applied to the suction port of the laryngoscope is also essential. When the nasotracheal route is used, the steps are

1. Have the patient lying supine or sitting comfortably in the semi-Fowler's position. (If the patient is sitting up, the operator should stand at the side of and facing the subject. If the patient is lying supine, the operator can stand at the subject's head or side.)

2. Advance the stem of the scope backward toward the nasopharynx through the nose until its tip has been positioned in the oropharynx.

3. Look through the scope and manipulate the tip of the stem as it is advanced in search of the epiglottis.

4. Ask an assistant to support the jaw and maneuver the tip of the scope to go past the epiglottis posteriorly in search of the glottis.

5. Advance the tip of the scope through the cords into the trachea. (Appearance of tracheal rings at this point will confirm that the tip of the scope is in the trachea. If the glottis has disappeared from view without the appearance of tracheal rings, the tip of the scope has advanced into the esophagus or lodged in the vallecula or piriform fossa. It should be withdrawn slowly until the epiglottis is again in view, and Steps 4 and 5 repeated.)

6. Once the tip of the scope is in place, advance the endotracheal tube into the trachea using the stem of the scope as guide.

7. Inflate the cuff of the endotracheal tube and verify its position, as described under "Orotracheal Intubation" above.

The method of intubation via the orotracheal route is essentially similar, but either the Williams, the Berman, or a similar intubating airway should be used as a conduit for the laryngoscope and to prevent the patient from biting on the fragile stem of the scope. When the Williams airway is used, an endotracheal tube that is large enough to accommodate the stem of the scope but small enough to slip through the lumen of the airway should be selected. When the Berman airway is used, the stem of the scope should be slid out of the airway through its opening on the side once the trachea is entered.

Another method of flexible fiberoptic orotracheal intubation is to use the laryngeal mask airway as the conduit. An uncut endotracheal tube matching the size of the laryngeal mask airway (see Table 13–1) should be used in this method. Although it is possible to get around the fenestrations at the distal end of the airway (at the point where the conduit enters the mask), cutting these fenestration will offer an unobstructed view of the glottis. Once intubation of the trachea is accomplished, both the laryngeal mask airway and the endotracheal tube should be fastened in place until the end of surgery.

Management of Unexpectedly Difficult Intubation

Difficulties in intubation can be related to poor exposure of the glottis during direct laryngoscopy. Four grades of exposure were described by Cormack and Lehane (Fig. 13–10): in Grade 1 view, the entire glotid inlet is visible; in Grade 2 view, only the posterior portion of the glottid inlet is seen; in Grade 3 view, only the tip of the epiglottis is in view; and in Grade 4 view, none of the glottid structures is visible. Tracheal intubation

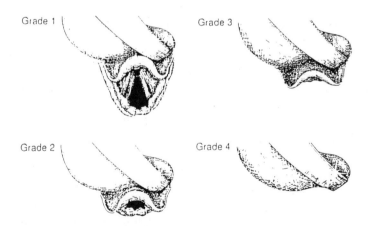

FIGURE 13–10. Classification of views of the glottis through a laryngoscope: Grade 1, the entire glottid inlet is visible; Grade 2, only the posterior portion of the glottid inlet is seen; Grade 3, only the tip of the epiglottis is in view; Grade 4, none of the glottid structures is visible. (From Cormack RS, Lehane J: Difficult tracheal intubation in obstetrics. Anaesthesia 39:1105, 1984; reprinted with permission.)

should be easy if the laryngoscopic view is Grade 1 and should not present any problem if it is Grade 2. However, tracheal intubation will be difficult if the laryngoscopic view is Grade 3 and may be impossible if it is Grade 4.

Because the signs of difficult intubation discussed under "The Airway" in Chapter 12 are relatively nonspecific and insensitive, unexpectedly *difficult* intubation following induction of general anesthesia is as high as 1–4%. Whereas the incidence of *impossible* intubation is approximately 1 in 2000 in general surgical patients, the incidence is said to be eight times higher in parturients. All anesthetic practitioners should have a well-developed plan to deal with unexpected difficulties when approaching tracheal intubations. A simple routine to make the procedure safer is preoxygenation before induction of anesthesia (see "Rapid-Sequence Induction" in Chapter 15). Unless contraindicated, the patient's lungs should also be ventilated with 100% oxygen via face mask and pharyngeal airway following induction while waiting for muscle relaxation to set in. These simple maneuvers will increase the oxygen concentration of alveolar gas and slow the development of hypoxemia during apnea. *A knowledge at this point of whether it is possible to ventilate the patient's lungs using face mask and pharyngeal airway is important.* What to do when tracheal intubation is unexpectedly difficult depends on whether ventilation of the the patient's lungs using face mask and pharyngeal airway is satisfactory.

Ventilation of Lungs with Face Mask and Airway Satisfactory

If tracheal intubation is unexpectedly difficult but manual ventilation of the patient's lungs using the face mask and pharyngeal airway combination is satisfactory, there is time to assess the problem at hand. Several alternatives can be tried in steps to overcome the difficulty, including

1. Ventilate the lungs with 100% oxygen between attempts at intubation.

2. Maintain anesthesia using an intravenous or inhalation agent and maintain muscle relaxation as necessary.

3. Reposition the patient's head and neck. (The head should be in the "sniffing" position with the neck flexed and the head extended on the neck at the atlanto-occipital joint. Malposition of the head and neck is the most common cause of a poor laryngoscopic view of the glottis.)

4. Instruct the assistant to apply backward, upward, rightward pressure (BURP) externally to the larynx. (It was shown by Dr. Richard Knill that this maneuver can improve the view of the larynx and make tracheal intubation easier.)

5. Use a malleable stylet to guide the tube into the anterior larynx.

6. If the above steps fail, consider using a laryngeal mask airway instead of tracheal intubation. (The laryngeal mask airway is an appropriate alternative if the following conditions are satisfied: the patient is not at risk of gastric aspiration, positive-pressure ventilation is required only for a short time, and peak airway pressure does not exceed 15–20 cm H_2O during controlled ventilation.)

7. If the laryngeal mask airway is not appropriate, consider using a Combitube (see "Emergency Airways" below) instead of tracheal intubation.

8. If neither the laryngeal mask airway nor the Combitube is an acceptable alternative, consider waking the patient and proceeding with surgery under regional anesthesia. If general anesthesia is required for the scheduled surgery, reanesthetize the patient only after "awake intubation" is successful using the fiberoptic technique under local anesthesia (see "Intubation under Local Anesthesia" and "Flexible Fiberoptic Laryngoscopy and Intubation" above).

9. If waking the patient is not necessary or not appropriate, insert a laryngeal mask airway of appropriate size. Use this device both to maintain ventilation and to act as a conduit to assist fiberoptic intubation as described under "Flexible Fiberoptic Laryngoscopy and Intubation" above.

Ventilation of Lungs Using Face Mask and Airway Unsatisfactory

If tracheal intubation is unexpectedly difficult after the first attempt and manual ventilation of the patient's lungs using the face mask and pharyngeal airway combination is impossible, the situation becomes critical. It calls for a cool head and a clear mind to re-establish the airway and maintain oxygenation. The appropriate steps to take include

1. Call for help from an experienced colleague and send for emergency airway equipment.

2. Try a two-operator approach to manual ventilation of the lungs using the face mask and pharyngeal airway combination; one operator maintains head tilt–jaw thrust and applys the face mask with both hands as illustrated in Figure 13–1B, the other applys positive-pressure ventilation by squeezing the reservoir bag. Go to Step 1 of the previous section if ventilation is satisfactory. Go to Step 3 below if it is not.

3. Attempt direct laryngoscopy and intubation one more time, provided the patient is not developing hypoxemia.

4. If the patient is developing hypoxemia or if Step 3 fails as well, insert a laryngeal mask airway, check its position, and institute positive-pressure ventilation. As an alternative, insert

a Combitube and use it as a conduit for ventilation. (If ventilation of the lungs is successful with either one of these methods, there is time to reevaluate the situation. The alternatives are (a) allow surgery to proceed by using the laryngeal mask or the Combitube as the airway if it is appropriate, (b) intubate the trachea via a patent laryngeal mask airway before allowing surgery to proceed, (c) allow the patient to emerge from anesthesia and perform the surgery under regional anesthesia, or (d) allow the patient to emerge from anesthesia and perform an "awake intubation" under local anesthesia before inducing general anesthesia again.)

5. If ventilation of the lungs is still unsatisfactory using the laryngeal mask airway or the Combitube, proceed to establish a subglottid airway by emergency cricothyrotomy or transtracheal jet ventilation. (Failure to establish an airway using the laryngeal mask airway and Combitube can only mean supraglottid or glottid obstruction by tumor, edema, or the like. In this situation, establishing a subglottid airway as described in the next section on "Emergency Airways" is the last resort.)

6. Re-evaluate the situation after establishing a subglottid airway and consider a formal surgical airway by tracheostomy before proceeding with surgery.

Emergency Airways

Because unexpected difficult intubation is a potential problem during direct laryngoscopy and tracheal intubation, certain emergency equipment should be readily available to meet such difficulties. The merits of the *laryngeal mask airway* have been described in a previous section. It can be used to provide a patent airway for ventilation of the lungs even when the face mask and pharngeal airway method fails, and it can be used as a conduit to assist fiberoptic tracheal intubation. Inability to protect the airway from gastric aspiration is its only shortcoming.

Combitube. The Combitube is a double-barrelled conduit (No. 1 and No. 2) with two cuffs (Fig. 13–11*A*). The larger pharngeal cuff has a capacity of 100 ml and the distal cuff a capacity of 15 ml. Conduit No. 1 communicates with eight ventilating eyes located between the two cuffs and conduit No. 2 communicates with the distal opening. This design allows ventilation of the lungs whether the distal portion of the tube is in the esophagus or in the trachea after placement. The method of insertion is

1. Check and deflate the cuffs; lubricate the tube well with water-soluble jelly.
2. Insert the tube blindly until the larger pharyngeal cuff is well within the oral cavity. (Normally the distal portion of the tube will enter the esophagus.)

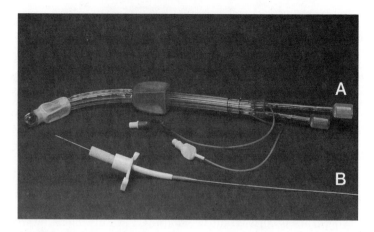

FIGURE 13–11. Emergency airways. *A*, The Combitube. *B*, A cricothyrotomy airway with the guidewire and obturator/dilator in place. (Refer to text for their function.)

3. Inflate the distal and then the proximal cuff to capacity.

4. Connect conduit No. 1 (color-coded blue) to the anesthetic circuit and ventilate the lungs using this conduit. (Successful placement of the Combitube in this "usual" position is confirmed by chest wall movements, breath sounds, and carbon dioxide waveform on the capnograph. Absence of these signs indicate the distal portion of the tube has entered the trachea.)

5. If signs of pulmonary ventilation are absent following Step 4, disconnect the anesthetic circuit from conduit No. 1 and reconnect it to conduit No. 2 and use this conduit to ventilate the lungs. (Successful ventilation of the lungs with the tube in this "unusual" position should be confirmed by chest wall movements, breath sounds and capnography.)

The Combitube is easy to use and is capable of isolating the trachea from the esophagus in either the "usual" or "unusual" position, thus preventing gastric aspiration.

Cricothyrotomy Airway. The percutaneous cricothyrotomy airway (Fig. 13–11*B*) is a device that can be used to provide a subglottid airway in an emergency. It comes with a curved airway together with a 15-mm connector, an obturator/dilator, and a guidewire. The method of insertion is

1. Assemble the airway and the obturator/dilator together and lubricate it well with water-soluble jelly.

2. Perform a cricothyroid membrane puncture in the midline using an 18-gauge intravenous (IV) cannula and aspirate for air. Thread the plastic cannula into the tracheal lumen and remove the metallic inner cannula.

3. Confirm that the plastic IV cannula is still in the tracheal lumen by aspirating for air again. Thread the guidewire into the trachea and remove the plastic IV cannula.

4. Enlarge the skin wound with a scalpel and advance the obturator/dilator together with the airway as one unit over the guidewire into the tracheal lumen.

5. Remove the guidewire and the obturator/dilator.

6. Connect the airway to the anesthetic circuit and use it to ventilate the lungs. (Because the airway is small in comparison to the trachea and does not have a cuff, a large retrograde leak through an open glottis will prevent effective ventilation of the lungs. The size of this leak can be decreased by depressing the patient's jaw so that the tongue will obstruct the glottis. Alternatively, the cricothyroid stoma can be dilated in steps with progressively larger obturator/dilators so that it will accept a cuffed airway. Another alternative is to use the cricothyrotomy airway for transtracheal jet ventilation as described in the next section.)

Transtracheal Jet Ventilation. The transtracheal jet ventilation device is another method of maintaining oxygenation using the subglottid route.

1. Perform a cricothyroid membrane puncture in the midline using a 14- or 16-gauge IV cannula and aspirate for air. Thread the plastic cannula into the tracheal lumen and discard the inner metal cannula.

2. Angle the plastic cannula caudad and into the long axis of the trachea. Confirm its position by aspiration for air again.

3. Use low-compliance tubing with compatible adaptors to connect the plastic cannula to the fresh gas outlet of the anesthetic machine. Achieve jet ventilation of the lungs by activating the Oxygen Flush Control of the anesthetic machine intermittently. (Effective jet ventilation is judged by excursions of the chest wall. It requires entrainment of air through an open glottis. This can be achieved by head tilt–jaw thrust and keeping the patient's mouth open at the same time.)

Transtracheal jet ventilation does not protect the trachea from gastric aspiration. It can also cause barotrauma to the tracheobronchial tree, pneumothorax and pneumomediastinum, and gross subcutaneous emphysema. It is not a method for the uninitiated.

Extubation

Extubation is usually a simple, uncomplicated procedure when done properly. As with intubation, a certain routine should be followed (see also "Emergence from Anesthesia" in Chapter 15):

1. Check that the patient has regained normal neuromuscular function if muscle relaxant was used (see "Monitoring Neuromuscular Function" in Chapter 14) and check that the patient is recovering from the effects of anesthesia and is breathing spontaneously with adequate volumes.

2. Allow the patient to breathe 100% oxygen at high flow for 2–3 minutes to wash out nitrous oxide.

3. Remove secretions accumulated in the pharynx by suction; remove them with a suction catheter introduced through the lumen of the endotracheal tube if secretions are suspected in the tracheobronchial tree.

4. Wait until the patient has regained protective laryngeal reflexes and can obey simple commands. (The patient should not be in a semiconscious state. Extubation at this plane can provoke laryngospasm.)

5. Deflate the cuff and remove the endotracheal tube quickly but smoothly during inspiration. Alternatively, turn the patient onto one side and extubate in the lateral position.

6. Continue to give the patient oxygen by face mask as required.

7. If direct laryngoscopy and tracheal intubation was difficult, extubate only after the patient has fully regained consciousness and is able to maintain his or her own airway. Alternatively, thread a long catheter into the trachea via the endotracheal tube and leave it in place after extubation. (This catheter can be used as a conduit for jet ventilation or as a guide for reintubation when necessary. It should not be removed until the patient can maintain a patent airway and adequate spontaneous ventilation.)

Complications of Laryngoscopy and Intubation

Complications following short-term tracheal intubation in the operating room are usually minor. The following problems may be encountered.

Trauma to Lips, Teeth, and Soft Tissues of the Airway. Constant awareness of the possibility of these complications and a gentle, meticulous technique will help to reduce their incidence.

Reflex Tachycardia and Hypertension, Ventricular Arrhythmias, Bronchospasm, and Chest Wall Spasm. These complications are common when the trachea is intubated with the patient at a light plane of general anesthesia. The pressor response is attenuated by increasing the depth of anesthesia or by applying topical lidocaine to the larynx and trachea. The administration of lidocaine, 1.5 mg/kg, intravenously 1.5–3 minutes before the procedure is another alternative. Bronchospasm and chest wall spasm are also associated with intubating the trachea under light anesthesia. Bronchospasm usually re-sponds to deepening of anesthesia and aerosolization of a bron-chodilator into the airway (e.g., two to three puffs of salbuta-mol); chest wall spasm usually responds to muscle relaxants.

Esophageal Intubation. This is not an uncommon compli-cation when the laryngoscopic view is Grade II and above. Aus-cultation of the chest and over the epigastrium does not always rule out esophageal intubation because air going down the esophagus can mimic breath sounds and air entering the stom-ach can be silent. Only the appearance of a carbon dioxide waveform on the capnograph can confirm tracheal and rule out esophageal intubation.

Bronchial Intubation. Inadvertent bronchial intubation (usually of the right main bronchus) is not an infrequent com-plication of tracheal intubation because methods of estimating the correct length of an endotracheal tube are only guides. Aus-cultation of the chest bilaterally for air entry is the only sure method for determining that the tube has been successfully placed in the trachea and not in a mainstem bronchus.

Laryngospasm following Extubation. This problem is com-mon when extubation is done with the patient in a semicon-scious state. Extubation in adults should be done either in a relatively deep plane of anesthesia or when the protective la-ryngeal reflex has returned; extubation in children and infants should be done when laryngeal reflex has returned.

Postintubation Hoarseness and Sore Throat. These un-pleasant side effects are due to the mechanical presence of the endotracheal tube. Use of low-pressure cuffs has not eliminated these problems entirely. In order to minimize them, unneces-sary movement of the head and neck should be avoided once the endotracheal tube is in place.

Postintubation Stridor or Croup. Pediatric patients are more prone to this complication than adults; it is due to edema of subglottic regions of the airway. These patients should be given humidified oxygen, and administration of racemic epi-nephrine by inhalation may be necessary. Selection of an en-dotracheal tube of the correct size will reduce the incidence of this complication.

Monitoring Principles and Practice

14

The primary goal of surgical anesthesia is to alleviate pain and stress. Unfortunately, the patient is also exposed to the systemic side effects of anesthetic drugs in the process and is rendered helpless against physiologic trespasses accompanying surgery. The patient's survival is totally dependent on the supportive care provided by the anesthesiologist. Therefore, careful monitoring of the patient's vital functions and of the effects of anesthesia and surgery is mandatory.

To exercise the clinical skills of inspection, palpation, percussion, and auscultation is the most basic means of monitoring. In an attempt to improve on human senses, industry has made available a large array of automated instruments to measure body functions, to monitor the anesthesiologist's action and the patient's response, to detect failure in the anesthetic machine and its circuit, and to sound an alarm when certain limits have been breached. What is an appropriate level of monitoring during anesthesia? To answer this question requires a knowledge of the methods available and an understanding of their capabilities and limitations.

Monitoring Depth of Anesthesia

Clinical Signs

Although they vary according to the agents used, clinical signs associated with surgical anesthesia remain a reliable gauge of the depth of anesthesia. When barbiturates or propofol are used for induction of anesthesia, loss of eyelash reflex (blinking in response to gentle stroking of the eyelash) marks the onset of unconsciousness. Some patients may yawn or take a deep breath just before falling into a deep sleep. When ketamine is used, unconsciousness is marked by the onset of a cataleptic state accompanied by profound analgesia. When volatile agents are used, the signs of surgical anesthesia include a central gaze, pupils that are small and reactive to light, and respiration that is regular in both rate and depth (automatic breathing).

The most critical test of depth of anesthesia is the patient's reaction to surgical stimulation. Somatic responses may take the form of frank movements of extremities or laryngospasm, or they may be subtle, as in wrinkling of the forehead, vocalization, irregular breathing, or breath holding. Sympathetic responses to surgical stimulation include hypertension, tachycardia, sweating, and lacrimation. Both somatic and sympathetic responses to surgical stimulation should be abolished by anesthesia in the patient who is breathing spontaneously. In the paralyzed patient, however, only sympathetic responses are available to help in gauging depth of anesthesia. In short, the patient who is adequately anesthetized is quiet, normotensive, warm, pink, and dry. A progressive fall in blood pressure and profound respiratory depression are signs of an excessive depth of anesthesia. Fixed, dilated pupils are an ominous sign; immediate investigation is called for, and gross overdose or profound hypoxia must be ruled out.

Electroencephalogram

Two types of rhythms can be identified on the classic 16-channel EEG in normal adults: sinusoidal alpha waves of 8–12 Hz present over the occipital and parietal regions in relaxed subjects whose eyes are closed but that disappear when the eyes are opened; and lower voltage beta waves of 13–30 Hz present over central and frontal regions. Slower theta rhythm (4–7 Hz), delta waves (less than 4 Hz), and electrical silence— present either focally or diffusely—are always abnormal in awake subjects and can be traced to destructive lesions. Certain general but nonspecific trends can be observed on the EEG following induction of surgical anesthesia. They include the spread of alpha waves anteriorly over all parts of the cerebral cortex and appearance of theta and delta rhythms. Alpha waves predominate during deep levels of anesthesia and coexist with delta rhythm. Finally electrical silence follows, coinciding with the onset of coma.

In order to facilitate the use of EEG monitoring by less experienced personnel in the operating suite, various electronic data-processing techniques have been introduced to remove artifacts, analyze frequencies, quantify amplitudes, and report trends (e.g., by power spectral analysis). Use of a computer-processed EEG to monitor depth of total intravenous anesthesia (TIVA) has been explored. However, EEG changes associated with anesthesia do not reflect the tissue level of anesthetic in the brain alone; differences in the intensity of surgical stimulation can cause varying patterns of EEG changes. Furthermore, EEG changes are dependent on the dose of anesthetic drug and vary among drugs, even drugs of the same class. In addition, hypothermia, hypoglycemia, hyponatremia, hypocapnia, and persistent hypoxemia can cause nonspecific slowing of EEG wave patterns. These pitfalls have combined to make observation of clinical signs still the only practical method of monitoring depth of anesthesia.

Note: Although use of the EEG to monitor anesthetic depth has remained an investigative tool, use of the EEG and evoked potentials to monitor central nervous system function and surgical trespass is well established in neurosurgery and neurovascular surgery. The student should refer to specialized textbooks for these monitoring modalities.

■ Monitoring Circulatory Function

Pulse and Blood Pressure

It is customary to record the patient's pulse rate and blood pressure regularly, at least every 5 minutes, during the course of anesthesia. Such importance is placed on these variables because of the following considerations:

1. Pulse rate and blood pressure are time-honored vital signs.
2. Pulse rate and blood pressure, in addition to other clinical signs, are used as indicators of anesthesia depth (e.g., tachycardia and hypertension at levels inadequate for surgery; progressive hypotension at inappropriately deep levels).
3. Changes in pulse and blood pressure are recognized outcomes of certain surgical maneuvers or undesirable trespasses (e.g., bradycardia in response to traction on visceral organs or extraocular muscles; hypotension and tachycardia following hemorrhage).
4. Some anesthetic agents can alter cardiac rhythm, which may be evidenced by changes in the mechanical rhythm of the pulse (e.g., sinus or nodal bradycardia or cardiac standstill following succinylcholine).

Pulse rate, pulse volume, and mechanical rhythm of the heart can be obtained by palpation of an artery. In an emergency, pulse volume may be used to estimate blood pressure. The radial pulse feels thready as blood pressure falls; it disappears when systolic blood pressure drops below 50 mm Hg, and the carotid or femoral pulse vanishes when systolic pressure drops to 30 mm Hg.

As an alternative to palpation, pulse can be monitored with a digital plethysmograph. Another method is auscultation using a mechanical or electronic precordial stethoscope positioned at the third interspace, just left of the sternum, or using an esophageal stethoscope placed at the midsternal level. When heart sounds are monitored, loudness of aortic valve closure (the second sound) can be used as a semiquantitative index of diastolic pressure.

Sphygmomanometry by auscultation of Korotkoff's sounds in the upper arm (the Riva-Rocci technique) is the traditional method of measuring blood pressure. When the upper extremity cannot be used, the cuff may be placed around the thigh. Accurate results are obtained only if the width of the cuff is approximately one third the circumference of the arm or thigh. A cuff that is too narrow will give falsely high readings; one that is too wide will give spuriously low readings. If this method of sphygmomanometry is difficult (e.g., during hypotension or in obese patients), placement of an ultrasound flow transducer (the Doppler) over an artery distal to the cuff (e.g., the radial or dorsalis pedis artery) is a useful adjunct for measuring systolic blood pressure. (Systolic blood pressure is indicated by return of flow signals during deflation of the cuff.)

In the last decade, monitoring pulse rate and blood pressure by automated sphygmomanometers that operate on the principle of oscillometry has become commonplace. During their operation, pressure in the bladder of the cuff is automatically increased to above systolic pressure and then is decreased slowly in steps. At pressures between the systolic and diastolic ranges, pulsation in the partially obstructed artery is transmitted to the bladder. The amplitude of these pulsations is sensed by a transducer and its relationship to bladder pressure is analyzed by a microprocessor that computes systolic, diastolic, and mean blood pressure as well as pulse rate. These devices can be programmed to make repeated measurements at regular intervals —as frequently as every 20 seconds—and to sound an alarm when the measured variables fall outside chosen limits, but these instruments should not be abused. Too-frequent determination of blood pressure using these devices has caused pressure injury to nerves. Measurements should not be made more frequently than every 5 minutes unless the patient's clinical condition warrants it.

In addition to automated oscillometric sphygmomanometers, there are devices purported to be capable of monitoring beat-to-beat blood pressure noninvasively. One of them is the arterial tonometer, in which an external pressure transducer is applied against the radial artery at the wrist. Pulsation in the artery is sensed by the transducer and transcribed by a microprocessor into blood pressure readings that are calibrated against readings from the contralateral arm using the oscillometric method. However, the necessity to obtain frequent calibrating pressures by the oscillometric method makes this tonometric technique less useful. A second device uses photometric pulse transducers to measure the time required by pulses to travel from one part of the body to a more distal part of the body (the pulse transit time) and exploits the inverse relationship between systolic blood pressure and pulse transit time. However, this relationship has not been fully evaluated. Another device uses the Peñaz technique, in which an inflatable cuff is fitted over the middle phalanx of a finger and an infrared beam transmitted across the thickness of the finger is used to monitor blood volume in that finger. Because blood volume in the finger increases over systole and decreases over diastole, absorption of the infrared beam increases over systole and decreases over diastole. During measurement of blood pressure, the light absorption signal is used in a servo-loop to control the pressure in the inflatable cuff and keep blood volume in the finger constant. That is, as blood pressure rises during systole, increases in blood volume and light absorbence act through the servo-controller to increase the cuff pressure instantaneously. Increase in cuff pressure compresses the digital arteries, thus maintaining the blood volume in the finger constant throughout systole. Conversely, as blood pressure falls during diastole, decreases in blood volume and light absorbence act through the controller to decrease the cuff pressure. As cuff pressure decreases, compression of the digital arteries decreases, thus allowing more blood to enter the digit to maintain blood volume unchanged. In this manner, the cuff pressures recorded during systole and diastole equal systolic and diastolic pressure. A major disadvantage of this technique is inaccuracy in hypoperfusion states, when continuous arterial blood pressure monitoring is most necessary. Despite advances in design and engineering, none of these three methods can supplant direct invasive arterial blood pressure monitoring at this stage (see "Invasive Hemodynamic Monitoring" below).

Electrocardiogram

Continuous monitoring of the electrocardiogram (ECG) was originally introduced to monitor cardiac rhythm. Because the vector of lead II (right arm to left leg) parallels the P-wave axis, it is the most useful lead for monitoring electrical activities of the heart.

In recent years the ECG has also been recommended as a monitor of myocardial ischemia. A 1-mm horizontal depression of the ST segment is accepted as a sign of subendocardial ischemia. Because more than 80% of ischemic changes occur in the left ventricle, precordial lead V_5 (left anterior axillary line at the fifth interspace) should be used for this purpose if it is available. If the ECG oscilloscope is equipped with bipolar leads only, modified precordial leads (CM_5 or CS_5) should be used. In the CM_5 modification, the right-arm electrode of lead I is placed over the manubrium, the left-arm electrode over the V_5 position, and the ground electrode over the left shoulder. Lead CS_5 is similar to CM_5, except that the right-arm electrode is positioned over the right shoulder.

Invasive Hemodynamic Monitoring

Availability of plastic cannulas and catheters as well as transducers has made invasive hemodynamic monitoring simple. It allows continuous monitoring of arterial pressure, central venous pressure, and pulmonary capillary wedge pressure. The presence of these catheters also allows access for sampling of blood for arterial and mixed venous blood gas analysis.

Direct measurement of arterial pressure can be made via a cannula in a peripheral artery (radial, brachial, dorsalis pedis, common femoral, or left axillary); insertion of a 20-gauge cannula into the radial artery is the most popular method. Before this artery is cannulated, adequate collateral circulation from the ulnar artery should be demonstrated by the modified Allen's test, in which the clinician occludes the radial and ulnar arteries with digital pressure while the patient clenches the fist. When the hand is exsanguinated, have the patient relax the fingers and hand in a neutral position. Adequate collateral circulation from the ulnar artery is confirmed by rapid capillary filling of the radial aspect of the hand when pressure on the ulnar artery alone is released.

Indications for the use of direct arterial pressure monitoring include the following:

1. Major cardiac, vascular, thoracic, and neurosurgical procedures.

2. Other surgical procedures during which large fluid shifts are anticipated.

3. Management of critically ill or high-risk patients.

4. Cases in which blood pressure cannot be determined accurately using indirect methods.

5. Use of "controlled hypotension" as part of the anesthetic technique.

Central venous pressure can be measured with a catheter introduced into the superior vena cava via the internal jugular, external jugular, subclavian, or basilic vein. Measurement of central venous pressure is indicated when massive hemorrhage or fluid shift is anticipated. Individual values of central venous pressure are poor reflections of blood volume, but when the trend of these values and that of pulse rate, blood pressure, and urine output are considered together, central venous pressure measurement is an invaluable guide to fluid replacement. (Normal values for patients lying supine are $0-10$ cm H_2O from the anterior axillary line or $4-14$ cm H_2O from the midaxillary line.)

Measurement of pulmonary capillary wedge pressure (a reflection of left atrial pressure) has been popularized by introduction of the flow-directed Swan-Ganz catheter. A triple-lumen version of this catheter with a thermistor near its tip is available for measurement of cardiac output by thermal dilution; another version has an optical fiber incorporated into its lumen for continuous monitoring of mixed venous oxygen saturation. Measurements of pulmonary capillary wedge pressure and cardiac output are generally indicated during cardiac, major vascular, and major neurosurgical operations, in surgical patients with severe heart disease, and in those who are gravely ill.

Measurement of Blood Loss

The topic of blood transfusion to replace loss beyond a certain limit is discussed in Chapter 22. Unfortunately, neither hemoglobin concentration nor hematocrit reflects the amount of blood loss during acute hemorrhage. The most simple and accurate method of measuring blood loss is to weigh discarded sponges and to measure the volume of blood in the suction apparatus. The difference in weight between blood-soaked and dry sponges in grams is equal to the volume of blood in the sponges in milliliters; the difference in volumes between fluid in the suction apparatus and irrigation fluid used is equal to the volume of blood removed by suction. Volume of blood spilled on surgical drapes is more difficult to measure, but with experience the amount can be estimated with fair accuracy by careful inspection.

Monitoring of Respiratory Function

Clinical Signs

Invaluable information about the patient's respiratory function can be obtained by observing the respiratory rate, movement of the chest wall and abdomen, and excursion of the reservoir bag. The anesthetized patient who is not in distress breathes quietly. The chest wall rises and falls in rhythm with the reservoir bag, and the respiratory pattern is regular in both depth and rate. Irregular breathing or breath holding indicates inadequate anesthesia; a slow respiratory rate or apnea indicates overdose of opioids or other respiratory depressants. Paradoxical movement of the chest wall and abdomen, suprasternal in-drawing, and tracheal tug (downward movement of the thyroid cartilage with each inspiratory effort), with or without stridor, are pathognomonic for upper airway obstruction. Unequal movement of the two sides of the thoracic cage during inspiration is a sign of endobronchial intubation.

Clues to the adequacy of oxygenation and carbon dioxide elimination can be obtained by observing the patient's pulse rate, blood pressure, and color. Both hypoxemia and hypercapnia can cause tachycardia and hypertension; cyanosis is seen when more than 5 g of deoxyhemoglobin is present in each 100 ml of blood; and a warm, flushed, moist skin is associated with hypercapnia. However, it must be stressed that the cardiovascular response to hypoxemia and hypercapnia is attenuated by anesthesia, and cyanosis may not be a reliable sign owing to the presence of natural pigmentation, poor lighting conditions, and cutaneous vasoconstriction. These are late signs that demand prompt action.

Ventilatory Volumes

During spontaneous ventilation, ventilatory function in healthy patients is usually judged by clinical signs alone and ventilatory volumes are seldom measured routinely. During controlled ventilation, the bellows of the ventilator is usually calibrated to indicate inspired tidal volume. When independent verification is warranted during spontaneous or controlled ventilation, expiratory tidal and minute volumes can be measured by spirometry using mechanical devices, the most popular versions being the Wright respirometer and Dräger volumeter.

In the Wright respirometer, gas flow is directed by a series of slots onto rotating vanes, and flow over time is registered as volume on a dial by the movement of a needle connected to the vanes by mechanical gears (Fig. 14–1*A*, *B*). It is basically a flow-sensing device designed for flow rates between 3 and 300 L/min. For accuracy, it is imperative to check that the vanes are free of water condensate before use. The Dräger volumeter is a similar device, but the flow-sensing mechanism is a pair of cogs that rotate in opposite directions (Fig. 14–1*C*). Again flow over time is transcribed by internal gears into movement of a

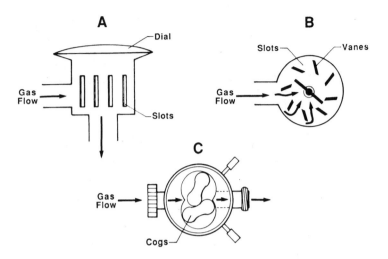

FIGURE 14–1. Mechanical volumeters: *A*, Wright respirometer, side view. *B*, Wright respirometer, cross-sectional view. In the Wright respirometer, gas flow is directed onto rotating vanes and flow over time is transcribed mechanically and registered as volume on a dial by the movement of a needle. *C*, Dräger volumeter, in which the flow-sensing mechanism is a pair of rotating cogs.

needle on a dial. Both devices underestimate volumes in low-flow conditions and overestimate when flow rate is high.

Ventilatory flow and volumes can also be measured electronically. In the pneumotachometer (Fig. 14–2*A*), pressure difference across a resistive element is measured by a differential pressure transducer. Because the magnitude of laminar flow across the element is directly proportional to the pressure difference, volume can be computed by the integration of flow over time. In the Pilot-tube flowmeter (Fig. 14–2*B*), the pressure difference between two ports, one perpendicular to the flow tube and the other facing the direction of air flow, is measured. Because the flow rate is proportional to the square root of the pressure difference in this device, volume can be computed by integrating flow over time.

Airway Pressure

Airway pressure can be measured by incorporating an aneroid pressure gauge into the anesthetic circuit. The mechanical aneroid pressure gauge is based on the Bourdon tube (Fig. 14–2*C*), which is a tubular coil blind at one end and exposed to the pressure to be measured at the other. When the pressure to

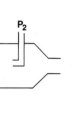

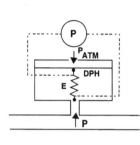

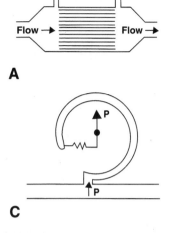

FIGURE 14–2. *A*, The pneumotachometer is an electronic flow and volume meter in which gas flow is directed across a laminar flow resistor and the pressure difference ($P_1 - P_2$) across the resistor is measured by a differential pressure transducer. Flow, which is directly proportional to the pressure difference, is computed electronically and volume is computed by the integration of flow over time. *B*, The Pilot tube is another electronic flow and volume meter in which the pressure difference ($P_2 - P_1$) between two ports (one perpendicular to and the other facing the direction of flow) is measured by a differential pressure transducer. Flow is proportional to the square root of the pressure difference in this instance. *C*, The mechanical aneroid pressure gauge is based on the Bourdon tube. Pressure (P) applied to the tube changes the dimension of the tube, and this change is transcribed by mechanical gears to register pressure (P) in a dial by the movement of a needle. *D*, The electronic pressure transducer (strain gauge) has a piezoresistive element (E) fixed at one end and attached to a flexible diaphragm (DPH) at the other. The pressure difference across the diaphragm, which equals the difference between the applied pressure (P) and atmospheric pressure (P_{ATM}), determines the shape of the diaphragm and the dimension of the piezoresistive element. Because atmospheric pressure can be regarded as constant, the shape of the diaphragm and the dimension of the element are determined only by the magnitude of the applied pressure. As a result, the resistance of the element, which is proportional to its dimension, can be transcribed electronically to reflect the applied pressure.

be measured increases, the tube uncoils, and its movement is transcribed by mechanical gears to an indicator needle.

Airway pressure can also be measured by an electronic pressure strain gauge (pressure transducer). The most common design consist of a piezoresistive element fixed at one end and attached to a flexible diaphragm at the other (Fig. 14–2*D*). The diaphragm is exposed to ambient pressure on one side and to the pressure to be measured on the other. When the pressure to be measured changes, the shape of the diaphragm changes, causing a change in the dimension of the element. This change in dimension causes a proportional change in the electrical resistance of the element, which is transcribed electronically into change in pressure.

Airway pressure fluctuates around zero during spontaneous ventilation and seldom exceeds 30 cm H_2O at its peak during positive-pressure ventilation. Monitoring airway pressure is important in both instances. During spontaneous ventilation, positive pressure in the airway usually indicates that the APL valve is not fully open (see "Adjustable Pressure-Limiting Valve" in Chapter 8). During controlled ventilation, an increase in peak inspiratory pressure may mean an increase in airway resistance (e.g., bronchospasm, kinked endotracheal tube) or a decrease in pulmonary compliance (e.g., pulmonary congestion). A large drop in peak inspiratory pressure to below normal values during positive-pressure ventilation, in contrast, always means a major leak in the circuit or complete disconnection. Current standards require that a low-airway-pressure alarm be incorporated into the breathing circuit during positive-pressure ventilation, to alert the anesthesiologist in case of such a disconnection (see "Pressure Monitor" and "Pressure Alarms" in Chapter 9).

Blood Gas Analysis

Information on PaO_2 and P_aCO_2, pH, and buffering capacity of arterial blood can be obtained by blood gas analysis. Normal PaO_2 is above 95 mm Hg, but it can be as low as 70 mm Hg in healthy geriatric patients. Normal P_aCO_2 is 35–45 mm Hg; normal arterial pH, 7.35–7.45; and normal standard bicarbonate concentration, 22–26 mEq/L. In general, blood gas analysis should be done at regular intervals during long procedures, in patients with cardiopulmonary disease, in seriously ill or severely injured patients, and during cardiovascular, intracranial, or thoracic operations. It must be stressed that blood gas analysis does not constitute continuous monitoring, even if it is done frequently, because results are always delayed and reflect past events. Intravascular electrodes with a rapid response time are available but require improvements before they can be recommended for general use.

Measurement of transcutaneous oxygen tension ($tcPO_2$) has been exploited as a noninvasive means of continuously monitoring oxygenation. In this method, vasodilation and arterialization of subepidermal capillary blood is produced by heat, and oxygen diffusing through the epidermis is measured by a polarographic oxygen analyzer (see "Galvanic Fuel Cell and Polarographic Oxygen Analyzers" below.) Although tcPO$_2$ approaches PaO$_2$ when it is measured with meticulous care, its accuracy suffers when vasodilation is less than maximum (e.g., in low cardiac output states), when the epidermis is thick, and when oxygen consumption of surrounding tissue is high. Its application is more popular among infants and young children than among adults.

Another alternative to monitoring oxygenation is noninvasive measurement of oxygen saturation (SpO$_2$) by pulse oximetry. This method is based on the differential absorption of red and infrared light by oxyhemoglobin and deoxyhemoglobin (Fig. 14–3A). While red light of wavelength 660 nm is absorbed strongly by deoxyhemoglobin and weakly by oxyhemoglobin, this difference is much less with infrared light of wavelength 940 nm. Light-emitting diodes (LEDs) in the pulse oximeter probe send light of these wavelengths through the test site (e.g., finger, earlobe, palm of neonates) and the intensities of transmitted lights are monitored continuously by sensors. During diastole, part of the incident light of both wavelengths is absorbed by a constant amount of tissue and blood in nonpulsatile capillaries (Fig. 14–3B). During systole, the pulse-added portion of arterial blood absorbs additional light. At the peak of the pulse, these additional absorptions (equal to the difference between the intensity of transmitted light at the trough

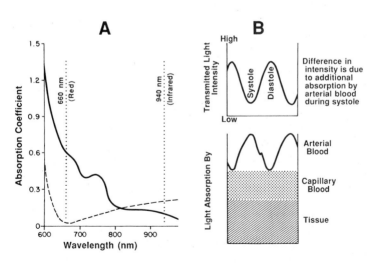

FIGURE 14–3. Principle of pulse oximetry. *A*, Absorption spectrum of oxyhemoglobin (broken line) and deoxyhemoglobin (solid line). *B*, Pulsatile variation in light absorption by arterial blood. (Refer to text for details.)

and that at the peak of the pulse) are related to the concentrations of oxyhemoglobin and deoxyhemoglobin in arterial blood alone. This difference in intensities is sensed by the photodetectors and fed into a microprocessor, which computes SpO_2 empirically:

$$SpO_2\% = \frac{\text{oxyHb conc.}}{\text{oxyHb conc.} + \text{deoxyHb conc.}} \times 100\%$$

In addition, a pulse oximeter can act as a pulse plethysmograph, and reproduce pulse waveforms on a monitor screen. Between saturation values of 60% and 100%, pulse oximeter measurements are accurate to ±2.5%. However, because other species of hemoglobin (carboxyhemoglobin, methemoglobin, sulfhemoglobin) have been ignored in the computation, the presence of a significant amount of abnormal hemoglobins in the patient's blood can yield erroneously high values of oxygen saturation. Although normal skin pigments do not interfere with measurements, the presence of bilirubin or dyes such as methylene blue and indocyanine green can produce errors. For accuracy, the probe and test site must be protected from excessive movement and shielded from bright ambient lights, particularly infrared heat lamps, which are used on infants and young children.

■ Monitoring Respiratory and Anesthetic Gases

In order to protect the patient from exposure to hypoxic gas mixtures, anesthetic machines are equipped with an oxygen failure safety valve and alarm (see Chapter 7). For similar reasons, continuous monitoring of inspired oxygen concentration has become a standard practice. Earlier models of these devices were based on galvanic fuel cell or polarographic principles; they had a slow response time and were suitable for monitoring only oxygen concentration in the anesthetic circuit. Monitors capable of measuring breath-to-breath concentrations of respiratory and anesthetic gases or vapors at the airway soon followed. They include paramagnetic oxygen analyzers, capnographs, nitrous oxide and halogenated vapor monitors, mass spectrometers, and Raman photospectrometers.

Galvanic Fuel Cell and Polarographic Oxygen Analyzers

The galvanic fuel cell oxygen analyzer is an electrochemical device consisting of one gold and one lead electrode immersed

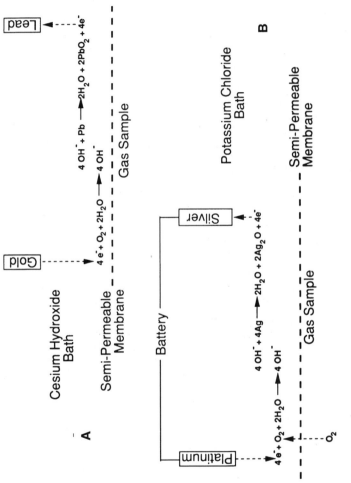

FIGURE 14-4. A, Galvanic fuel cell oxygen analyzer. B, Polarographic oxygen analyzer. (Refer to text for details.)

in a cesium hydroxide bath and separated from the gas sample by a semipermeable membrane (Fig. 4–4A). As it diffuses into the bath, each oxygen molecule combines with four electrons from the gold cathode and water molecules to form hydroxyl ions:

$$O_2 + 2H_2O + 4e^- \rightarrow 4OH^-$$

In turn, these hydroxyl ions migrate toward the lead anode and react with it to form lead oxide and water, surrendering four electrons in the process:

$$4OH^- + Pb \rightarrow PbO_2 + 2H_2O + 4e^-$$

Constant diffusion of oxygen into the bath would mean a constant flow of electrons between the gold and lead electrodes and build-up of a potential difference that can be measured on a meter as oxygen concentration.

The polarographic (Clark-type electrode) oxygen analyzer is similar to the fuel cell model, but the silver–silver chloride and platinum electrodes are kept polarized with the help of a battery (Fig. 14–4B). Negatively charged hydroxyl ions formed by oxygen diffusing across the membrane are actively attracted toward the positively charged silver–silver chloride electrode, thus improving the response time of this device. Nevertheless, both the fuel cell and polarographic analyzers are designed for monitoring oxygen concentration in the anesthetic circuit only; their relatively slow response time precludes use for breath-to-breath measurement.

In order to make them true monitors, these instruments are equipped with low concentration alarms that warn the operator when oxygen concentration falls below a chosen limit. Common sense dictates that the lower limit should be set no lower than 21%. Because water condensate on the semipermeable membrane can interfere with oxygen diffusion, these sensors should be positioned at the fresh gas outlet of the anesthetic machine or at the inspiratory limb of the circle system proximal to the mouthpiece. Two-point calibration, at 21% and 100% oxygen, must be performed on these instruments daily before use.

Paramagnetic Oxygen Analyzers

Unlike other gases, oxygen is paramagnetic—that is, it has magnet-like properties. When exposed to a strong magnet, oxygen molecules align with and enhance the applied magnetic field. In the paramagnetic oxygen analyzer, a dehumidified test sample and a reference gas of known oxygen concentration (room air) are fed through tubings into adjacent test chambers between the two poles of an electromagnet that is being

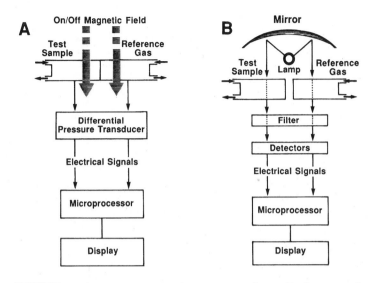

FIGURE 14–5. *A*, Paramagnetic oxygen analyzer. *B*, Capnograph. (Refer to text for details.)

switched on and off repeatedly at a frequency of 110 Hz (Fig. 14–5*A*). Because forces acting on oxygen molecules in the on again–off again magnetic field will vary according to their concentration, an alternating pressure difference is generated between the test and reference chambers. This pressure difference is sensed by a differential pressure transducer, the signals are fed into a microprocessor, and oxygen concentration in the test sample is computed and displayed. In the magnetoacoustic version of the paramagnetic oxygen analyzer, pressure changes are converted to changes in the volume of a sound wave, which is detected by a sensitive microphone and processed and displayed as oxygen concentration. Paramagnetic oxygen analyzers have a response time on the order of 200 msec and are capable of breath-to-breath measurement of inspiratory and expiratory oxygen concentration at the airway.

Capnographs

These devices measure instantaneous changes in carbon dioxide (CO_2) tension or concentration at the airway using infrared light absorption technology. A dehumidified test sample is drawn into a test chamber lying next to a reference chamber containing air, and identical beams of infrared light from an incandescent lamp are shined through both (Fig. 14–5*B*). After passing through these chambers, the two beams are filtered to allow only a narrow band of light with wavelengths around 4.3 μm to pass through. Infrared light of this wavelength is strongly absorbed by CO_2. The difference in intensities of these filtered beams is directly related to the difference in CO_2 concentrations between test sample and reference gas. This difference in intensities is sensed by infrared sensors, the signals are processed, and instantaneous CO_2 tension or concentration is displayed graphically on a monitor screen. With mainstream devices, the sensor is positioned close to the airway in line with the anesthetic circuit and response time is almost instantaneous (about 10 msec). With sidestream devices, test samples are withdrawn continuously from the airway via a pilot line and directed to a distantly located sensor. In this instance, response time is dependent on the length of the pilot line and the rate of sample flow (usually around 150 msec).

Three major landmarks can be identified on a normal airway CO_2 waveform (Fig. 14–6A): an inspiratory phase and an expiratory slope, which rises rapidly to a well-developed endtidal plateau. Because there is very little alveolar-arterial CO_2 gradient in healthy subjects, the end-tidal carbon dioxide ($ETCO_2$) level approximates P_aCO_2 of 35–45 mm Hg. However, if development of the $ETCO_2$ plateau is cut off prematurely, as in tachypnea or bronchospasm (Fig. 14–6B), peak CO_2 levels in these instances are less than $ETCO_2$ values.

Inspiratory and $ETCO_2$ values and the shape of the waveform yield many clues to the functional status of the patient, the

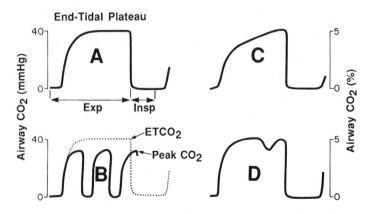

FIGURE 14–6. Airway CO_2 waveforms. *A*, Normal waveform. *B*, Difference between peak CO_2 level during tachypnea and normal $ETCO_2$ level during a normal breath. *C*, Airway CO_2 waveform in partial airway obstruction or severe ventilation-perfusion abnormalities. *D*, Spontaneous tidal breath shows as indentation of the end-tidal plateau of a ventilated breath.

adequacy of ventilation, and the integrity of the anesthetic circuit. (Capnometers, which do not display an airway CO_2 waveform, are not as versatile as capnographs.) During inspiration the CO_2 tension of the inspired gas mixture should be near zero. If it is elevated to any degree, immediate investigation and correction are imperative. Common causes of CO_2 appearing in the inspired gas mixture when the circle system is in use are (1) exhaustion of the CO_2 absorption canister, (2) unintentional switching off of the canister, and (3) leak or backflow in unidirectional valves. When the Bain, Magill, or T-piece circuit is in use, the cause is always inadequate fresh gas flow.

In the absence of CO_2 rebreathing, $ETCO_2$ values depend on (1) adequacy of alveolar ventilation, (2) CO_2 production, and (3) state of pulmonary circulation. Proper interpretation of $ETCO_2$ values in anesthetized patients requires an awareness of the mode of ventilation and the trend of development of these values:

1. A mild degree of hypercapnia ($ETCO_2$ up to 55 mm Hg) during spontaneous ventilation is usually due to central respiratory depression by anesthetic drugs.

2. Gradual development of hypercapnia during controlled mechanical ventilation should raise the possibility of alveolar hypoventilation, a result of either inappropriate ventilator settings or leaks in the system.

3. Rapid development of hypercapnia during adequate mechanical ventilation is associated with excessive CO_2 production in hypermetabolic states (e.g., hyperthermic crisis or thyroid storm). Checking the patient's body temperature and acid-base status and reviewing the medical history will help to clarify these issues.

4. Sudden development of hypercapnia during intra-abdominal CO_2 insufflation (e.g., in laparoscopic surgery) means CO_2 embolism.

5. A mild degree of hypocapnia during controlled ventilation is usually due to alveolar hyperventilation. If hypocapnia is inappropriate, hypometabolic states (e.g., inadvertent hypothermia and hypothyroidism) or large drops in cardiac output (e.g., hypovolemia and acute myocardial infarction) should be considered. In the former, CO_2 production is reduced; in the latter, diminished pulmonary perfusion leads to increase in physiologic dead space and arterial-alveolar CO_2 tension gradient.

6. Sudden and unexpected falls in $ETCO_2$ should raise the possibility of mechanical obstruction to the pulmonary circulation, as in pulmonary embolism (blood clot, air, amniotic fluid) or cardiac arrest.

In addition to inspired CO_2 and $ETCO_2$ values, the airway CO_2 waveform can be used as a diagnostic tool. In partial airway obstruction (e.g., bronchospasm or kinked endotracheal tube) or severe ventilation-perfusion abnormalities, the latter half of the expiratory slope rises slowly and continuously to merge with an ill-defined plateau (Fig. 14–6C). Partial recovery from muscle relaxants during mechanical ventilation may show up as indentations in the end-tidal plateau resulting from spontaneous respiratory efforts (Fig. 14–6D). Total disconnection of the anesthetic circuit is characterized by sudden disappearance of a pre-existing waveform, and esophageal intubation by absence of the waveform following an assisted breath.

Nitrous Oxide and Anesthetic Vapor Monitors

Like capnographs, these monitors are based on infrared light absorption technology. Nitrous oxide strongly absorbs infrared light in a narrow band around 3.9 μm; the filters in nitrous oxide monitors are adjusted to this bandwidth accordingly.

When it is applied to measuring anesthetic vapor concentrations, the operative infrared light absorption wavelength of 3.3 μm is not specific for the halogenated volatile agents. Older version of these halometers cannot be relied on to distinguish one agent from another, they cannot recognize inadvertent admixture or substitution of agents. Unless the operator selects the correct setting for the agent in use, the displayed concentration is erroneous. With some new models, agent recognition is possible using advanced technology. One version uses the pattern of light absorption at wavelengths slightly above and slightly below 3.3 μm to identify the agent; another uses light absorption at wavelengths between 9 and 11 μm to identify the agent.

Mass Spectrometers

These instruments can distinguish and measure the concentration of all respiratory, anesthetic, and atmospheric gases and vapors. The test sample is injected into an ionization chamber, where all gas molecules become ionized through bombardment by electrons (Fig. 14–7A). The ionized molecules are then propelled through a magnetic field in the test chamber, in which each molecular species will follow a unique circular path depending on its charge-to–molecular weight ratio. These ion flows are registered as electric currents by sensors on the collecting plate, and the concentration of a gas is computed according to the following formulas:

Total current = O_2 current + N_2O current + CO_2 current + others

$$O_2\% = (O_2 \text{ current/total current}) \times 100\%$$

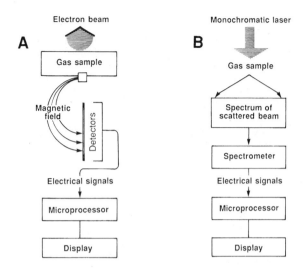

FIGURE 14–7. *A*, Mass spectrometer. *B*, Photospectrometer. (Refer to text for details.)

Mass spectrometers have a response time of the order of 60 msec and can be used to monitor breath-to-breath inspiratory and end-tidal concentrations. Because they can measure nitrogen concentration, these devices have unique applications not available to dedicated monitors described previously:

1. End-tidal nitrogen concentration can be used to follow denitrogenation of the lungs during preoxygenation before rapid-sequence induction (see "Rapid-Sequence Induction" in Chapter 15).

2. After denitrogenation is complete, the reappearance of end-tidal nitrogen is a sensitive indicator of air embolism.

3. Once nitrogen has been eliminated, reappearance of nitrogen during inspiration means the presence of an air leak.

Most of the mass spectrometers work on a time-shared basis between multiple locations. Depending on the number of locations in operation, intervals between sampling at any one location can vary from 1 to 5 minutes. That is, monitoring is intermittent rather than continuous; mishap and harm to the patient can occur without warning between samples. Dedicated single-user units will eliminate this danger.

Raman Photospectrometers

Like mass spectrometers, Raman photospectrometers can measure the concentration of all respiratory, anesthetic, and atmospheric gases and vapors. In these instruments, a monochromatic (single-wavelength) visible laser beam is directed at and scattered by molecules in the gas sample (Fig. 14–7B). Some of the photons (light particles) of the incident beam continue on without change in wavelength, and some emerge at different wavelengths, having gained energy from or lost it to the scattering molecules. Thus the emergent beam acquires a spectrum of wavelengths that is unique to the composition of the gas sample. Spectral analysis of the scattered beam is used to determine the concentration of each component.

■ Monitoring Renal Function

Kidneys with normal concentrating function can excrete their daily solute load in as little as 600 ml of urine, but this is possible only if renal blood flow is normal. In general, a minimal hourly urine output of 25 ml is accepted as a sign of normal renal blood flow. Moreover, the ability of the kidneys to maintain this minimum hourly output has also been regarded as a sign of normovolemia and normal cardiac output. It is customary to monitor urine output via an indwelling urinary catheter when large fluid shifts or blood loss is anticipated during surgical procedures. Unfortunately opioids and stress can stimulate the secretion of antidiuretic hormone (ADH), and oliguria alone is not a reliable sign of hypovolemia or low cardiac output during surgery. A rational interpretation of urinary output can be made only if hemodynamic variables (pulse rate, blood pressure, and central venous pressure) and volume of blood lost during the operation are also taken into consideration.

■ Monitoring Neuromuscular Function

The popularity of muscle relaxants in current anesthesia practice has made it necessary to monitor neuromuscular function whenever these agents are used. Although clinical signs are helpful, an objective evaluation can be made only by using the peripheral nerve stimulator.

Clinical Signs

During abdominal surgery, a quiet operative field is a reliable sign of adequate muscle relaxation. Twitching of the diaphragm, appearance of bowel at the edge of the surgical wound, and appearance of skeletal muscle myopotentials on the ECG oscilloscope are indications for an additional dose of muscle relaxant.

At the end of the operation, return of neuromuscular function is signaled by the onset of spontaneous ventilation. The signs of adequate tidal exchange are quiet respiration, normal respiratory excursions that involve the apical regions of the chest wall, and absence of tracheal tug; however, they do not necessarily mean full recovery of neuromuscular function. The ability of the patient to exhale a vital capacity of at least 15 ml/kg, to generate a negative pressure of at least -25 cm H_2O on inspiration, to protrude the tongue, to lift the head off the pillow for 5 seconds, and to maintain a powerful hand grip are more helpful signs, but these tests are possible only when the patient is awake and can obey commands. Thrashing movements of the extremities and the trunk (like those of a "fish out of water"), inspiratory stridor, and muted coughs are signs of partial paralysis.

Peripheral Nerve Stimulation

Apnea may be due to central respiratory depression rather than paralysis, and the patient who is partially paralyzed may have an adequate tidal volume but will not be able to cope with increases in demand. In these situations, objective evidence of normal neuromuscular function should be sought by electrical stimulation of the ulnar nerve. Stimulation of the facial or lateral popliteal nerve has been used also for convenience. Many anesthesiologists advocate routine use of the peripheral nerve stimulator as an adjunct to observation of clinical signs whenever muscle relaxants are employed.

The peripheral nerve stimulator is designed to deliver a supramaximal electrical stimulus that, when applied to a peripheral nerve, will elicit a muscle twitch. This stimulus can be delivered in three different modes: at a frequency of 1 Hz (single-twitch stimulus), at a frequency of 2 Hz for 2 seconds (train-of-four stimulus), or at a frequency of 50 or 100 Hz (tetanic stimulus). The use of the peripheral nerve stimulator serves three purposes:

1. To differentiate the type of neuromuscular block
2. To determine the magnitude of the block
3. To determine the degree of recovery at the end of a procedure

In the presence of a nondepolarizing neuromuscular block, stimulation of the ulnar nerve elicits the following motor responses in muscles of the hand (Fig. 14–8):

MONITORING DURING ANESTHESIA

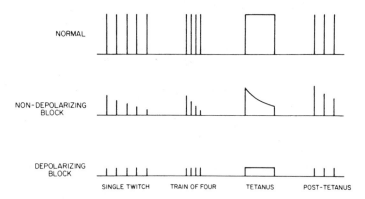

FIGURE 14–8. Illustrations of muscle twitches in response to the electrical stimulation of a peripheral nerve in normal subject and to subjects under the influence of nondepolarizing and depolarizing blocks. (Refer to text for details.)

1. Lower-than-normal twitch height that fades gradually when the single-twitch stimulus is applied repeatedly
2. Similar fade in twitch height when the train-of-four stimulus is applied
3. Unsustained response when the tetanic stimulus is applied
4. Transient increase in twitch response when the single-twitch stimulus is applied following tetany (a phenomenon called post-tetanic facilitation)
5. Disappearance of fade and of post-tetanic facilitation and return of twitch heights toward normal following administration of an adequate dose of anticholinesterase

When a depolarizing muscle relaxant is used, the characteristic motor response to ulnar nerve stimulation during a Phase 1 block is as follows (see Fig. 14–8):

1. Decreased twitch height that does not fade when the single-twitch stimulus is applied repeatedly
2. Absence of fade when the train-of-four stimulus is applied
3. Tetany that is sustained
4. Absence of post-tetanic facilitation

The characteristic response to stimulation during a Phase II depolarizing block is similar to that during a nondepolarizing block.

It must be stressed at this point that these responses are seen only in the presence of partial blockade. When neuromuscular blockade is complete, no twitch response is seen; however, complete neuromuscular blockade is rarely necessary in anesthesia practice. A 90% reduction in single-twitch height is adequate for most abdominal procedures, and a reduction in twitch height of only 70% is required when an inhalation agent with muscle-relaxant action (e.g., enflurane or isoflurane) is used concurrently.

Since its introduction in 1975, the train-of-four stimulus has been used extensively as a semiquantitative method of determining the magnitude of nondepolarizing block. When only the last of the four twitches is abolished, the degree of blockade correlates with a 70% reduction in single-twitch height; when the last two twitches are not detectable, reduction in single-twitch height is 80%; and when the last three twitches are not observable, reduction is 90%. Neuromuscular blockade is complete or 100% only when all four twitches are abolished. This method of assessing neuromuscular blockade requires no recording instrument. By counting the number of twitches in the train-of-four response, the degree of neuromuscular blockade can easily be ascertained. Uneventful reversal of nondepolarizing blocks with an anticholinergic agent can be expected when three or more twitches are present. Reversal of nondepolarizing block should not be regarded as adequate until all four twitches in the train-of-four stimulus have returned and when the strength of the last twitch approximates that of the first. As a diagnostic test for adequacy of reversing nondepolarizing blocks, sustained contraction in response to 50-Hz tetanic simulation is even more reliable than the train-of-four stimulus, but the former procedure is painful and cannot be used in patients who have regained consciousness.

Data correlating degree of neuromuscular blockade and its reversal to twitch heights were obtained by stimulation of the ulnar nerve. In clinical practice, stimulation of the facial nerve is often used for convenience to monitor neuromuscular blockade. It must be emphasized that facial muscles recover from nondepolarization blocks earlier than muscles of the hand. Recovery of twitch heights in facial muscles when the train-of-four stimulus is applied does not guarantee similar recovery in muscles of the hand.

■ Monitoring Body Temperature

Use of thermometry to detect changes in body temperature during anesthesia should be practiced routinely. Hypothermia is a common complication during the course of anesthesia and surgery, and the drop in body temperature can be particularly severe in infants and children, in critically ill patients, and when large volumes of fluid or blood are given. Hyperthermia, in comparison, is much less common. It usually occurs during febrile illness or when waterproof surgical drapes are used in infants and small children. An unexpected rise in core temperature following induction of anesthesia in a cool operating room should raise the possibility of malignant hyperthermia (see "Malignant Hyperthermia" in Chapter 16).

Temperature can be measured with thermistors or thermocouples at many sites: midesophagus, nasopharynx, rectum, axilla, tympanic membrane, and skin. Usually esophageal or nasopharyngeal probes are used to measure core temperature in adults, and rectal probes are used in infants.

▰ Monitoring Other Systemic Functions

Frequently it is necessary to monitor other physiologic variables during the perioperative period, owing either to existence of concurrent illness or to complications of surgery. Blood sugar concentration should be determined periodically in diabetic patients, and electrolytes as well as buffer base should be followed in critically ill patients or in those who have had large fluid and electrolyte shifts. Furthermore, the need to monitor hemoglobin concentration and coagulation in patients who have received large volumes of stored blood should not be overlooked.

▰ Basic Intraoperative Monitoring

To monitor is to observe for changes so that the practitioner can be forewarned. In this role, the anesthesiologist is the master monitor: absorbing information and correlating and integrating all input data before dispensing an appropriate response. Therefore, continuous presence of the anesthesiologist at the patient's side throughout the course of the procedure is the first cardinal rule of monitoring. If a temporary absence is necessitated by extenuating circumstances (e.g., attendance at life-threatening emergency), the anesthesiologist should transfer his or her duty to a surrogate who has the ability and agrees to take on the responsibility. During transfer of duty, the anesthesiologist should summarize for the colleague the patient's medical history and findings, mode of ventilation under anesthesia, dosage of drugs received, and progress to date. In the event that momentary absence from the patient's side is required (e.g., due to radiation hazards), the anesthesiologist should remain in visual contact with the patient and the monitors and should return to the patient's side as soon as conditions permit.

Obviously the choice of monitors should be appropriate for the patient's medical condition and the planned operation. Nevertheless, a minimum level of monitoring should be practiced during the course of anesthesia even if the subject is an American Society of Anesthesiologists Class I patient undergoing a simple surgical procedure. Many institutions and national organizations have published guidelines regularly on this topic. In general, monitoring of the following parameters and functions during all anesthetic procedures are mandatory:

1. Display cardiac rhythm continuously on ECG.

2. Record blood pressure and heart rate at least every 5 minutes and check circulatory function more frequently by palpation of the pulse, auscultation of the heart, or other instrumentation.

3. If patient is breathing spontaneously, monitor ventilation by clinical signs and expiratory volumes using a mechanical or electronic respirometer. If ventilation is controlled, monitor tidal volume and respiratory rate as well as airway pressure.

4. Monitor the respiratory cycle and $ETCO_2$ by capnography.

5. Measure oxygen concentration of the anesthetic fresh gas using an oxygen analyzer with alarm, and monitor the patient's oxygenation by clinical signs as well as pulse oximetry.

6. Monitor integrity of the anesthetic circuit during controlled ventilation using a low-pressure alarm or similar device.

7. Monitor depth of anesthesia by clinical signs.

In addition to these monitors, it is the consensus of many anesthesiologists that the automated sphygmomanometer, peripheral nerve stimulator, and electronic thermometer are indispensable. They have proved to be cost effective and will become standard tools as guidelines for basic monitoring evolve.

In summary, vigilance is the cornerstone of monitoring. Emphasis should not be placed on the measurement of a single variable. Changes in all measured variables should be correlated and examined from the perspective of the patient's clinical condition.

Techniques of General Anesthesia

15

There are four phases in all techniques of general anesthesia: induction, maintenance, emergence, and recovery. Each phase requires skill and attention to details. Meticulous preparation and planning should be part of each anesthetic procedure. A little time well spent in preparation will save anxiety afterward.

A Practical Guide to Preparation

Preparation in the operating room before arrival of the patient should include the following steps:

1. Fill syringes with appropriate intravenous agents and label them clearly.
2. Check that endotracheal equipment is available and in working order (see "Techniques of Intubation" in Chapter 13); this is necessary even if endotracheal anesthesia has not been planned because tracheal intubation may be required if complications develop.
3. Check that the pharyngeal suction apparatus is available on demand.
4. Switch on, set up, and calibrate all monitors.
5. Check the anesthetic machine and its functions as described under "Checking the Anesthetic Machine" in Chapter 7.
6. Check the anesthetic circuit and its integrity as described under "Checking the Anesthetic Circuit" in Chapter 8.
7. Attach a face mask of appropriate size to the anesthetic circuit.
8. Check the mechanical ventilator and its functions as described under "Checking the Ventilator" in Chapter 9.

When the patient is in the operating room, his or her identity and the nature and site of the scheduled operation should be checked once more. This is the last chance to avoid disasters of mistaken identity and misdirected surgery. Before induction of anesthesia, the anesthesiologist should establish a freely running intravenous infusion, attach all monitoring devices, and record baseline values.

■ Induction of Anesthesia

The phase of induction begins when the anesthetic is first given to the patient and ends when surgical anesthesia is established. The trachea is intubated during this phase if endotracheal anesthesia is planned.

Before commencing induction, it is important to ascertain that the patient is secure on the operating table and that the arms are well supported. With onset of anesthesia and loss of muscle tone, poorly supported arms can fall off the edge of the table, producing shoulder dislocation or traction injury of the brachial plexus. Such accidents are preventable.

Intravenous Induction

Of all the intravenous induction agents (see Chapter 2), thiopental is the most established, but the method of induction is similar for all of them. Only the method for thiopental is described below.

Although the average induction dose of thiopental is 4–5 mg/kg, there is a wide variation in the requirement among individual patients. Therefore, its dose should be titrated against observed effects. It is good practice to administer a test dose of 2 ml before giving the full dose. Pain at the site of injection following the test dose suggests a leak into perivenous space; pain distal to the site of injection in the digits should raise the possibility of intra-arterial injection (an accident that is complicated by thrombosis and gangrene). In either case, position of the intravenous cannula should be checked.

When thiopental is used for induction, most patients experience a taste of onion or garlic before onset of anesthesia. Some patients may yawn or take a deep breath at this point, but the most reliable sign of loss of consciousness is loss of eyelash reflex (blinking in response to stroking of the eyelash). Once unconsciousness is established, the next steps depend on whether tracheal intubation is planned. If it is, a muscle relaxant is usually given at this point and the trachea intubated as described under "Tracheal Intubation" and "Rapid-Sequence Induction" below.

Note: Many factors can influence the choice of face mask, laryngeal mask, or tracheal intubation as the method to manage the airway. These factors are detailed under "Direct Laryngoscopy and Tracheal Intubation" in Chapter 13.

If tracheal intubation is not planned, a nitrous oxide–oxygen mixture should be given via face mask. The concentration of nitrous oxide should not exceed 70%, and total fresh gas flow should be consistent with that recommended for the anesthetic circuit being used (see Chapter 8). A volatile agent should be added, and its concentration increased in increments to a value equal to 2 MAC, so that an anesthetic level of alveolar concentration can be achieved quickly (see "Inspired Concentration" in Chapter 3). Once surgical anesthesia is established, the concentration of the volatile agent can be returned to lower levels for maintenance. Some patients become apneic following an induction dose of thiopental; if this is the case, ventilation should be assisted until spontaneous respiration returns. Some others may develop signs of airway obstruction as a result of the tongue falling backward into the hypopharynx. In these instances, the head tilt–jaw thrust maneuver with or without a pharyngeal airway should be used to keep the airway patent as described in Chapter 13.

For very short procedures, managing the airway using the face mask and pharyngeal airway combination would suffice. For longer procedures, particularly when both hands of the anesthesiologist are required for other chores, the laryngeal mask airway is indicated. Thiopental does not inhibit airway reflexes; after thiopental induction, it is best to insert the laryngeal mask airway after establishment of surgical anesthesia using a volatile agent. After propofol induction, in contrast, the laryngeal mask airway can be inserted soon after loss of consciousness without provoking laryngospasm.

It must be emphasized that patients are only lightly anesthetized during induction. Unnecessary stimulation (e.g., catheterization of urinary bladder, manipulation of limbs) can provoke laryngospasm. No procedure, no matter how minor, should be allowed until surgical anesthesia is established.

Inhalation Induction

Inhalation induction via face mask with selected volatile anesthetics is both rapid and pleasant. Except for transient movement of the extremities, breath holding, nystagmus, and a divergent gaze, the second stage described for ether is not seen. A technique using halothane is described below.

At the beginning of the procedure, only oxygen or a nitrous oxide–oxygen mixture without halothane should be given. When the patient has become accustomed to breathing through the mask, halothane should be added in 0.5% increments until its concentration is 3–4%. The patient should be allowed to take three or four breaths before each increase in concentration. Too rapid an increase can induce coughing and laryngospasm.

Onset of surgical anesthesia is marked by disappearance of both nystagmus and divergent gaze, by midsized pupils that react to light, and by a breathing pattern that is regular in rate and depth. When this stage is reached, the concentration of halothane can be returned to lower levels for maintenance. Once surgical anesthesia is established, induction can continue with tracheal intubation or the use of a face mask or laryngeal mask airway as described in the previous section.

All the other inhalation agents can be used to induce surgical anesthesia in the manner described for halothane. However, enflurane is a more potent respiratory depressant than halothane, and isoflurane is rather pungent. These properties can make inhalation induction somewhat more difficult. Of the new insoluble agents, desflurane is also irritating to the airway but sevoflurane is not. Induction of anesthesia with sevoflurane is a pleasant experience for both adults and children because of its nonpungent smell and low solubility (see "Solubility of Anesthetic Agent" in Chapter 3).

Tracheal Intubation

If endotracheal anesthesia is planned, the trachea should be intubated soon after unconsciousness is established. Intubation is usually facilitated by administration of succinylcholine, 1 mg/kg, intravenously (1.5–2 mg/kg if precurarization is practiced). After onset of paralysis, the lungs should be ventilated gently with 100% oxygen for approximately 1 minute. This measure is necessary to fill the lungs with oxygen so that the patient can tolerate apnea during intubation without developing hypoxemia. (The technique of tracheal intubation is described in Chapter 13.) After tracheal intubation, manual ventilation of the lungs should continue with a mixture of nitrous oxide, oxygen, and a volatile agent until adequate spontaneous respiration has returned or mechanical ventilation is instituted.

Rapid-Sequence Induction

Rapid-sequence induction (crash induction) is a technique in which the trachea is intubated during induction of anesthesia without manual ventilation of the lungs with pure oxygen beforehand. It is designed to minimize the risk of aspiration pneumonitis and is indicated in all clinical situations that predispose the patient to regurgitation or vomiting (e.g., obesity, pregnancy, bowel obstruction, acute abdomen, hiatus hernia, emergency operations). During this procedure, the presence of an assistant is absolutely necessary. The technique is as follows:

1. Check the anesthetic machine, anesthetic circuit, ventilator, and endotracheal equipment as described earlier. Be prepared for unforeseen difficulties and have at hand a backup laryngoscope, endotracheal tubes of different sizes, and emergency airways.

2. Turn on the pharyngeal suction apparatus, which should be easily accessible.

3. Have the patient breathe 100% oxygen at high flow from a form-fitting mask for 3–5 minutes before induction of anesthesia. Alternatively have the patient breathe in four to five vital-capacity breaths of 100% oxygen just before induction of anesthesia. (This period of preoxygenation will eliminate the necessity for manual ventilation of the lungs with oxygen following onset of paralysis.)

4. Position the patient's head in the "sniffing" position.

5. With due consideration given to the patient's size, age, and state of health, determine the ideal induction dose of thiopental or other agents. Give this dose and 1 mg/kg of succinylcholine in quick succession. Give rocuronium, 1.2 mg/kg, instead of succinylcholine in patients in whom succinylcholine is contraindicated.

6. As soon as the patient has lost consciousness, have the assistant apply pressure to the cricoid cartilage and direct it posteriorly. (The cricoid cartilage is the only tracheal ring that is complete. Pressure directed posteriorly on this cartilage will compress the esophagus against the sixth cervical vetebra and prevent regurgitation of stomach contents into the larynx and pharynx. This procedure is often referred to as "Sellick's maneuver.")

7. Reconfirm the posture of the patient's head and neck and intubate the trachea at onset of paralysis.

8. Inflate the cuff of the endotracheal tube before pressure on the cricoid cartilage is released.

9. Check the position of the endotracheal tube (see "Orotracheal Intubation" in Chapter 13), make any necessary adjustment, and secure it in place.

After tracheal intubation, the course of anesthesia can proceed as described in the previous section.

In addition to these basic steps, some anesthesiologists recommend other measures to minimize the risk of regurgitation and aspiration. These measures include positioning the patient in a head-up position to prevent regurgitation or in a head-down or left lateral position to prevent aspiration. Unfortunately, none of these measures is foolproof and all can make intubation difficult. One popular measure is precurarization (see "Precurarization" in Chapter 5). Succinylcholine-induced muscle fasciculation can cause a large increase in intra-abdominal pressure. Pretreatment of the patient with 3–6 mg of *d*-tubocurarine (or an equivalent dose of another nondepolarizing agent) given 3–4 minutes before succinylcholine can abolish this fasciculation and reduce the risk of regurgitation. It should be remembered, however, that precurarization reduces the potency and delays the action of succinylcholine. In order to obtain maximal muscle relaxation for intubation, the succinylcholine dose should be increased to 1.5–2 mg/kg following precurarization.

■ Positioning the Patient on the Operating Table

Following induction of anesthesia, a change in the position of the patient may be required for the operation. Although the choice of intraoperative position is made by the surgeon, every member of the surgical team should play an active role in ensuring that the patient is secure on the table. Improper postures and support can cause injuries and cardiovascular instability. Certain precautions should routinely be followed in positioning patients:

1. Make sure that the eyes are shut and protected. Pressure against the eyeballs can cause retinal vein thrombosis and blindness.

2. Protect the elbows. Allowing them to lie unpadded against the edge of the table can cause ulnar nerve palsy.

3. Do not abduct the arms farther than 90 degrees. Excessive abduction can cause traction injury of the brachial plexus.

4. Flex both knees and hips simultaneously during movement to the lithotomy position to avoid causing traction injury to the sciatic nerve.

5. Protect the knees in the lithotomy position. Allowing the lateral aspect of the knee to rest unpadded against the lithotomy post can cause lateral popliteal nerve palsy.

6. Make sure that the abdomen is free if the patient is in the prone position. Pressure against the abdomen can obstruct venous return and restrict excursion of the diaphragm.

7. Monitor vital signs closely when a sudden change in posture is made. Such changes can cause venous pooling, interfere with cardiac output, and result in disconnection of the anesthetic circuit or inadvertent extubation.

8. Do not allow bare metal parts of the operating table to come into contact with the patient. Electric currents used for cauterization running through these high-resistance pathways can cause electrical burns.

▓▓▓ Maintenance of General Anesthesia

After the patient is properly positioned, the operation may commence. When the operation is concluded, the depth of anesthesia should be lightened and the patient should be allowed to emerge. The phase of maintenance refers to the period beginning with the onset of surgical anesthesia and ending with emergence. One or more drugs can be given to maintain unconsciousness, analgesia, and muscle relaxation during this period. Whether a patient should be allowed to breathe spontaneously or controlled ventilation should be used during this period is not always easy to judge. Indications for controlled ventilation include the following:

1. Procedures requiring muscle relaxant to provide profound muscle relaxation for surgical access.
2. Instances in which muscle relaxant is part of the anesthetic plan (e.g., balanced anesthesia or total intravenous anesthesia).
3. Intraoperative positions that restrict the respiratory excursion of the rib cage or diaphragm (e.g., prone, steep Trendelenburg tilt, jackknife).
4. Presence of cardiorespiratory disease or other severe systemic illness.
5. Cases in which hyperventilation is desirable (e.g., to reduce intracranial pressure).

Aside from these indications, the chosen mode of ventilation is a matter of the anesthesiologist's preference. In general, healthy patients are allowed to breathe spontaneously during short procedures, provided profound muscle relaxation is not required.

Spontaneous Ventilation

With operations that require only a mild degree of muscle relaxation (e.g., operations on extremities and the head and neck), spontaneous ventilation is usually allowed. With this technique, a mixture of nitrous oxide and oxygen (usually in a 2:1 ratio) is given for basal anesthesia and analgesia, a volatile agent is added as an adjunct to maintain unconsciousness, and an opioid is given as analgesic supplement when required. Because the combined respiratory depressant effects of the volatile agent and the opioid can cause apnea, the narcotic analgesic should be given in small increments only.

As a result of ventilatory depression (see Chapter 10), hypercapnia is always a complication of this technique; however, in healthy patients the degree of hypercapnia is usually mild when the correct fresh gas flow is used.

Controlled Ventilation

A neuromuscular blocking drug is used whenever profound muscle relaxation is required. Frequently it is also used in the nitrous oxide–narcotic-relaxant technique or total intravenous anesthesia (TIVA) technique, even when profound muscle relaxation is not required for the operation. When use of a muscle relaxant is part of the technique, the patient's trachea is always intubated and controlled ventilation is instituted. The choice of agent is usually governed by the duration of the operation. When duration of the operation is to be less than half an hour, succinylcholine given intermittently or as a continuous infusion or mivacurium can be given. When duration of the operation is to be well under an hour, atracurium, vecuronium, or rocuronium given when necessary is suitable. When duration of the operation is to be an hour or longer, intermittent doses of d-tubocurarine, metocurine, alcuronium, or pancuronium are more appropriate. In addition to muscle relaxant, nitrous oxide and oxygen, together with a volatile anesthetic and a narcotic analgesic, should be given to maintain unconsciousness and analgesia. Alternatively, a continuous infusion of propofol can replace the volatile anesthetic for maintenance in the TIVA technique.

It is important to avoid hypoventilation and hyperventilation during controlled ventilation. This can usually be achieved by using a fresh gas flow and ventilatory volume recommended for the anesthetic circuit being used (see Chapter 8).

Controlled ventilation also can be achieved without muscle relaxants by using a volatile agent that has good muscle-relaxant properties to supplement nitrous oxide. With the availability of the relatively insoluble agents enflurane and isoflurane and the insoluble agents desflurane and sevoflurane, use of this technique has become popular in cases when controlled ventilation is indicated but profound muscle relaxation is not required.

■ Emergence from Anesthesia

At the conclusion of the anesthetic, the patient is allowed to emerge from the stage of surgical anesthesia. The emergence phase is different for patients who are breathing spontaneously and for those whose ventilation is controlled.

The patient who is breathing spontaneously will emerge from surgical anesthesia as soon as administration of nitrous oxide and volatile agent is discontinued. If intubation was performed, the endotracheal tube can be removed, with the precautions previously described (see "Extubation" in Chapter 13). Extubation can be done either while the patient is still in the plane of surgical anesthesia or after protective laryngeal reflex has returned. (If aspiration of stomach contents, blood, debris, or pus is a potential complication, extubation should always be delayed until gag and cough reflex have returned.) If extubation is done at the plane of surgical anesthesia, the patient will probably require assistance in maintaining a patent airway (see "Airway Obstruction" in Chapter 16) and should be turned to a lateral position to prevent aspiration. If extubation is done after laryngeal reflex has been regained, a phase of breath holding and coughing (which is to be avoided after procedures such as intraocular and intracranial surgery) is likely. Because extubation while the patient is in a semiconscious state can result in laryngospasm, it should be avoided.

During emergence, the patient who has received succinylcholine should be allowed to recover from muscle paralysis spontaneously; the patient who has received a nondepolarizing muscle relaxant should be given an anticholinesterase together with an anticholinergic agent (e.g., neostigmine, 2.5 mg, and atropine, 1.2 mg). As soon as neuromuscular function returns and ventilation is adequate, the patient should be allowed to emerge, as described above. It is recommended that a peripheral nerve stimulator be used to monitor neuromuscular function at this stage (see "Peripheral Nerve Stimulation" in Chapter 14). It is important not to let the patient regain consciousness before adequate recovery of neuromuscular function. The experience of being awake but half-paralyzed is unpleasant.

A potential complication in all patients during emergence is diffusion hypoxia, resulting from dilution of alveolar oxygen content by the large amount of nitrous oxide leaving pulmonary capillary blood during this phase. It can be prevented by having the patient breathe pure oxygen at high flow for at least 2 minutes before being allowed to breathe room air. The risk is also minimized if care is exercised to avoid hypoventilation and airway obstruction during this period.

At the end of the operation, the patient should be admitted to a postanesthesia recovery area for continuing observation and care. The recovery phase of anesthesia begins with admission of the patient to this area, and emergence continues into this phase. The management of the patient during recovery is discussed in Chapter 18.

Management of Complications during Anesthesia

16

There are several complications that are common or important during the course of general anesthesia. Some are due to an inappropriate level of anesthesia, others are part of the side effects of anesthetic drugs, and still others are complications of pre-existing illnesses. As long as the patient is under his or her care, the anesthesiologist must be prepared to cope with these events without delay.

Respiratory Complications

Hypoxemia, with or without hypercapnia, is a consequence of all respiratory complications. Even a mild degree of hypoxemia has the potential to cause harm. Cyanosis is a late sign of impaired oxygenation seen only when more than 5 g of deoxyhemoglobin is present in each 100 ml of arterial blood. Poor lighting and increased skin pigmentation can make cyanosis even harder to detect. Observing the color of blood in the operation site instead of color of skin, although more sensitive, is a haphazard method of detecting arterial desaturation. Monitoring by pulse oximetry is by far the most reliable. In order to prevent hypoxemia, inspired oxygen concentration should always be increased when respiratory complications develop in a patient under anesthesia.

Coughing

Coughing is a protective reflex in response to irritants in the airway. It is a complication seen at light levels of anesthesia. Irritation may be caused by the vapor of a volatile agent, the

223

pharyngeal airway, saliva or mucus, or even gastric contents. Treatment should be directed at removing the irritant. The concentration of volatile agents should be increased only gradually during induction, a pharyngeal airway should be inserted only when the level of anesthesia is appropriate, and fluid contents in the pharynx should be cleared by suction. If gastric fluid is suspected, tracheal intubation is indicated, and the patient should be examined for signs of aspiration (see also "Aspiration of Gastric Contents" below).

Breath Holding

Breath holding is seen not infrequently during inhalation induction. It may also be seen in patients who are breathing spontaneously during maintenance. During inhalation induction, breath holding is a transient phenomenon. During maintenance, breath holding, with or without laryngospasm, can occur when a painful stimulus is applied and the level of anesthesia is inadequate. Spontaneous respiration will return when the painful stimulus is withdrawn, but surgery should not be allowed to proceed until depth of anesthesia is increased. If breath holding persists, attempts should be made to ventilate the lungs manually, but care should be exercised not to inflate the stomach with overzealous efforts. Manual ventilation is not a problem when an endotracheal tube is in place and it is usually successful with a face mask or laryngeal mask if laryngospasm is absent. The management of breath holding with laryngospasm is discussed later in this chapter.

Airway Obstruction

The most common cause of airway obstruction in an unconscious patient lying supine is the tongue falling backward to lie on the posterior pharyngeal wall. In addition to signs of airway obstruction discussed earlier (see "Clinical Signs" under "Monitoring Respiratory Function" in Chapter 14), snoring occurs during inspiration and grunting during expiration. This problem is easily corrected by flexing the neck, extending the head, and supporting the angles of the jaw. In some cases placement of a pharyngeal airway, either oral or nasal, may be necessary (see also "Head-Tilt–Jaw Thrust Maneuver" and "Pharyngeal Airways" in Chapter 13). If improvement does not follow, tracheal intubation is indicated.

Kinking or compression of the endotracheal tube can cause airway obstruction in the intubated patient. Presence of a kinked or compressed segment can be checked by direct inspection or digital exploration. It is confirmed if a well-lubricated suction catheter threaded down the lumen of the endotracheal tube fails to reach beyond the tip of the tube. Correction of the defect is usually simple, but reintubation with a new endotracheal tube may be necessary. Using reinforced tubes can eliminate this problem.

Obstruction of the distal lumen of the endotracheal tube by a herniated cuff is a rarer cause of airway obstruction in intubated patients. This problem should be suspected if a suction catheter cannot be passed beyond the end of the tube (see above). Deflating the cuff should resolve the problem.

Laryngospasm

Laryngospasm is a serious complication when the patient is breathing spontaneously via a face mask and pharyngeal airway combination or laryngeal mask airway. Normally the vocal cords move apart on inspiration. During laryngospasm the cords are fixed in apposition, resulting in respiratory obstruction. If laryngospasm is only partial, stridor is heard during inspiration; in addition, exaggerated activities of the diaphragm, in-drawing, tracheal tug, and paradoxical movements of the abdomen and chest wall may be noted. If laryngospasm is complete, no stridor is heard. If laryngospasm and breath holding are both present, there is neither respiratory movement nor stridor. Like coughing, laryngospasm may be precipitated by irritation of the airway. It may also be caused by surgical stimulation applied at a light level of anesthesia.

Prolonged spasm can result in asphyxiation. Treatment should be directed at removing irritation or withholding stimulation, improving ventilation and oxygenation, and increasing the depth of anesthesia. If laryngospasm is only partial, assisted ventilation is usually successful; the spasm resolves spontaneously when depth of anesthesia is increased. When laryngospasm is complete, vigorous attempts at assisted ventilation only inflate the stomach and so should be avoided. When laryngospasm persists and attempts at assisted ventilation fail, 10–20 mg of succinylcholine should be given intravenously. This small dose is enough to relax the intrinsic muscles of the larynx. When the cords are paralyzed, manual ventilation should be instituted, and tracheal intubation may be indicated.

Hypoventilation

There are many reasons for hypoventilation during anesthesia, including respiratory depression by anesthetic drugs, inadequate recovery from muscle relaxants, and airway obstruction. The consequence of hypoventilation is carbon dioxide retention and hypercapnia. Hypercapnia can coexist with hypoxemia, but it also can exist alone if high inspired oxygen concentration is administered. An elevated $ETCO_2$ by capnography is the more reliable sign of inadequate ventilation, but certain clinical signs are also helpful: warm, flushed, and moist skin; tachycardia and hypertension; and increased oozing in the surgical field. In addition, careful observation may detect other clinical signs associated with the underlying cause of hypoventilation (e.g., apnea following intravenous barbiturates, shallow breaths in patients receiving a volatile agent, slow respiratory rate in patients receiving an opioid, signs of partial paralysis, and signs of airway obstruction).

Severe hypoventilation is a potentially fatal emergency. The patient who is hypoventilating should be given ventilatory assistance immediately, and the inspired atmosphere should be enriched with oxygen. When the emergency is brought under control, definitive treatment should be directed at eliminating the precipitating cause. Sometimes it is more appropriate to assist or control ventilation until the end of the operation, when the patient's ability to maintain adequate tidal exchange can be reassessed. In severe illness, sensitivity to the effects of anesthetics, opioids, or muscle relaxants may be increased and ventilatory support may be needed well into the postoperative period.

Bronchospasm

Many anesthetic agents (e.g., thiopental, morphine, *d*-tubocurarine) can release histamine from mast cells and trigger the onset of bronchospasm in patients with asthma or bronchitis. Both ketamine and halothane have bronchodilating properties and are agents of choice in these patients. Halothane is also useful in the treatment of mild bronchospasm, but intravenous aminophylline and nebulization of salbutamol into the airway are indicated if the attack is severe.

Bronchospasm can also be precipitated in lightly anesthetized patients by noxious stimuli (e.g., tracheal intubation). The spasm will subside if depth of anesthesia is increased. Halothane is again a useful agent for this purpose.

Aspiration of gastric contents may be the cause of bronchospasm that develops when the patient is under anesthesia. Aspiration may go unrecognized at the time of the incident. When it is diagnosed, prompt attention is crucial (see "Aspiration of Gastric Contents" below).

▨ Circulatory Complications

Hypotension

It is not uncommon to see blood pressure fall by 10–15% following induction of anesthesia in healthy persons; also it is not unusual for anesthetized patients with cardiovascular disease (e.g., atherosclerosis or hypertension) to have markedly lower pressures during periods when they receive little surgical stimulation. In addition, many other factors can cause hypotension during the course of an operation: circulatory depression by anesthetic agents, hypovolemia, interference with venous return or cardiac output by surgical packings and retractors, cardiac arrhythmias, acute myocardial infarction, underlying organic heart disease, and anesthetic accidents (e.g., hypoxemia, excessive airway pressure, tension pneumothorax, and transfusion of mismatched blood). Perfusion of the brain, heart, kidneys, and liver is reduced during profound hypotension. The absolute lower limit of blood pressure required to maintain perfusion of these organs varies according to the patient's physical status and health. In general, a fall in blood pressure greater than 20% should be investigated and treated accordingly.

In the face of severe hypotension, decisive actions are called for. Inspired oxygen concentration should be increased immediately, and specific treatment should be directed at elimination of the underlying cause: decreasing the depth of anesthesia if possible, replacing volume deficit, rectifying mechanical interference of venous return or cardiac output, treating cardiac arrhythmias, ruling out acute myocardial infarction, draining a pneumothorax, and treating mismatched transfusion. For severe myocardial disease, circulatory support with an inotropic agent is indicated (e.g., dopamine, 5–50 μg/kg/min, or dobutamine, 2.5–40 μg/kg/min).

Hypertension

Hypertension during anesthesia is as common as hypotension. It usually occurs as a response to noxious stimuli (e.g., tracheal intubation and traction on visceral organs) and is a sign of inadequate anesthesia. Other causes of intraoperative hypertension include hypercapnia and hypoxemia, pre-existing arterial hypertension, fluid overload, and undiagnosed and untreated pheochromocytoma.

The pressor response to tracheal intubation is preventable by increasing the depth of anesthesia, although this may not be appropriate in ill patients. An alternative is to apply lidocaine to the pharynx, larynx, and trachea before intubation or to administer lidocaine, 1.5 mg/kg, 1.5–3 minutes before the procedure is attempted. The rise in blood pressure is also minimal if intubation is done gently, skillfully, and swiftly.

Hypertension in response to surgical stimulation should be treated either by increasing the concentration of the volatile agent or by an additional dose of an opioid. Patients with cardiovascular disease are prone not only to have low blood pressure during periods when stimulation is minimal but also to react to stimulation with a marked increase in blood pressure. Depth of anesthesia should be carefully monitored in these patients. As described earlier, hypertension may be secondary to hypercapnia or hypoxemia and should be treated accordingly.

Arrhythmias

The incidence of cardiac arrhythmias during anesthesia is extremely high, even in patients without organic heart disease. Arrhythmias may be precipitated by anesthetic agents in use or by manipulation during anesthetic and surgical procedures. Fortunately, most of these disturbances are benign.

Sinus tachycardia following administration of atropine, pancuronium, gallamine, or ketamine is benign in patients without organic heart disease and requires no treatment. Sinus tachycardia in response to tracheal intubation or surgical stimulation is a sign of inadequate anesthesia and will disappear when depth of anesthesia is increased. Hypoxemia, hypercapnia, or hypovolemia can also cause sinus tachycardia and should be corrected promptly.

Atrial flutter or fibrillation is rare but always serious. The abnormality may be precipitated by manipulation of the heart during thoracic operations, particularly in geriatric patients and those with organic heart disease. In the operating room, atrial flutter or fibrillation of acute onset should be treated by direct-current cardioversion. If this is unsuccessful, digitalization may be necessary to control the ventricular rate.

A *lower-than-normal heart rate* is common in patients receiving halothane or large doses of morphine or fentanyl and its congeners for maintenance. Treatment with atropine is not necessary unless there is a concurrent fall in blood pressure. However, profound bradycardia and transient asystole require immediate attention. These disturbances are frequently associated with repeated doses of succinylcholine or traction on extraocular muscles. They can be prevented or treated with atropine, 0.6 mg, given intravenously.

A *slow nodal rhythm*, another common complication in patients receiving halothane for maintenance, is usually benign. However, sequential atrioventricular contractions can account for as much as 25% of stroke volume in a small number of patients. If nodal bradycardia causes hypotension, it should be treated with atropine.

A third rhythm disturbance often found in patients receiving halothane is *ventricular premature beats*. They are particularly common if hypercapnia is allowed to develop or if epinephrine is used to infiltrate the surgical field. Ventricular arrhythmias caused by interaction of halothane and hypercapnia will disappear if P_aCO_2 is returned to normal by increasing ventilation. Arrhythmias caused by interaction of halothane and epinephrine, in contrast, can be bizarre and alarming. The dose of epinephrine used to infiltrate the operative site should be limited to 10 ml of 1:100,000 concentration in 10 minutes or 30 ml in 1 hour. Lidocaine, 1 mg/kg or 30 μg/kg/min, may be necessary to treat ventricular premature beats that are frequent (more than five per minute), those that come in runs of three or more, those that are multifocal in origin, and those that fall on the T wave of the preceding beat.

Patients who have organic heart disease, hypokalemia, or acidemia are more prone to develop serious arrhythmias during anesthesia. In these patients, careful evaluation should be carried out and the abnormalities should be treated in the preoperative period.

▀ Aspiration of Gastric Contents

Aspiration of gastric contents is a potentially fatal complication of anesthesia. Patients who are at risk include those who have bowel obstruction, acute abdomen, or disease of the stomach or esophagus; those who are pregnant or obese; those who have sustained severe injuries; and those who require emergency operations. The consequences of aspiration vary according to the physical characteristics of the inhaled material. Solids, by obstructing the tracheobronchial tree, cause atelectasis. Gastric juice with a pH of less than 2.5 will cause acid pneumonitis (Mendelson's syndrome). Clinical signs of acid pneumonitis are cyanosis, tachycardia, tachypnea, rales, and rhonchi. In a florid case, signs of pulmonary edema and circulatory collapse may be seen. Whereas clinical signs of atelectasis are usually obvious immediately following aspiration of solids, those of acid pneumonitis may be delayed for several hours.

Aspiration pneumonitis is a preventable complication. In patients predisposed to regurgitation, the airway should be protected with a cuffed endotracheal tube. Use of the rapid-sequence induction technique and delay of extubation until return of laryngeal reflex are advised in these patients. Should aspiration occur, solids should be removed by bronchoscopy and liquids by postural drainage and tracheobronchial toilet. Some degree of pneumonitis occurs after any acid aspiration. The sequelae of a minor episode are usually mild and require only symptomatic treatment, but pulmonary edema and severe hypoxemia resulting from massive aspiration require intensive therapy.

The most effective means of improving arterial oxygenation following massive aspiration is to control ventilation and to apply PEEP. The level of PEEP should be adjusted to yield the best oxygenation without decreasing blood pressure or cardiac output. Because a large portion of the circulating volume may be lost as pulmonary edema fluid, aggressive replacement is indicated. Continuous measurement of arterial and central venous or pulmonary capillary wedge pressure, as well as intermittent sampling of arterial blood for blood gas analysis, is necessary to guide therapy. With optimal supportive care, the disease process is self-limiting and recovery is spontaneous. There is litle indication that steroids will alter the course of acid pneumonitis. However, antibiotics should be used when there is evidence of secondary bacterial infection.

■ Anaphylactic and Anaphylactoid Reactions

In anesthesia practice, the incidence of "allergic" reactions is as high as 1 in 4000 anesthetic procedures. Depending on whether an immunologic mechanism is involved, two separate entities can be identified.

Anaphylactic reaction (anaphylactic shock or anaphylaxis) is an immune reaction in which an antigen (a foreign substance such as an intravenous anesthetic) combines with immunoglobulin antibodies located on the surfaces of mast cells or basophils. This antigen-antibody complex activates these cells to release histamine, leukotrienes (formerly called slow-reacting substance of anaphylaxis), prostaglandins, and kinins—all of which can cause bronchoconstriction, vasodilation, and increase in capillary permeability. The hallmark of anaphylaxis is previous exposure to the antigenic foreign substance and sensitization to that substance. Cross-sensitization can occur from a different substance that has a structure similar to that of the antigen.

Anaphylactoid reaction, in contrast, is one in which a foreign substance (e.g., an intravenous anesthetic) activates mast cells by an ill-understood non−immunologically mediated mechanism to release histamine. No previous sensitization is necessary. Anaphylactoid reaction also differs from anaphylactic reaction in that only mast cells are involved and only histamine is released. Yet the clinical manifestations of both are similar. They include urticaria, facial and laryngeal edema, laryngo-spasm, bronchospasm, tachycardia, and hypotension. Death is usually attributable to respiratory failure or cardiovascular collapse; the morbidity rate is as high as 3−4%.

Many anesthetic drugs can precipitate an anaphylactic or anyphylactoid reaction, or both. They include

Intravenous anesthetics	Barbiturates, etomidate, propofol
Muscle relaxants	Succinylcholine, d-tubocurarine, gallamine, metocurine, pancuronium, atracurium, vecuronium, mivacurium, doxacurium
Opioids	Codeine, meperidine, morphine, fentanyl
Local anesthetics	Procaine, (?) other aminoesters

In recent years, latex rubber allergy has become common-place. Because ordinary surgical gloves, syringes, intravenous cannulas, intravenous solution containers and delivery sets, an-esthetic machines and accessories, masks, and ventilators have rubber components, the possibility of these components causing a reaction should not be overlooked.

Anaphylatic and anaphylactoid reactions can occur within minutes of an injection of the offending antigen, although re-action to latex rubber is often delayed. It is impossible to differentiate the two types of reaction on clinical grounds, but the treatment of both is the same:

1. Discontinue administration of the offending agent if it is known. Switch all anesthetic drugs to agents in a different class if the offending agent is unknown. Switch to glass syringes and equipment using plastic rather than rubber components if latex rubber allergy is suspected.

2. Inform the surgeon and request that the operation be concluded as soon as possible.

3. Administer oxygen supplement by face mask if there is no sign of upper airway obstruction (from laryngospasm or edema); intubate the trachea and control ventilation if there is.

4. Administer epinephrine intravenously in 50 to 100 μg increments to correct hypotension. Start an infusion at 0.05 μg/kg/min and titrate the rate to blood pressure. Treat as cardiac arrest and institute advanced cardiac life support if hypotension is profound. (Epinephrine is the mainstay in the treatment of anaphylactic/anaphylactoid reaction. Its alpha action causes vasoconstriction; its beta$_1$ action improves myocardial contractility; and its beta$_2$ action relieves bronchospasm and inhibits the release of broncho- and vasoactive substances by mast cells and basophils.)

5. Give 20 ml/kg of normal saline or lactated Ringer's solution intravenously quickly and assess volume status by checking jugular venous filling or central venous pressure. Give incremental boluses of crystalloid if indicated. (Large volumes of fluid can be lost into the interstitial space because of increase in capillary permeability. Epinephrine together with aggressive volume expansion is the best way to treat hypotension.)

6. Give diphenhydramine, 50 mg, and cimetidine, 300 mg, intravenously. (Diphenhydramine and cimetidine are H_1 and H_2 histamine antagonists, respectively. Ranitidine, 50 mg, may be used in place of cimetidine. Antihistamines do not inhibit the release of histamine by mast cells or basophils and cannot reverse an ongoing anaphylactic or anaphylactoid reaction, but they can block the effects of released histamine at receptor sites.)

7. Give hydrocortisone, 250 mg, intravenously every 6 hours for 24 hours. (Hydrocortisone may be substituted with methylprednisolone, 125 mg. The place for a glucocorticoid is ill-defined. It may take 6–12 hours to work and prevents relapses seen in the late phase of some reactions.)

In addition to the above steps, the following second-line measures should be considered:

8. Give salbutamol, 0.5 ml, or metaproterenol, 0.3 ml, in 2.5 ml of normal saline by inhalation to treat bronchospasm. Alternatively, nebulize these agents directly into the airway if the patient is intubated.

9. Give aminophylline, 6 mg/kg, intravenously over 20 minutes as a loading dose to be followed by an infusion of 0.5 mg/kg/hr. (Aminophylline, a phosphodiesterase inhibitor with beta-like actions, can by itself improve cardiac contractility, relieve bronchospasm, and inhibit the release of broncho- and vasoactive mediators by mast cells or basophils. It can also potentiate the action of epinephrine.)

10. Give glucagon, 5–10 mg, intravenously and start an infusion at 1–5 mg/hr, which can be adjusted according to blood pressure. (Glucagon has inotropic and chronotropic effects even in the presence of beta-adrenergic blockade. It has a special place in the treatment of hypotension in patients who are on beta-adrenergic antagonists.)

11. Give sodium bicarbonate, 50 mEq, to correct metabolic acidosis and additional doses according to the formula described under "Acid-Base Abnormalities" in Chapter 21.

Anaphylactic and anaphylactoid reactions are critical events that demand prompt actions. If response to treatment is not immediately favorable, direct arterial blood pressure measurement and monitoring of central venous pressure are indicated. If these reactions are refractory to treatment, measurement of pulmonary artery pressures should be considered. All patients should have an indwelling catheter to monitor urine flow. Blood samples for laboratory analysis to guide the treatment of acid-base and electrolyte abnormalities are indicated.

Malignant Hyperthermia

Malignant hyperthermia is caused by a rare skeletal muscle disease. The victims, usually children or young adults, are prone to develop life-threatening hyperpyrexia under anesthesia. There appears to be a large regional variation in the prevalence of this disease; incidence of malignant hyperthermic crisis has been reported to be as high as 1 in 20,000 anesthetic procedures and as low as 1 in 100,000. The syndrome is characterized by a hypermetabolic, hyperthermic state precipitated by succinylcholine and volatile anesthetics, and occasionally by physical or emotional stress. The pathologic mechanism is believed to be initiated by loss of control over calcium ion sequestration and reuptake in skeletal muscle fibers, leading to contracture, increase in oxygen consumption, and increase in lactate and heat production.

Pedigrees of affected persons suggest that the trait is inherited in an autosomal dominant pattern with reduced penetrance and variable expressivity. In 3–5% of victims, a defect has been traced to chromosome 19 at a locus close to the gene responsible for the skeletal muscle ryanodine receptor. In others, the abnormality has been traced to chromosome 17. Many patients who have the malignant hyperthermia trait have abnormal muscle morphology (excessive bulk), other skeletal muscle abnormalities (e.g., strabismus, inguinal hernia, clubfoot), cardiomyopathy, or elevated serum creatine kinase. All patients who are first-degree relatives of a person known to have had malignant hyperthermia or to have tested positive should be regarded as potential victims until proven otherwise, as should all members of an affected family who have skeletal muscle abnormalities or elevated serum creatine kinase.

Contrary to previous belief, masseter muscle spasm, which occurs in 1% of children given succinylcholine against a background of halothane anesthesia, is not necessarily a sign of imminent hyperthermic crisis. A full spectrum of increase in masseter muscle tension can occur in normal subjects, varying from simply tight to solidly rigid. The approach to patients who develop masseter muscle spasm following succinylcholine should be

1. If masseter muscle spasm occurs in isolation and can be overcome with effort, it is safe to continue with anesthesia and surgery, albeit increased vigilance is required. It is also prudent to switch to nontriggering agents.

2. If masseter muscle spasm occurs in conjunction with other muscle rigidity or if spasm cannot be overcome with effort, a crisis may be in the offing and should be treated accordingly.

Muscle biopsy and determination in vitro of contracture response to caffeine and halothane is the only reliable diagnostic test for malignant hyperthermia to date. Serum creatine kinase level has no diagnostic value as a screening test in the general population, nor does a normal serum creatine kinase level rule out susceptibility in members of a family known to have malignant hyperthermia. However, elevated values in members of an affected family demand further investigation. Halothane-induced depletion of platelet adenosine triphosphate and calcium uptake by muscle strips have been suggested also as diagnostic tests but have been found to be unreliable. Other noninvasive tests are under investigation, including measurement of ankle torque and its modification by dantrolene, halothane-induced changes in ionized calcium within lymphocytes, and phosphorus nuclear magnetic resonance spectroscopy. Results are still pending.

Whether patients suspected to have the malignant hyperthermia trait should receive dantrolene for prophylaxis is a matter of conjecture. If it is used, the dose is 2 mg/kg intravenously given before induction of anesthesia for best effects. In addition, these patients should not be exposed to agents that can trigger a crisis, including all volatile agents and succinylcholine. Because only a trace of volatile anesthetic can precipitate an attack, an anesthetic machine without a vaporizer that is reserved for this purpose should be employed. A machine that has been purged for several hours with oxygen *after its vaporizers have been removed* is also suitable. There is evidence to suggest that purging the machine with high flows of oxygen for several minutes is sufficient. Similarly, an uncontaminated fresh gas hose, anesthetic circuit, mask and ventilator bellows, and fresh carbon dioxide absorption canister should be used.

Because inappropriate hypercapnia and hypoxemia are early signs, the capnograph and pulse oximeter have been recognized as the best monitors to give early warning of an impending crisis. Other signs of an attack include tachycardia, tachypnea, ventricular arrhythmia, muscle rigidity, cyanosis, mottled skin, profuse sweating, inappropriate increase in body temperature (as much as 1° C every 5 minutes), arterial and mixed venous desaturation, respiratory and metabolic acidosis, electrolyte abnormalities, myoglobinemia, myoglobinuria, and elevated serum creatine kinase. Late complications include disseminated intravascular coagulation, renal failure, muscle necrosis, and coma.

The mortality rate following an acute crisis is 10%. Successful treatment depends on early recognition and intensive therapy. The onset of a crisis requires immediate institution of the following measures:

1. Stop administration of all offending agents. Maintain anesthesia with intravenous anesthetics if necessary.

2. Inform the surgeon and request that the operation be concluded as soon as possible.

3. Call for help to obtain central venous access, to cannulate an artery for blood samples and pressure monitoring, and to introduce an indwelling urinary catheter.

4. Hyperventilate the patient with 100% oxygen at a high flow rate.

5. Administer dantrolene, 2–3 mg/kg, intravenously in a bolus. Repeat the dose if necessary until the total dose is 10 mg/kg. (Dantrolene can abort a crisis; the dose of 10 mg/kg may have to be exceeded if the crisis is fulminant. Treatment with dantrolene, 1–2 mg/kg every 6 hours, should be continued for 1–3 days after the crisis is arrested.)

6. Cool the patient if body temperature is 39° C or above by using ice packs on the body surface and irrigating body cavities with ice-cold saline. Stop the process once body temperature has fallen to 38° C. (Continued cooling can cause hypothermia. Remember, dantrolene is the mainstay of treatment. Elevated body temperature will subside as dantrolene takes effect.)

7. Give sodium bicarbonate, 2–4 mEq/kg, initially to correct metabolic acidosis. If pH remains below 7.2, give more according to the result of blood gas analysis as described under "Acid-Base Abnormalities" in Chapter 21. (Sodium bicarbonate reacts with hydrogen ions to release more carbon dioxide and can cause hypernatremia and hyperosmolarity. The current trend is to use sodium bicarbonate more conservatively than was previously recommended. Remember that hyperventilation can increase pH to some extent by inducing respiratory alkalosis.)

8. Treat hyperkalemia with a glucose-insulin infusion of 10 units of regular insulin in 50 ml of 50% dextrose and give it by titration according to serum potassium level. Be prepared to give potassium chloride intravenously at a later stage if hypokalemia develops. (Potassium leaking out of skeletal muscle cells during the initial stage of a crisis can cause cardiac standstill. Correction of respiratory and metabolic acidosis will also help to reverse hyperkalemia. Although the use of calcium chloride in malignant hyperthermia is controversial, 2–4 mg/kg may be given to counteract life-threatening hyperkalemia. As the crisis subsides and diuresis is induced, hyperkalemia can give way to hypokalemia. Potassium replacement should be undertaken cautiously because potassium chloride itself can trigger a crisis. Therapy should be guided by frequent measurements of serum electrolyte concentrations.)

9. Treat sinus tachycardia with propranolol and ventricular arrhythmias with procainamide. (Procainamide, 15 mg/kg,

given intravenously can abort an attack. Unfortunately, it also can cause cardiotoxicity and hypotension. The use of calcium channel blockers is contraindicated because verapamil has been shown to cause hyperkalemia and cardiovascular collapse in the presence of dantrolene.)

10. Induce diuresis when indicated. (Dantrolene preparation contains 3 g of mannitol per 20-mg vial, which is enough to induce a moderate degree of osmotic diuresis. If the patient is hypernatremic or if hyperkalemia persists, furosemide should be given intravenously to increase urinary excretion of sodium and potassium.)

In the event of a crisis, time is crucial in aborting an attack. Therefore, all drugs and equipment mentioned above should be readily available before a potential victim is anesthetized. (At least thirty-six 20-mg vials of dantrolene should be available on site in institutions in which anesthesia is practiced.)

Techniques of Local and Regional Anesthesia

17

In skilled hands, local and regional techniques provide excellent anesthesia for many surgical procedures. Although the systemic actions of local and general anesthetic agents are different, patients merit the same attention whether they are scheduled for local or for general anesthesia. General preoperative assessment should be performed, and it is also important to establish that these patients are willing subjects, that they do not have a history of bleeding diathesis, and that there is no infection at the site of injection. Pre-existing neurologic deficits should be regarded as a relative contraindication to nerve blocks and spinal or epidural anesthesia. Because most patients are anxious about being awake during the operation, an anxiolytic agent should be included in the premedication. In the operating room, a freely running intravenous infusion should be established, and equipment for resuscitation should be checked before major blocks are attempted. During the entire course of the operation, vital functions should be monitored.

Introduction of pathogenic organisms via the needle is always a potential danger with all regional techniques. Therefore, major regional blocks should be attempted only in a sterile setting: long hair at the site of injection should be shaved off, the site of needle entry should be cleansed and draped; the anesthesiologist should wear cap, mask and gloves; and sterile equipment should be used. Because injection of the anesthetic solution into an intravascular space is a potential complication, thorough aspiration before injection is mandatory. In the sections that follow, some common techniques of local and regional anesthesia using lidocaine as an example are described. (Equivalent doses for other local anesthetic agents appear in Chapter 6.) Unless otherwise specified, use of a 22-gauge needle is appropriate in the following procedures.

Local Infiltration

Local infiltration is suitable for suturing superficial wounds and excising cutaneous or subcutaneous lesions. Epinephrine may be added to prolong the action of the anesthetic agent in this technique, but its concentration must be limited to 1:200,000 because necrosis of skin edges is a potential complication.

The technique of local infiltration is as follows:

1. Pierce the skin with the needle and raise a wheal by injecting a small amount of 0.5% lidocaine.

2. Advance the needle to deposit most lidocaine on either side of and beneath the lesion (Fig. 17–1A).

3. Make subsequent entries with the needle at sites already anesthetized, and deposit more lidocaine solution until the lesion is encircled.

Digital Nerve Block

Each finger or toe is supplied by two dorsal and two palmar digital nerves alongside the digit. A digital nerve block is satisfactory for simple operations such as suturing wounds and

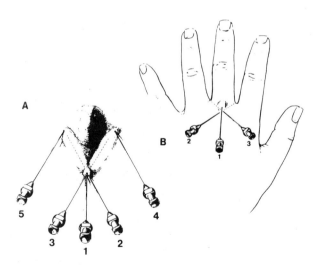

FIGURE 17–1. Technique of local and regional anesthesia. *A*, Local infiltration, *B*, Digital nerve block.

excising nails. The technique of digital nerve block is as follows:

1. Approach the digital nerves from the dorsal aspect of the hand or foot.
2. Raise a skin wheal close to the base of the digit (see Fig. 17–1B).
3. Advance the needle to deposit 1–1.5 ml of 1.5% lidocaine without epinephrine on both sides of the digit.

Injection of a large volume of anesthetic solution and addition of a vasoconstrictor should be avoided in this technique. Both can compromise the circulation of the digit, either by mechanical compression or by constriction of the digital arteries.

■ Infiltration of Fracture Hematoma

Both the periosteum and soft tissue at the site of a fracture can be anesthetized adequately by infiltrating the fracture hematoma. The technique is both simple and safe, and onset of anesthesia is usually obvious within 5 minutes. The technique is as follows:

1. Raise a skin wheal over the fracture site.
2. Advance the needle into the hematoma.
3. Verify the position of the needle by aspirating for blood.
4. Deposit 10–15 ml of 1.5% lidocaine with epinephrine in the hematoma. (The injection should be made slowly because rapid injection can cause pain.)

A major disadvantage of this technique is lack of muscle relaxation. It should be used only for closed reduction of simple fractures (e.g., Colles' fracture).

■ Intravenous Regional Anesthesia

Intravenous regional anesthesia is a simple technique that provides excellent anesthesia and muscle relaxation for operations on the extremities. The technique is as follows:

1. Cannulate a peripheral vein on the limb to be anesthetized with a plastic cannula.
2. Exsanguinate the limb by simple elevation or by using an Esmarch bandage. (Proper exsanguination of the limb reduces the volume of anesthetic solution required.)
3. Place an arterial tourniquet around the arm or thigh and inflate it to a pressure of 100 mm Hg above the patient's systolic pressure.

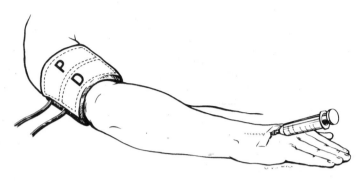

FIGURE 17–2. Intravenous regional anesthesia of the upper extremity using a double arterial tourniquet. The proximal cuff is *P* and the distal cuff *D*.

4. Inject 0.6 ml/kg of 0.5% lidocaine without epinephrine intravenously via the indwelling cannula for anesthesia in an upper extremity. Increase the volume to 1–1.2 ml/kg for a lower extremity.

5. Remove the venous cannual when anesthesia is established. (The onset of warmth and a tingling sensation should be immediate, and anesthesia should be complete within 15 minutes.)

A major limitation of this technique is the large dose of lidocaine required, particularly for the lower limbs. The arterial tourniquet should not be deflated for at least 15 minutes after injection of the local anesthetic solution; otherwise rapid uptake of lidocaine can cause systemic toxicity. Because sensation will return within 2–5 minutes following deflation of the tourniquet, a second limitation is restriction on the duration of the operation imposed by the maximum period of interrupted circulation considered safe (usually not more than 90 minutes). A third limitation is pain at the site of the tourniquet. Pain can be prevented by using the double-tourniquet technique (Fig. 17–2), in which anesthesia is induced with the proximal cuff inflated. When discomfort develops at the site of this cuff, the distal cuff is inflated and the proximal cuff is deflated, in that order. Because the distal cuff lies over an anesthetized area, tourniquet pain is minimized.

▨ Brachial Plexus Block

The brachial plexus arises from the anterior rami of spinal nerves C5–C8 and T1, with contributions from C4 and T2.

These segmental nerves join to form trunks, divisions, and cords that emerge between the scalenus anterior and scalenus medius to lie between the clavicle and the first rib, lateral and posterior to the subclavian artery. In the axilla and beyond, they divide to form the major nerves supplying the arm and the forearm. Together with the subclavian artery and vein, the plexus is ensheathed in connective tissue to form the neurovascular bundle. There are three different approaches to brachial plexus block. Whereas the interscalene approach is suitable for surgery on the shoulder and upper arm, the supraclavicular or axillary approach is more suitable for surgery on the forearm and hand.

The classical approach to locate major nerves and their branches is to seek paresthesia in the territory to be anesthetized with the exploring needle. This approach is associated with a potential risk of intraneural injection causing neuropathy. When this technique is used, a small test dose should be injected initially. If the patient complains of a cramp or an ache in the territory to be anesthetized, the position of the needle should be adjusted and the test injection repeated. The full dose should be given only if the test dose is not causing distress.

Another approach is to use a nerve stimulator in combination with an insulated needle. The nerve stimulator should be capable of generating a pulsatile current with these characteristics: an amplitude variable in steps between 0.1 and 10 mA, a pulse width of 200 ms, and a pulse frequency of 1 Hz. In this approach, the negative terminal should be connected to the insulated needle and the nerves to be anesthetized are located by seeking motor response in the territory supplied by these nerves. The general location of the nerves to be anesthetized can be identified initially with a current of 5 mA, but the current should be decreased in steps as the tip of the needle approaches the nerves. Injection should be made only at a site where a current of 0.5 mA or less is eliciting the desired motor response. However, injections at sites where a current of less than 0.3 mA is eliciting a response should be made with care because intraneural injection has also been reported in these instances.

Interscalene Approach

This approach blocks the brachial plexus near its roots. The technique is as follows:

1. Position the patient supine with the arm by the side and the head in a neutral position but turned to the opposite side.

2. Locate the interscalene groove between the anterior and middle scalene muscles at the level of the cricoid ring by palpating the neck and rolling the index and middle fingers of one

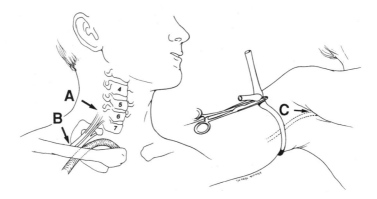

FIGURE 17–3. Brachial plexus blocks. *A*, Interscalene approach. *B*, Supraclavicular approach. *C*, Axillary approach.

hand posterolaterally off the lateral border of the sternocleidomastoid muscle, onto the anterior scalene muscle, and into the interscalene groove. (This can be made easier by asking the patient to raise his or her head off the table, tensing the sternocleidomastoid and scalene muscles.)

3. With the patient relaxed again, raise a skin wheal at this point and advance the needle perpendicular to the skin with the other hand, pointing it mediad (toward midline), slightly caudad (toward the patient's foot), and slightly posteriorly (toward the patient's back), as illustrated in Figure 17–3*A*. Locate the plexus either by seeking paresthesia or using a nerve stimulator. Redirect the needle without changing its angles in an anteroposterior plane if required.

4. Inject 30–35 ml of 1.5% lidocaine with epinephrine when the needle position is satisfactory.

Inadequate spread of lidocaine to involve the C8 and T1 roots can lead to inadequate anesthesia in the ulnar nerve territory. Potential complications of this approach include subarachnoid or epidural injection, neuropathy involving the C6 nerve root, injection into the vertebral artery, phrenic nerve block, and, rarely, pneumothorax.

Supraclavicular Approach

For brachial plexus block using the supraclavicular approach, anesthetic solution is deposited in the sheath of the neurovascular bundle as it crosses the first rib. The technique is as follows:

1. Position the patient supine with the arm by the side and the head turned to the opposite side.

2. Locate the subclavian artery and depress it with the index finger of one hand. (The artery can usually be located just behind the midpoint of the clavicle.)

3. Raise a skin wheal at this point with the other hand and advance the needle toward a site immediately behind the artery, pointing it in a caudad and slightly medial and posterior direction as illustrated in Figure 17−3B. Continue to advance the needle and locate the plexus by seeking parasthesia or using a nerve stimulator. If the needle touches the first rib without signs that it is in the neurovascular bundle, withdraw it partially and "walk" it across the first rib anteriorly or posteriorly until these signs are elicited.

4. Inject 20−25 ml of 1.5% lidocaine with epinephrine into the neurovascular sheath when the needle is satisfactorily positioned.

A serious complication of supraclavicular brachial plexus block is pneumothorax. This problem should be suspected if the patient coughs while the needle is being advanced, if air is aspirated during the procedure, or if the patient complains of respiratory distress. When the suspicion is confirmed, the patient's respiration and oxygenation should be monitored and the size of the pneumothorax assessed on chest films. A patient who has symptoms should be given oxygen by face mask. Drainage of the pleural space by a catheter connected to an underwater seal may be necessary. Owing to the proximity of the phrenic nerve, the recurrent laryngeal nerve, and the stellate ganglion, paralysis of these nerves and Horner's syndrome are occasional complications.

Axillary Approach

The axillary approach to the brachial plexus block offers little or no anesthesia on the lateral aspect of the arm, but it is an excellent technique for use in operations on the hand and forearm. The technique is as follows:

1. Position the patient supine with the arm abducted 90 degrees at the shoulder and the forearm flexed 90 degrees at the elbow.

2. Apply a venous tourniquet to the arm just beyond the axilla, as shown in Figure 17−3C. (In some patients, the musculocutaneous nerve leaves the lateral cord of the plexus high up in the axilla. The venous tourniquet helps to spread the anesthetic solution cephalad to include this nerve. Digital compression of the neurovascular sheath during injection is an alternative.)

3. Identify the axillary artery at the highest point in the axilla.

4. Raise a skin wheal at this point and advance the needle toward a site adjacent to the artery until a click is felt by the operator as the needle punctures the neurovascular sheath. (Either paresthesia or a nerve stimulator may be used to help in locating the plexus.)

5. Inject 30 ml of 1.5% lidocaine with epinephrine into this neurovascular space when the needle is satisfactorily positioned. Alternatively, inject 10 ml of the lidocaine solution into each of the four quadrants around the artery.

The axillary route is a popular approach because there is no risk of pneumothorax. However, the musculocutaneous nerve is often missed and the time of onset may be delayed for up to 30 minutes. Because a near-toxic dose of lidocaine is required, the risk of systemic toxicity is proportionally increased.

■ Spinal Anesthesia

The spinal cord extends down to the second lumbar vertebra (L2) and the dural sac to the second sacral vertebra (S2). Therefore, the subarachnoid space between L2 and S2 contains only cerebrospinal fluid and lumbar and sacral nerve roots (the cauda equina). Local anesthetic solution deposited in the lumbar subarachnoid space can travel caudad and cephalad to provide anesthesia for operations on the perineum, the external genitalia, the lower extremities, and abdominal organs.

Dural puncture for spinal anesthesia requires both care and skill. The technique is as follows:

1. Position the patient on the side with the spine flexed.

2. Identify the L3-4 interspace on an imaginary line joining both iliac crests.

3. Raise a skin wheal at the center of the interspace.

4. Advance the spinal needle with its stylet in place in a direction perpendicular to the skin but pointed slightly cephalad. (An introducer should be used to help direct 24-gauge or finer needles.) Note the changes in resistance to advancement of the needle as it traverses the subcutaneous tissue, supraspinous ligament, interspinous ligament, ligamentum flavum, epidural space, and dura (Fig. 17–4). (A click may be felt as the dura is pierced, and the patient may complain of paresthesia in the lower extremities at the same time).

In elderly patients with calcified ligaments, a paramedian approach to the subarachoid space may be easier. The technique is

1. Position the patient on the side with the spine flexed.
2. Identify the L3-4 interspace on an imaginary line joining both iliac crests.
3. Raise a skin wheal 1 fingerbreadth off the midline and infiltrate widely and deeply in a mediad and cephalad direction.
4. Advance the spinal needle with the stylet in place, pointing it medially at an angle of 10–15 degrees to the sagittal plane and slightly cephalad. (A click may be felt as the needle pierces the dura.)

The subarachnoid space is approximately 6 cm from the skin surface in a person of average build. If bone is encountered before the space is entered, the needle should be withdrawn, the landmarks redefined, and the needle redirected accordingly. Dural puncture at lower spaces may be successful when those at L3-4 fail. A clear flow of cerebrospinal fluid when the stylet is removed confirms that the tip of the needle is in the subarachnoid space. Persistent paresthesia and grossly bloody spinal fluid that does not clear are indications for readjusting the position of the needle. Local anesthetic should be injected only when there is free flow of clear spinal fluid. After deposition of the local anesthetic, the needle is withdrawn and the patient is turned carefully to the supine position with hips and knees flexed and head resting comfortably on a pillow. Onset of anesthesia is rapid and is preceded by a feeling of warmth in the lower extremities.

The agents most commonly used for spinal anesthesia are hyperbaric solutions (heavier than cerebrospinal fluid): 0.5%

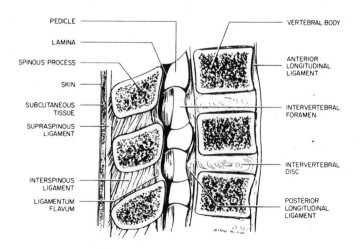

PEDICLE

LAMINA

SPINOUS PROCESS

SKIN

SUBCUTANEOUS TISSUE

SUPRASPINOUS LIGAMENT

INTERSPINOUS LIGAMENT

LIGAMENTUM FLAVUM

VERTEBRAL BODY

ANTERIOR LONGITUDINAL LIGAMENT

INTERVERTEBRAL FORAMEN

INTERVERTEBRAL DISC

POSTERIOR LONGITUDINAL LIGAMENT

FIGURE 17–4. Sagittal section of the spinal canal with its contents removed.

tetracaine in 5% dextrose 0.75% bupivacaine in 8.25% dextrose, and 5% lidocaine in 7.5% dextrose. The dose of local anesthetic is governed by the spinal level of anesthesia required for surgery. If tetracaine is used in a patient of average height, 5 mg is required for anal operations (anesthesia of sacral segments only), 10 mg for operations on external genitalia or lower extremities (anesthesia to T12), and 15 mg for intra-abdominal operations (anesthesia to T6). Each of these doses should be increased by 2 mg in taller than average patients. A similar dose guideline applies to hyperbaric 0.75% bupivacaine solution. If hyperbaric 5% lidocaine is used, the dose in milligrams described for tetracaine should be increased fivefold. The choice of agent depends on the duration of the surgical procedure. Whereas lidocaine is suitable for operations lasting up to 1 hour and bupivacaine up to 2 hours, tetracaine lasts for 3 hours.

Many factors other than dose can increase the number of spinal segments affected in spinal anesthesia using hyperbaric solutions, an important one being pregnancy. The aforementioned dose should be reduced by one quarter in parturients. Other factors include a large volume of anesthetic solution, increases in intra-abdominal pressure, head-down tilt of the patient, coughing or straining by the patient during or immediately following injection, injection at higher segmental levels, a rapid rate of injection, and barbotage (a technique in which cerebrospinal fluid is repeatedly drawn into the syringe during the course of injection to promote mixing).

The most common immediate complication seen following spinal anesthesia is a drop in blood pressure without increase in heart rate. Hypotention is usually mild in young adults but can be severe in parturients and geriatric patients. The cause of hypotension is loss of sympathetic tone. It can be prevented by giving a 1- to 1.5-liter bolus of lactated Ringer's solution or normal saline before the onset of anesthesia, and ephedrine in increments of 5 mg can be given intravenously when necessary. Profound hypotension and bradycardia together with loss of consciousness and apnea are signs of total spinal anesthesia. In addition to circulatory support, tracheal intubation and controlled ventilation with 100% oxygen are indicated. Recovery should be complete if action is taken promptly.

Sudden and unexpected cardiac arrest during spinal anesthesia has been reported recently, always in patients who have received sedation to supplement an otherwise uneventful spinal anesthetic. It is postulated that loss of sensory input following the onset of spinal anesthesia increases the sensitivity of these patients to sedatives. Unrecognized progressive hypoventilation and hypoxemia may have been the cause of these arrests.

Spinal headache (postdural puncture headache), occasionally accompanied by auditory and visual disturbances, is an unpleasant side effect of dural puncture. The headache is typically postural in nature—brought on by assuming the erect posture and relieved by lying supine. It is due to intracranial hypotension from leakage of cerebrospinal fluid. The incidence of headache is highest in women and least in geriatric patients, and it decreases with the size of the spinal needle used. Needle design also influences the incidence of spinal headache: with the needle size being equal, it is higher with the beveled Quincke needle (Fig. 17–5A) and lower with the pencil-point Sprotte (Fig. 17–5B) or Whitaker (Fig. 17–5C) needle.

Treatment of spinal headache should be directed at keeping the patient resting flat in bed, relieving headache with analgesics, and hydrating the patient with liberal fluid intake. Caffeine sodium benzoate, 500 mg, intravenously or caffeine, 300 mg, orally can relieve spinal headache in some patients, but its salutary effect may be transient. If headache is protracted, injection of 10–15 ml of autologous blood into the epidural space at the level of the original lumbar puncture to seal the dural leak is curative in over 90% of the patients. This procedure,

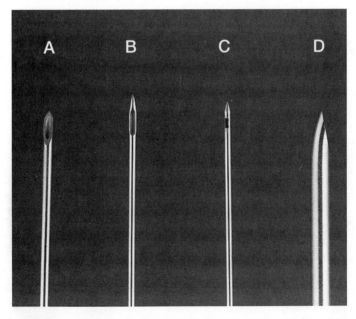

FIGURE 17–5. Spinal and epidural needles. *A*, A 22-gauge Quincke spinal needle with a beveled tip. *B*, A 24-gauge Sprotte spinal needle with a pencil-point tip. *C*, A 25-gauge Whitaker spinal needle with a pencil-point tip. *D*, Side view of a 17-gauge Tuohy needle. The directional bevel can be used to direct an epidural catheter cephalad or caudad.

known as autologous blood patch, has become an alternative to conservative therapy.

Radicular-like leg pain without neurologic deficit that lasts for up to 1 week has been reported following spinal anesthesia. It is limited to cases in which hyperbaric 5% lidocaine was used and may be due to sequestration of the concentrated lidocaine solution in the subarachnoid space. The current recommendation is to dilute the 5% solution with an equal volume of cerebrospinal fluid or normal saline before subarachnoid injection. Focal neurologic deficits following spinal anesthesia have also been reported occasionally. Fortunately, they are both minor and transient. The most dreaded, although rare, complication is adhesive arachnoiditis, characterized by nonspecific inflammation of the meninges and the spinal cord. The end result is paraplegia. There is no known treatment, only supportive care.

Spinal and epidural hematoma also are rare complications. They usually follow repeated traumatic attempts at lumbar puncture. Bacterial meningitis as a result of poor aseptic technique has also been reported. These complications are preventable.

■ Lumbar Epidural Anesthesia

The epidural space is a potential space outside the spinal dural sac. It extends from the foramen magnum to the sacrococcygeal membrane and is bounded by the posterior longitudinal ligament anteriorly, the ligamentum flavum posteriorly, and the vertebral laminae, vertebral pedicles, and intervertebral foramina laterally (Fig. 17–4). Local anesthetics deposited into this space can block neural transmission by diffusing intrathecally, by anesthetizing spinal nerve roots, and by blocking spinal nerves as they emerge from the intervertebral foramina.

Epidural anesthesia is suitable for intra-abdominal operations and for those on the perineum and the lower extremities. The most popular approach to the epidural space is the lumbar route using a 16- or 18-gauge Tuohy needle. Careful placement of the needle is essential. For better control of anesthetic dose and for repeat injections in long procedures, a thin catheter is threaded into the space via the Tuohy needle (Fig. 17–5D). The epidural space can be cannulated by the following method:

1. Position the patient in the lateral decubitus position with the spine well flexed.

2. Raise a skin wheal at an interspace between L2 and S1.

3. Advance the Tuohy needle with its stylet in place, as described for dural puncture. (The bevel of the needle can be pointed cephalad or caudad, depending on the direction the

catheter is to be fed. The paramedian approach described for spinal anesthesia also applies to epidural puncture.)

4. When the needle is firmly planted deep in the interspinous ligament, remove the stylet and attach a 5-ml glass syringe half-filled with air to the hub of the needle.

5. Advance the needle slowly with one hand while applying gentle pressure to the plunger of the syringe with the other. Note the loss of resistance as the needle enters the epidural space. (When the tip of the needle is in the interspinous ligament or the ligamentum flavum, there is resistance to both advancement of the needle and depression of the plunger. As the needle pierces the ligamentum flavum to enter the epidural space, resistance to both disappears and a click may be felt by the operator.)

6. Detach the syringe and feed the catheter into the epidural space for 3−5 cm and remove the needle over the catheter, taking care not to remove the catheter with it. (Most epidural needles are 10 cm in length, and all catheters have centimeter markings between 5 cm and 20 cm from the tip.)

7. Support the catheter at the site of skin puncture and secure it in place using tapes.

> **Note:** The appearance of clear fluid or blood through the needle or catheter means the subarachnoid space or an epidural vein has been entered. In either case, the needle and catheter should be withdrawn as one unit and the attempt repeated. Never extract the catheter through the needle; it can shear off the catheter.

Despite an apparently, uneventful placement of the catheter, it is customary practice to rule out subarachnoid or intravenous cannulation by injecting a test dose through the catheter: 3 ml of either 1.5% lidocaine or 0.5% bupivacaine with 1:200,000 adrenaline added. If the catheter is in the subarachnoid space, onset of spinal anesthesia would be obvious in the patient within 2−3 minutes; if the catheter is in a vein, the patient's heart rate would go up by at least 20 beats per minute within 30 seconds. However, even this method is not foolproof. Because a full dose of local anesthetic solution for epidural anesthesia can cause catastrophic total spinal anesthesia when injected into the subarachnoid space and an equally catastrophic toxic reaction when injected intravascularly, it is recommended that the full dose should always be given in divided increments, and the level of anesthesia checked after each increment.

> **Precaution:** The use of adrenaline as a test to rule out epidural vein cannulation is contraindicated in patients who are on beta-blocking drugs. By blocking the beta action of adrenaline, beta-blocking drugs will leave the alpha action of adrenaline unopposed, leading to severe systemic hypertension.

The full dose of lidocaine varies according to the level of anesthesia required and the age of the patient. It is approximately 1.5 ml of 2% lidocaine per spinal segment for a patient of 20 years, 1.25 ml per segment at age 40, 1 ml per segment at age 60, and 0.75 ml per segment at age 80. These volumes also apply to 0.5% bupivacaine. The onset of anesthesia is usually rapid, but maximum effect is not seen for 10–15 minutes. Unlike spinal anesthesia, the spread of local anesthetic solution in the epidural space is relatively independent of the force of gravity, the position of the patient, or the mode of injection, however, the dose of anesthetic solution should be reduced by one third in parturients, owing to engorgement of epidural veins.

In epidural as well as spinal anesthesia, arterial hypotension is a potential complication and should be managed accordingly. Owing to the large size of the epidural needle, transient backache is also a common complaint. Systemic toxicity, inadvertent dural puncture followed by headache, accidental total spinal anesthesia, and epidural hematoma are relatively rare complications.

Neither spinal nor epidural anesthesia is effective in alleviating ischemic pain associated with an arterial torniquet used on extremities during surgery. Such pain can be excruciating, but supplementation of the spinal or epidural anesthesia with intrathecal or epidural opioids can ameliorate this problem.

■ Treatment of Systemic Toxicity

Systemic toxicity is caused by a high blood level of local anesthetic agent from administration of a toxic dose, rapid absorption of a nontoxic dose, or accidental intravascular injection. Subtle signs of systemic toxicity include feelings of euphoria, apprehension, restlessness, nausea and vomiting, sensations of heat or cold, and tremor. Signs of frank toxicity are convulsion, postictal coma, respiratory arrest, and circulatory collapse. Most toxic reactions are preventable by keeping the dose within the nontoxic range. If nearly toxic doses are required, addition of epinephrine is indicated. It should be pointed out that systemic effects of epinephrine (pallor, sweating, tachycardia) may mimic the toxic effects of the local anesthetic agent.

Diazepam, given as a preoperative sedative, can increase the convulsion threshold of local anesthetics. It is also the drug of choice in the treatment of central nervous system toxicity. A dose of 5 mg should be given intravenously and repeated as required. Thiopental is also effective in treating convulsions. Because it is not a specific anticonvulsant, an anesthetic dose may be required.

Hypoxemia is always a complication of generalized convulsions because not only does the oxygen requirement of skeletal muscle rise sharply but ventilatory exchange also becomes inadequate as a result of the convulsive activity. If hypoxemia cannot be corrected by administration of oxygen alone, the trachea should be intubated and ventilation should be controlled. Succinylcholine should be used to facilitate tracheal intubation. By inducing muscle paralysis, it also returns oxygen consumption toward normal. It is a very useful agent in the event of such an emergency.

Circulatory collapse may be due to vasomotor paralysis following a massive overdose or to the vasodilating and myocardial depressant effects of local anesthetic agents. It is a grave complication. In addition to controlled ventilation, the patient will require expansion of intravascular volume and possibly myocardial support (e.g., dopamine, 5–50 µg/kg/min.)

Care of the Patient during Recovery

18

Responsibility of the anesthesiologist to the patient extends beyond the phase of emergence, because in most cases the patient is not fully conscious on leaving the operating room. Many of the intraoperative complications, anesthetic as well as surgical, can occur during the early postoperative period. Before being returned to the ward, the patient should be allowed to recover from the anesthetic in a postanesthesia care unit (PACU) for close monitoring and care by an experienced nursing staff. Discharge to the ward should be delayed until recovery from the effects of anesthesia is complete and complications are ruled out.

▉ Transporting the Anesthetized Patient

The means for monitoring and resuscitation are not readily available en route between the operating room and recovery area. Therefore, the decision to transfer the patient should not be made unless it is absolutely certain that

1. A patent airway can be maintained
2. Ventilation is adequate
3. Cardiovascular function is stable

During transfer, the patient should be positioned in the lateral decubitus position on the stretcher, and the anesthesiologist should be in attendance to look after the airway. If there is any doubt about the adequacy of ventilation, the problem should be corrected before the patient leaves the operating room. Alternatively, an endotracheal tube should be left in place so that ventilation can be controlled. Portable oxygen equipment to enrich the inspired atmosphere, a pulse oximeter to check oxygenation, and an ECG equipped with a defibrillator to monitor cardiac rhythm should be employed during transport when indicated by the patient's condition.

■ Arrival in the Postanesthesia Care Unit

On arrival in the PACU, responsibility for the patient's care should be transferred formally to a nurse. During this transfer, the anesthesiologist should supply information essential to proper nursing care as follows:

1. Identify the patient to the nurse.
2. Give a brief summary of the patient's medical history and indicate the nature of the operation.
3. Give a brief summary of the anesthetic technique, the course of the operation, the patient's intake and output in the operating room, and the patient's condition at the end of the operation.
4. Leave instructions on the management of pain, fluid therapy, oxygen therapy, and settings of the ventilator if one is in use.
5. Leave instructions on monitoring and laboratory investigation.

To complete the transfer, the nurse should check the patient's vital signs and state of consciousness and report these to the anesthesiologist. Unless it is contraindicated, the patient should be left lying on one side until fully conscious.

■ Monitoring the Patient during Recovery

Patients in need of different levels of care are admitted to the PACU. Therefore, the level of monitoring should be graded according to the needs of the patient. It is the duty of the attending anesthesiologist to leave clear instructions for the nursing staff to do so. For healthy patients who are breathing spontaneously and are stable with respect to respiratory and cardiac functions, the following standard suffices:

1. Monitor ECG continuously and check pulse rate, blood pressure, respiratory rate and pattern, and level of consciousness every 5 minutes for 15 minutes, then every 15 minutes thereafter if stable.
2. Monitor oxygenation continuously by pulse oximetry until oxygen supplement is discontinued for 15 minutes.

3. Ask the patient about pain and nausea and vomiting each time vital signs are checked.

For ill patients, additional monitoring is required:

4. Monitor capnography continuously for patients who are intubated and whose ventilation is controlled.

5. Continue invasive hemodynamic monitoring modalities if they have been instituted intraoperatively.

6. Sample blood for laboratory tests and order a 12-lead ECG and chest film as indicated by history of concurrent illness, surgical trespass, and the patient's condition.

■ Management of Common Postanesthetic Problems

Airway Obstruction

During recovery, the tongue lying against the posterior pharyngeal wall is the most common cause of upper airway obstruction in the supine unconscious patient. This problem will correct itself if the patient is turned onto one side. Occasionally it is necessary to support the jaw and insert a pharyngeal airway (see "Head Tilt–Jaw Thrust Maneuver" and "Pharyngeal Airways" in Chapter 13).

Laryngospasm, a less common cause of airway obstruction during this period, is almost always due to irritation of the pharynx or larynx during the "twilight zone" of emergence and recovery (e.g., by the presence of a pharyngeal airway, secretion, debris, or blood). Although the condition is usually self-limiting provided the irritant is removed, it can lead to life-threatening complete airway obstruction requiring the administration of succinylcholine and tracheal intubation. Occasionally healthy young patients can develop severe hypoxemia from negative-pressure pulmonary edema secondary to upper airway obstruction. Treatment is supportive: tracheal intubation and positive-pressure ventilation together with PEEP.

Airway obstruction, from whatever cause, is always an emergency because the end result is hypoventilation and hypoxemia. The precipitating cause must be treated, and the patient should be given oxygen by face mask. If the problem is not readily corrected, tracheal intubation should be considered.

Hypoventilation

Splinting of painful abdominal or chest wounds, narcotic analgesics given for pain, residual neuromuscular paralysis, and airway obstruction are some of the more common causes of hypoventilation seen in the recovery room. The patient who is hypoventilating should be given ventilatory assistance immediately, and airway obstruction should be corrected as described above. Although appropriate treatment of pain prevents hypoventilation resulting from splinting, an excessive dose of narcotic analgesic can cause unacceptable respiratory depression, particularly in a patient who has not yet fully recovered from the anesthetic. Naloxone given intravenously is the drug of choice in this last instance. By giving naloxone in increments of 50 µg, an endpoint at which the patient is breathing adequately and yet is pain free can be established.

Perhaps one of the most common causes of hypoventilation seen in the recovery room in modern anesthetic practice is residual neuromuscular blockade. When a nondepolarizing muscle relaxant is the cause of residual paralysis, an additional dose of anticholinesterase together with a vagolytic agent (e.g., neostigmine and atropine) is indicated. If improvement is not forthcoming, the patient should be reintubated and his or her ventilation should be controlled. When residual paralysis is due to Phase II succinylcholine block, the problem is pharmacologically more complicated. Although an anticholinesterase such as neostigmine will antagonize the Phase II block, it will also enhance any residual Phase I block. Therefore, it is simpler to ventilate the lungs mechanically until the neuromuscular junction has regained sensitivity to acetylcholine. In the patient with atypical plasma cholinesterase, the problem is prolonged apnea; in this case ventilation should be controlled until recovery is complete.

Hypoxemia

Cyanosis is a late sign of hypoxemia, of which hypoventilation, airway obstruction, ventilation-perfusion abnormalities, pulmonary edema, and aspiration of gastric contents are some of the causes. The cyanotic patient should be given oxygen by face mask; assisted ventilation should be instituted if indicated. (Management of airway obstruction and hypoventilation is discussed earlier in this chapter, and management of aspiration of gastric contents in Chapter 16.) Hypoxemia caused by ventilation-perfusion inequalities can be succesfully treated with an increase in inspired oxygen concentration (see Chapter 10), but arterial desaturation resulting from pulmonary edema requires treatment of the underlying cause. When pulmonary congestion is the result of fluid overload, treatment with a diuretic is indicated. When congestive heart failure is the cause of poor oxygenation, myocardial support using an isotropic agent is necessary.

Hypotension

The same factors that cause hypotension during surgery can cause hypotension in the recovery phase (see "Hypotension" in Chapter 16). Although hypovolemia is without a doubt the most common cause of hypotension, narcotic analgesics given for pain are a precipitating factor to be considered in the PACU. All hypotensive patients should receive oxygen supplement, and specific attention should be directed to elimination of the underlying cause.

Hypertension

Arterial hypertension is a not infrequent problem seen in the recovery room. It is particularly common in patients with hypertensive heart disease and systemic atherosclerosis. The more common precipitating factors are pain, distention of the urinary bladder, hypoxemia, hypercapnia, and fluid overload. The more serious consequences of uncontrolled hypertension are intracerebral hemorrhage and myocardial ischemia. Obviously treatment should be directed at elimination of the precipitating cause. In the event of a crisis, administration of an antihypertensive agent is indicated (e.g., nifedipine, 10 mg, sublingually; labetalol in 5- to 10-mg increments intravenously).

Shivering

Shivering—ranging from fine muscle tremors to frank convulsion-like clonic contractions—is a common problem during the recovery phase with many anesthetic techniques. The incidence of shivering following halothane anesthesia has been reported to be as high as 50%. Following induction of anesthesia, there is dilation of cutaneous vessels and a fall in the core body temperature. However, shivering is only partly explained by this phenomenon. A second contributing factor is loss of cortical inhibition of spinal reflexes during recovery.

Shivering produces a large increase in oxygen demand, which can be met only by similar increases in alveolar ventilation and cardiac output. Because the respiratory and circulatory depressant effects of anesthetic agents last well into the postoperative period, patients recovering from anesthesia may not be able to cope with these demands and may succumb to hypoxemia. Therefore, the patient who is shivering should receive oxygen by face mask. Keeping the patient warm could reduce the severity of shivering, and meperidine, 25 mg, given intravenously can abort an attack precipitated by abrupt arousal as a result of pain. Methylphenidate, 10–20 mg, intravenously is also effective, but this agent should not be given to patients in pain. (Methylphenidate is an analeptic without metabolic effects.)

Somnolence

Although somnolence is mostly due to the residual effect of anesthetic agents and to idiosyncrasy, many pre-existing disorders can cause delay in regaining consciousness following general anesthesia—organic disease of the central nervous system (e.g., cerebrovascular accident, head injury, increased intracranial pressure caused by space-occupying lesions); acute intoxication resulting from alcohol or other central nervous system depressants; and disorders of metabolic origin (e.g., myxedema, hepatic encephalopathy, hypoglycemia). Somnolence may also be caused by disorders that develop during the course of the operation. For example, diabetic patients can become hypoglycemic, and hypertensive patients may sustain a cerebrovascular accident. Therefore, both organic and anesthetic causes of delay in regaining consciousness should be sought and corrected in all somnolent patients.

Because elimination of inhalation agents via the respiratory trace is slower than normal if alveolar ventilation is inadequate (see "Elimination" in Chapter 3), attention should be directed to keeping the airway clear and maintaining adequate ventilation in somnolent patients. Hyoscine, droperidol, phenothiazines, and benzodiazepines (drugs often included as premedication) can also cause delays in regaining consciousness, particularly in geriatric patients. Usually in these cases it is necessary only to maintain adequate ventilation and allow recovery to occur spontaneously. Flumazenil, up to 1 mg, can be given intravenously in 0.1-mg increments until the desired level of consciousness has returned, if the offending agent is a benzodiazepine. Physostigmine, 0.5–2 mg, given intravenously can be used to reverse the hypnotic effect of the other agents. (Physostigmine is a tertiary amine and the only anticholinesterase that can cross the blood-brain barrier to act on cholinergic sites within the central nervous system.) Narcotic analgesics can also enhance the residual effect of intravenous or inhalation anesthetics to cause somnolence in the recovery phase. If this is the case, careful administration of naloxone in 50-μg increments can lead to a dramatic arousal.

Delirium

Postoperative delirium is a disconcerting problem. The restless patient can be violent and harm self and attendant. Hypoxemia may not be the most common cause of postoperative delirium, but it is certainly the most dangerous for the patient. It must be ruled out or corrected without delay. Some other causes of postoperative restlessness and excitement are pain, bladder distention, use of ketamine for induction or maintenance, inclusion of hyoscine or phenothiazines in the premedication (particularly in geriatric patients), alcohol or drug withdrawal, and hallucinogen intoxication in the unsuspected addict.

As in treatment of other postoperative complications, attention should be directed to eliminating the precipitating cause of delirium. Narcotic analgesics should be given for pain, and the full bladder should be relieved by catheterization. The patient who has received ketamine should be allowed to recover undisturbed in a darkened corner of the recovery area; diazepam, 5–10 mg given intravenously, is the agent of choice for prevention or treatment of unpleasant dreams associated with ketamine. Conversely, physostigmine, 0.5–2 mg, given intravenously is more effective in the treatment of delirium associated with hyoscine or phenothiazines. Restlessness and excitement resulting from acute alcohol or drug withdrawal or acute intoxication may be extremely difficult to diagnose and treat. A trial of methadone can prove successful with the heroin addict, and large doses of diazepam may be necessary to subdue the patient who is intoxicated with LSD or other hallucinogens.

Nausea and Vomiting

Next to pain, nausea and vomiting is the most common complaint in the postoperative period. Although it is a well-known side effect of narcotic analgesics used in treating pain, other factors are known to be associated with increased incidence and severity of this problem: intra-abdominal or ophthalmic operations, operations on the upper airway during which blood is swallowed, gastric distention from insufflation of air during vigorous positive-pressure ventilation via a face mask, and presence of foreign bodies in the pharynx (e.g., the nasogastric tube). Nausea and vomiting are better prevented than treated. The following points are helpful:

1. Use a posterior pharyngeal pack to minimize the amount of blood swallowed during nose and throat operations.
2. Decompress the stomach by orogastric suction if air has been forced down the esophagus inadvertently.

3. Include an antiemetic premedication for patients undergoing intra-abdominal or ophthalmic operations and patients known to have had severe nausea and vomiting following anesthesia. (Severe postoperative nausea and vomiting is amenable to pre-emptive treatment. Many anesthesiologists administer ondansetron, a selective antagonist of the $5HT_3$ subtype of serontonin receptors, at the time of induction to patients considered to be at high risk for postoperative nausea and vomiting, either because of the type of surgical procedure or because of past experience.)

In the postoperative period, prochlorperazine, 5–10 mg, or dimenhydrinate, 25–50 mg, given intramuscularly or intravenously may be used to control troublesome nausea and vomiting; droperiodol, 2.5 mg, or metoclopramide, 10 mg, given intravenously are also effective. If nausea and vomiting is refractory to the more traditional measures described above, ondansetron, 4–8 mg, intravenously should be effective.

Pain

Unrelieved pain can be the cause of many postoperative complications. Splinting of abdominal or chest wounds can lead to hypoventilation, sputum retention, atelectasis, and pneumonia; hypertension and tachycardia in response to pain can be the cause of myocardial ischemia and heart failure; and neurohumoral responses to pain can prolong the catabolic phase following surgical trauma and interfere with wound healing. Evidence is emerging that adequate relief of postoperative pain can shorten the hospital stay. Better pain management came about through improved understanding of the neurophysiology of pain and improved methods of delivering old drugs. This topic is covered separately in Chapter 19.

■ Care of Patients Recovering from Regional Anesthesia

The patient who has received regional anesthesia is free from the problems of general anesthesia and also from pain well into the postoperative period. However, other problems may be encountered:

1. Many patients have been given sedatives from which they must recover.
2. Hypotension accentuated by sudden postural changes is a known complication of spinal or epidural anesthesia.

3. Delays in recovery of motor and sensory functions following nerve blocks and spinal or epidural anesthesia are serious and require immediate attention.

4. Patients still under the effects of regional anesthesia may injure parts of the body without feeling pain (e.g., cigarette burns to fingers that are still numb from brachial plexus block).

Therefore, patients should be admitted to the recovery area for observation and protection after regional anesthesia as well.

Following major nerve blocks in the upper extremity, the arm and forearm should be protected in a sling. Following major nerve blocks to the lower extremity, the leg should be allowed to rest comfortably on a pillow. In order to avoid postural hypotension as a result of extensive sympathetic blockade, the patient who has had spinal or epidural anesthesia should be nursed supine. The patient who has a large intra-abdominal tumor should lie on the side to avoid caval compression. The supine position minimizes leakage of cerebrospinal fluid following dural puncture and decreases the incidence of spinal headache. In general, patients who have had regional anesthesia should not be discharged from the PACU until they have regained both motor and sensory functions or are showing signs of progressive recovery.

■ Fitness for Discharge from the Postanesthesia Care Unit

During the patient's stay in the PACU, an objective method should be used to assess the patient's physical and mental status and progress in recovery. The most popular method is that proposed by Aldrete and Kroulik. In this system, the recovery room nurse assigns a score of 0, 1, or 2 for each of five objective signs: activity, respiration, circulation, level of consciousness, and color (Table 18–1). The number of points scored by the patient is recorded every 15 minutes during the first hour of stay in the PACU and at longer intervals subsequently if vital signs are stable. Usually discharge from the PACU should be delayed until the patient has obtained a full score of 10. At the end of the stay, the anesthesiologist in charge or his or her deputy should make a final postoperative visit to assess the patient's condition. Like admission, discharge from the recovery room should be formalized. The anesthesiologist should sign a discharge order after he or she is satisfied that the patient has recovered fully from the anesthetic.

TABLE 18–1. Postanesthetic Recovery Score*

SIGN	CRITERIA	SCORE
Activity	Able to move 4 extremities voluntarily or on command	2
	Able to move 2 extremities voluntarily or on command	1
	Able to move 0 extremities voluntarily or on command	0
Respiration	Able to deep-breathe and cough freely	2
	Dyspnea or with limited breathing	1
	Apneic	0
Circulation	Blood pressure ± 20% of preanesthetic level	2
	Blood pressure ± 20–50% of preanesthetic level	1
	Blood pressure ± 50% of preanesthetic level	0
Consciousness	Fully awake	2
	Arousable on calling	1
	Not responding	0
Color	Pink	2
	Pale, dusky, blotchy, jaundiced, other	1
	Cyanotic	0

*From Aldrete JA, Kroulik D: A postanesthetic recovery score. Anesth Analg 49:924, 1970; reprinted by permission.

Management of Acute Postoperative Pain

19

Unrelieved pain can be the cause of many postoperative complications, but its management has been neglected by surgeons and anesthesiologists alike until some 10 years ago. Several convergent factors have contributed to make the management of acute postoperative pain more efficacious and efficient. They include a better understanding of the pharmacodynamics and pharmacokinetics of analgesic drugs, an improved knowledge of the physiology and pharmacology of pain and pain control pathways, the technology to safeguard the self-dispensing of opioid drugs, and the spare manpower to exploit these assets. By training and experience, anesthesiologists are playing a leadership role in "acute pain management teams" that have evolved in many institutions.

Pain and Pain Control Pathways

Somatic and Parietal Pain Pathways

Pain receptors, which are free nerve endings, are abundant in somatic structures such as skin, fascia, tendons, joints, and walls of blood vessels and on parietal surfaces such as parietal pleura, peritoneum, and pericardium. Impulses from these receptors are transmitted to the central nervous system via dual pathways: sharp pain associated with pinprick or knife cut via a fast pathway and dull, aching pain associated with tissue destruction via a slower pathway.

Receptors of sharp pain are thermomechanoreceptors or pure mechanoreceptors. Impulses from these receptors are conducted from the periphery to the spinal cord by small myelinated Aδ fibers at a velocity of 6–30 m/sec. The cell bodies of these fibers are found in the dorsal root ganglions. On entering the spinal cord, these fibers ascend or descend one to three segments in the tract of Lissauer to synapse with second-order neurons in the lamina I region of the dorsal horn (Fig. 19–1A). The second-order neurons then cross the midline at the anterior commissure and ascend toward the brain in the neospinothalamic tract of the anterolateral column of white matter in the spinal cord. These second-order neurons of the neospinothalamic tract end in the posterior nuclei and ventrobasal complex of the thalamus, from which third-order neurons relay the impulses to the somatic sensory cortex. Projections are also sent to the reticular formation and the periaqueductal gray area. This system is responsible for the localization of pain stimulus and appreciation of the intensity and duration of the stimulus. Through its projections to the periaqueductal gray area, it is also responsible for the activation of the descending pain control system (see below).

Receptors of dull, aching pain are polymodal receptors sensitive to mechanical deformity, heat, and a variety of chemicals released by tissue injury and inflammation. They include potassium and hydrogen ions, lactic acid, histamine, serotonin, and bradykinin. Prostaglandins are also released in tissue injury and inflammation. Although they do not themselves mediate pain, they enhance the action of other chemical pain me-

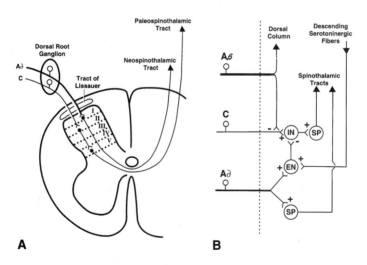

FIGURE 19–1. *A*, Somatic and parietal pain pathways. *B*, Organization of descending pain control and segmental pain modulation signals in the substantia gelatinosa region of the dorsal horn; IN = short interneuron, SP = second-order spinothalamic neuron, EN = enkephalinergic neuron, + = excitatory or facilitatory synapse, and (−)-inhibitory synapse. (Refer to text for details.)

diators. Impulses of dull, aching pain are conducted from the periphery to the spinal cord by nonmyelinated C fibers at a speed of only 0.5–2 m/sec. Their cell bodies are also found in the dorsal root ganglions (Fig. 19–1A). After entering the spinal cord and making their way in the tract of Lissauer, these C fibers terminate in laminae II and III (substantia gelatinosa region) of the dorsal horn, where they are connected by one or more short interneurons to second-order neurons in lamina V. After crossing the midline in the anterior commissure, these second-order neurons ascend toward the brain in the paleospinothalamic tract, also part of the anterolateral column of the spinal cord. Only a fraction of the fibers in this tract end directly in the intralaminar nuclei of the thalamus, while the majority terminate at various levels within the reticular formation, from which impulses are relayed through multiple synapses to the thalamus, hypothalamus, and other areas of the brain stem. (This spinoreticular portion of the paleospinothalamic tract is also called the spinoreticular tract.) The cortical projection of the paleospinothalamic tract from the thalamus is diffuse, but with prefrontal dominance. This system is concerned with the autonomic and emotional response to pain as well as the phenomenon of arousal.

Visceral Pain Pathways

In general, visceral organs are only sparsely endowed with pain receptors and their nerve fibers. A highly localized noxious stimulus like cutting or clamping usually produces little pain, but a diffuse stimulus like bowel distention, inflammation, or ischemia produces excruciating pain. Pain impulses are conducted from these organs toward the spinal cord in afferent fibers that are mixed with sympathetic efferent fibers. Some of these afferent fibers are mixed with parasympathetic fibers. On reaching the paravertebral sympathetic chains and ganglions, these afferent sensory fibers join the segmental sensory nerves by way of the rami communicans. Their cell bodies reside in the dorsal root ganglions, and they synapse in the dorsal horn of the spinal cord with second-order neurons that relay these pain impulses to higher centers and the cortex.

In some instances, visceral and somatic pain fibers share the same second-order neurons of the spinothalamic tracts. This convergence of peripheral pain pathways from visceral and somatic territories explains in part the phenomenon of *referred pain*. That is, pain originated in a visceral organ is localized to a part of the body surface whose pain fibers share with those from the viscera the same second-order spinothalamic neurons.

Descending Pain Control Pathways

The central nervous system is well endowed with opioid receptors, particularly in the mesolimbic system (including the periventricular and periaqueductal gray areas) and the substantia gelatinosa region of the spinal cord. A serotoninergic-enkephalinergic descending pain control pathway originates in the periventricular and periaqueductal gray areas. Its axons synapse in the midline nucleus raphe magnus of the medullary reticular formation, from which serotoninergic fibers descend in the dorsolateral column of white matter in the spinal cord to terminate in the substantia gelatinosa area of the dorsal horn (Fig. 19–1B). In the substantia gelatinosa, these serotoninergic fibers activate inhibitory enkephalinergic neurons, which in turn synapse with short interneurons that connect C fibers to second-order neurons of the spinothalamic tract. Activation of the enkephalinergic neurons inhibits the short interneurons, thus suppressing the conduction of pain impulses centrally. As mentioned in the previous section, this descending pain control pathway is activated by projections to the periaqueductal gray area from the neospinothalamic tract. In addition, the cortex can exercise influence on this pathway through projections to the thalamus, the periaqueductal gray area, the reticular formation, and other structures of the brain stem. It is well known that the emotional state and behavior of an individual can influence the perception of pain. For example, stress, relaxation, and autohypnosis can increase pain threshold, and fear and depression can decrease pain threshold. It is more than likely that these factors influence this descending pain control pathway through higher and other centers of the brain.

Besides this descending serontoninergic-enkephalinergic pathway, there is evidence that a descending adrenergic inhibitory pathway exists. Alpha$_2$ agonists can act both at the spinal level and supraspinally to produce analgesia. However, the anatomic projection and function of this andrenergic pathway has not been fully characterized.

Segmental Pain Modulation Pathways

According to the gate control hypothesis of Melzack and Wall, central transmission of pain impulses can be blocked at the spinal cord level without invoking descending pain control mechanisms. These segmental pain modulation pathways involve both the larger myelinated Aβ fibers responsible for conduction of tactile impulses and the smaller myelinated Aδ fibers responsible for fast sharp pain afferents.

After entering the spinal cord and before their ascent in the dorsal column, Aβ fibers sprout collaterals that terminate in a presynaptic inhibitory relationship with C fibers in the sub-stantia gelatinosa region (Fig. 19–1*B*). Activation of these Aβ fibers suppresses presynaptically the transmission of pain im-pulses from C-fiber terminals to short interneurons that relay information to second-order neurons of the paleospinothalmic tract. The Aδ fibers, in contrast, send collaterals to synapse with inhibitory enkephalinergic neurons in the substantia gelati-nosa, the same inhibitory neurons that are under the influence of the descending serontoninergic pain control pathway (Fig. 19–1*B*). Afferent impulses in Aδ fibers can activate these in-hibitory neurons, which in turn suppress the relay function of the short interneurons. Thus activation of both the Aβ and Aδ fibers can modulate the central transmission of C-fiber pain im-pulses at spinal cord levels.

Pathophysiology of Pain

Postoperative pain causes functional changes in many organ systems. Although they are normal responses to stress, these changes can become pathologic if left uncontrolled.

Respiratory System

Splinting of an abdominal or chest wound as a result of un-relieved pain decreases diaphragmatic excursion and the ability to cough effectively, thus leading to hypoventilation and spu-tum retention. Hypoventilation gives rise to ventilation-perfu-sion inequalities, hypoxemia, and hypercarbia, and sputum re-tention sets the stage for atelactasis and pneumonia. Even when the operative site is far from the thorax or abdomen, fear of aggravating pain can bring on hypoventilation and retention of secretions.

Cardiovascular System

Unrelieved pain increases sympathetic outflow; it releases antidiuretic hormone (ADH) from the hypothalamus–posterior pituitary complex, cortisol and aldosterone from the adrenal cortex, and catecholamines from the adrenal medulla; and it activates the renin-angiotension system. Together these re-sponses cause salt and water retention as well as tachycardia and hypertension, all of which can precipitate heart failure and myocardial ischemia in the susceptible patient.

Gastrointestinal and Genitourinary System

Pain inhibits smooth muscle contractility of abdominal and pelvic organs. The clinical manifestation is ileus and urinary retention.

Endocrine System

The stress of pain increases the release of the catabolic hormones catecholamine, cortisol, aldosterone, growth hormone, and glucagon and inhibits the release of the anabolic hormones insulin and testosterone. As a result of increased gluconeogenesis through protein catabolism and lipolysis, the catabolic phase following surgery is prolonged and wound healing is delayed.

Immune System

Unrelieved pain is associated with suppression of the cellular components of the immune system. This is reflected in lymphopenia and decreased activities of neutrophils and killer T cells.

Coagulation System

The stress of pain increases platelet adhesiveness and decreases fibrinolysin activity. Increased platelet adhesiveness and venous stasis as a result of physical inactivity are important factors contributing to the increased thromboembolic incidence seen in the postoperative period.

▬ Treating Acute Postoperative Pain

Pain is an inevitable sequela of surgery, but the initiation, transmission, and perception of pain impulses can be modulated by drugs or other measures at many levels, from the site of the wound to the cerebral cortex. They include

1. Modifying the action of chemical pain mediators at the site of injury using nonsteroidal anti-inflammatory drugs (NSAIDs)

2. Blocking pain impulse transmission in peripheral nerves and the neuroaxis (local anesthetic drugs)

3. Using drugs that act on receptor sites in pain control pathways at both the spinal and supraspinal levels (opioids and alpha$_2$-agonists)

4. Invoking the gate control mechanism of pain modulation (transcutaneous electrical nerve stimulation and acupuncture)

5. Exploiting the cortical influence on pain perception (cognitive and behavioral manipulations)

General Measures

Patients differ in their tolerance for pain, and its intensity can vary according to the patient's emotional state and physical activity. Other than administration of an analgesic, certain general measures can help to reduce the intensity of pain and improve the patient's well-being.

1. Address the patient's emotional state, which is best done during the preoperative visit. The patient should be given the chance to explain personal concerns and any questions should be answered. The pain treatment plan should be explained to reinforce confidence and alleviate fear.

2. Administer analgesic drugs before the beginning of surgery. There is evidence that pre-emptive treatment improves the quality of pain control and decreases the requirement of analgesics.

3. Dress wounds on extremities with bulk dressings but avoid restrictive bandages. Restriction of venous return can cause excruciating pain at the site of operation that throbs with arterial pulsation.

4. Similarly, be sure that plaster casts are not restrictive. Circulation to parts of the extremity distal to the cast should be checked frequently in the immediate postoperative period. Cyanosis and swelling of these parts are signs of restricted venous return; pallor should raise the possibility of arterial obstruction.

5. Support the extremity that has been operated on with pillows so that it is elevated above the patient's heart. Dependency can cause throbbing pain.

6. Instruct the patient who has had an abdominal operation to hug a pillow against the abdomen during coughing and deep breathing exercises but to avoid the use of abdominal binders. By restricting diaphragmatic excursion, these binders can cause basal atelectasis.

7. Treat anxiety with psychological support as well as a tranquilizer if necessary. Unrelieved anxiety can lower pain tolerance.

8. Do not prescribe a hypnotic if sleeplessness is the result of pain. The semiconscious patient who is still experiencing pain will become delirious.

Nonopioid Analgesics

Prostaglandins are produced at sites of tissue injury from cell membrane phospholipids, which involves the enzyme cyclo-oxygenase. Although they do not themselves produce pain, the prostaglandins sensitize pain receptors and potentiate the action of other pain medicators. Indomethacin, ibuprofen, and naproxen are NSAIDs that exert their analgesic action peripherally by inhibition of cyclo-oxygenase and decreasing the synthesis of prostaglandins. They are given orally and sometimes rectally for the treatment of minor to moderate pain. They are also useful as adjuncts to potentiate the analgesic effect of opioids given by any route. The recommended doses are

Indomethacin	25–75 mg per os every 8 hours as necessary or a 50 to 100-mg suppository per rectum every 12 hours; the maximum dose should be limited to 200 mg/day
Ibuprofen	400–800 mg per os every 6–8 hours as necessary; the maximum dose should be limited to 2400 mg/day
Naproxen	250–500 mg per os every 12 hours as necessary or a 500-mg suppository per rectum every 12 hours; the maximum dose should be limited to 1000 mg/day

Ketorolac, a new NSAID, is said to be as potent as morphine and can be given intramuscularly. A dose of 10 mg is given orally every 4–6 hours as necessary to treat minor to moderate pain, but the total dose should not exceed 40 mg/day. For severe pain after major surgery (e.g., abdominal procedures), the intramuscular route is more suitable and a dose of 30 mg should be given every 4–6 hours as needed. It is recommended that the total daily dose should not exceed 120 mg and the treatment duration should not exceed 5 days.

All NSAIDs are associated with systemic complications. The common ones include the following:

1. Peptic ulceration, gastric perforation, and massive gastrointestinal bleeding have been associated with all NSAIDs. These drugs are contraindicated in patients who have active peptic ulcer disease or inflammatory disease of the gastrointestinal tract.

2. Through inhibition of prostaglandin synthesis, NSAIDs have the potential to cause prerenal azotemia because real per-

fusion is dependent on a facilitative role played by prostaglandins. Elderly patients who have impaired renal or hepatic function and those who are taking diuretics are particularly susceptible. In addition, long-term administration of NSAIDs has resulted in renal papillary necrosis, interstitial nephritis, and nephrotic syndrome. They should be prescribed with caution in patients who have renal insufficiency.

3. Precipitation of congestive heart failure, possibly from fluid retention, has been reported. NSAIDs are contraindicated in patients who are in heart failure and relatively contraindicated in those whose failure is controlled.

4. Like acetylsalicylic acid (ASA), all NSAIDs can interfere with platelet function by inhibition of aggregation. However, the effect is less and the duration shorter than that seen with ASA. There has been no report of increased postoperative bleeding associated with NSAIDs. In this respect, NSAIDs appear to be safe to use in the postoperative period. However, caution is advised in patients who are on anticoagulants, including low-dose heparin for antithrombotic therapy.

5. Cross-hypersensitivity exists among all NSAIDs and between NSAIDs and ASA. Use of NSAIDs is contraindicated in patients who have the triad of nasal polyps, bronchospasm, and angioedema associated with ASA.

Acetaminophen, an antipyretic analgesic, is a weak inhibitor of prostaglandin biosynthesis that does not have the anti-inflammatory activity seen with NSAIDs. It is free of the complications associated with NSAIDs and there is no cross-hypersensitivity between it and these agents. A dose of 650–1000 mg can be given alone every 4–6 hours for treating postoperative pain of low intensity, but it is more common to give it as an adjunct to potentiate the analgesic effect of oral codeine (see next section). The maximum daily dose should be limited to 4000 mg in 24 hours. Acute poisoning from ingestion of more than 7.5 g of acetaminophen can cause hepatic necrosis and death; the hepatotoxin is an intermediate metabolite of hepatic biotransformation. Because acetaminophen is broken down in the liver by microsomal enzymes, chronic consumption of enzyme-inducing substances (e.g, barbiturates, alcohol) will enhance the hepatotoxicity of acetaminophen.

Opioid Analgesics

Oral Opioids

Codeine, usually combined with acetaminophen to improve the quality of analgesia, is the most common oral opioid used for treating postoperative pain of low to moderate intensity.

One to two tablets (containing 300 mg of acetaminophen, 15 mg of caffeine, and 8, 15, or 30 mg of codeine each) are given per os every 4–6 hours as needed after minor surgery on the body surface or extremities. It is used also for pain relief in the later stages after major surgery. As an alternative to codeine, the following opioids are also suitable as oral analgesics: morphine, 15–30 mg, every 4 hours; meperidine, 50–150 mg, every 4 hours; or pentazocine, 50–100 mg, every 4 hours.

Intramuscular Opioids

Intramuscular injection of meperidine, 1–2 mg/kg, or morphine, 0.1–0.2 mg/kg, every 3–4 hours when necessary, has been the mainstay of treating severe postoperative pain for decades. Although it has the benefit of simplicity, this form of pain relief has several limitations:

1. Dose requirement varies widely among patients, and calculation of dose according to body weight does not take into account the different pain thresholds that exist among patients.
2. Dose requirement can vary in any given patient, depending on physical activity. A dose that is adequate when the patient is at rest may be far from adequate when this same patient is active (e.g., during physiotherapy).
3. Drug absorption from an intramuscular site is dependent on muscle blood flow. Depending on the hemodynamic status, plasma drug concentration and time to peak plasma concentration can vary from patient to patient and from time to time in the same patient.
4. Even under ideal conditions, intermittent intramuscular injection will produce peaks and troughs in plasma drug concentration between injections (Fig. 19–2A). Drug concentration at the peaks, being higher than the plasma concentration required for analgesia, will be associated with unwanted sedation and respiratory depression; drug concentration at the troughs, having fallen below the plasma concentration required for analgesia, will be associated with unrelieved pain. In order to improve on the safety of intramuscular opioids, agonist-antagonists with a ceiling effect on respiratory depression have been introduced (e.g., pentazocine, butorphanol, nalbuphine, buprenorphine), but these agents also have limited analgesic potency.
5. In practice, the dose prescribed is often far from optimum because of the fear of unwanted side effects mentioned in point 4. Furthermore, the "when necessary" or "as needed" part of the order is taken by many to mean "only when absolutely necessary or needed." Nursing protocol can cause even more delays between the time when the patient makes a request and the time the patient receives the injection. It is little wonder that close to 75% of surgical patients find this intermittent on-

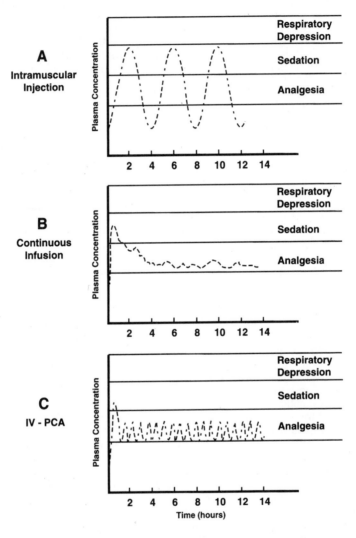

FIGURE 19–2. Plasma concentration of an opioid (*A*) following intermittent intramuscular injection, (*B*) during continuous infusion after the administration of a loading dose, and (*C*) during IV-PCA after the administration of a loading dose.

demand method of intramuscular opioids unsatisfactory for pain relief.

Despite the limitations mentioned above, intramuscular opioids still have a role in the treatment of acute postoperative pain. Their efficacy and safety can be improved if the dose and dosing interval are constantly reviewed to meet the patient's need. It should not be assumed that a prescribed dose will be effective just because it is ordered on an "as needed" basis. Patients receiving opioids by newer dispensing techniques described below are given constant attention. Patients receiving intramuscular opioids for postoperative pain relief would benefit from the same attention.

Intravenous Opioid

The quality of analgesia following intermittent boluses of intravenous opioids is far superior to that after intermittent intramuscular injection. Meperidine, 10–30 mg, or morphine, 1–3 mg, is given every 5–10 minutes when necessary in this technique. Unfortunately, this method of pain relief requires constant nursing attention and is practical only in the PACU or intensive care unit. In order to overcome the manpower-intensive nature of this technique, a continuous infusion of opioids can be used.

In any continuous infusion technique, the time to reach steady-state plasma drug concentration is typically delayed and requires a latent period equal to four to five times the half-life of the drug being infused. Therefore, enough meperidine or morphine (a loading dose) should be given in increments at the beginning until an analgesic plasma concentration is obtained. Once analgesia is optimum, a continuous infusion of meperidine (up to 50 mg/hr) or morphine (up to 5 mg/hr) is set up to maintain the analgesic plasma concentration. A typical plasma concentration of the opioid given by this technique is illustrated in Figure 19–2B. Without doubt, continuous infusion is superior to intermittent intramuscular injection in providing analgesia, but it still lacks flexibility in the following ways:

1. The plasma drug level sufficient to provide analgesia varies with the patient's activity. An infusion rate sufficient to keep the patient who is sleeping pain free may be totally inadequate when the patient is awake. Conversly, an infusion rate set high enough to provide pain relief for a patient who is active may cause respiratory depression when the patient is resting.

2. Following prolonged infusion, lipophilic drugs can accumulate in tissue depots. When tissue depots are saturated, the plasma drug concentration can rise rapidly to dangerously high levels.

Therefore patients receiving continuous intravenous infusion of opioids for pain relief should be monitored regularly and the infusion rate should be reset from time to time to match the needs of the patient.

Intravenous Patient-Controlled Analgesia

In intravenous patient-controlled analgesia (IV-PCA), a computer-controlled pump is used to dispense small intermittent boluses of intravenous opioids on demand by the patient. This method of postoperative pain relief eliminates the large fluctuation in plasma drug concentrations seen with intermittent intramuscular injections of much larger doses of opioids (Fig. 19–2C). Because the patient is in control, it has the flexibility of meeting the varied needs of the patient resulting from changing levels of physical activity. Without the manpower-intensive nature of the nurse-dispensed intravenous boluses described in the previous section, patients on IV-PCA can be nursed in general wards instead of acute care units. Most IV-PCA devices offer some or all of the following options to be programmed into the memory of the device before use. Attention should be paid to define these options during the set-up procedure.

1. *Opioid selection.* When this option is offered, the generic name of the chosen opioid should be identified. This option is not absolutely essential for the device to function safely, so long as the opioid concentration and dose values are clearly defined.

2. *Opioid concentration.* This refers to the concentration of the opioid solution being used. It should be entered accurately for the device to deliver the proper dose.

3. *Loading dose.* Patients who are in pain when IV-PCA is being set up should be given the chosen opioid intravenously until satisfactory pain relief is obtained. The desired dose should be given in repeated increments by titration using this option (e.g., 10–30 mg of meperidine or 1–3 mg of morphine every 5 minutes). This option can also be used to give additional increments of opioids for breakthrough pain or when increased pain is anticipated (e.g., in preparation for physiotherapy). The loading dose bolus must be programmed and dispensed by the practitioner each time it is required. It cannot be preprogrammed into the device for the patient to dispense it on demand.

4. *Bolus dose.* Also called "incremental dose," this option defines the dose to be given on demand by the patient, if the demand is made outside the lockout interval. A typical example is 10 mg of meperidine or 1 mg of morphine; the usual range is 5–20 mg of meperidine or 0.5–2 mg of morphine.

5. *Lockout interval.* This option limits the dosing interval. Typical settings are between 5 and 10 minutes. If the patient presses the demand switch within this lockout interval, the device will register the demand but will not dispense a bolus dose. A large discrepancy between the number of demands

made by the patient and the number of bolus doses dispensed is a sign of inadequate pain relief.

6. *Continuous infusion.* All IV-PCA devices offer the option of continuous background infusion in addition to the PCA-only mode. Continuous infusion has the theoretical advantage of providing a background level of analgesia to which the patient can add only when needed. If this background level of analgesia is adequate, it allows the patient to rest for long periods without the need to activate the pump. However, such a high rate of background infusion can cause unwanted respiratory depression. It is not necessary to set a background infusion for the IV-PCA device to function. If this option is chosen, the infusion rate per hour should be limited to one quarter of the anticipated hourly opioid requirement of the patient. Adjustment may be required when the patient is sleeping and when the intensity of pain recedes as the patient continues to recover in the postoperative period.

7. *Maximum dose limit.* The option of setting a 1-hour or 4-hour maximum dose limit is offered by some IV-PCA devices. Setting this option is not essential to the function of the device, but it acts to safeguard against programming errors and to alert the practitioner to the unsatisfied needs of the patient.

In the first few hours after starting IV-PCA, the patient should be visited regularly to check on the quality of pain relief and the occurrence of unwanted complications. The size of the bolus dose, the lockout period, and the rate of continuous infusion (if one is being used) may have to be adjusted to meet the patient's needs. After the patient has settled, the number of visits can be reduced to twice daily to check on progress. Continuous infusion should be weaned after 1 or 2 days, and oral analgesics prescribed if the number of demands made is less than 1 per hour. Most patients require IV-PCA for 1–3 days after abdominal or major joint surgery.

Other than intrathecal or epidural analgesia, IV-PCA is the most effective method of dispensing opioids parenterally. Compared to patients on intermittent intramuscular injection, patients on IV-PCA consistently report better quality of analgesia with smaller doses of opioids.

Intrathecal Opioids

With the discovery of opioid receptors in the substantia gelatinosa of the spinal cord, treating pain by injecting opioids intrathecally or epidurally became firmly established in 1979. The quality of analgesia by these routes is far superior to that obtained by intramuscular, intravenous, or IV-PCA opioids. When they are given intrathecally, both the onset time and the duration of action of intrathecal opioids are shorter for agents that have a high lipid solubility and longer for agents that have a low lipid solubility. For example, the onset time and duration of action of the lipid-soluble agent fentanyl are 5 minutes and 3–6 hours, respectively, whereas the onset time and duration of action of the less soluble agent morphine are 15 minutes and 12–24 hours, respectively. Preservative-free morphine, 0.25–0.5 mg, is the most popular intrathecal opioid in clinical use today. Fentanyl, 10–20 μg, can be added for rapidity of action if desired.

When an agent that has low lipid solubility, such as morphine, is injected intrathecally at the lumbar level, its analgesic action can spread to include thoracic dermatomes through rostral circulation of cerebrospinal fluid. Rostral circulation of intrathecal morphine can reach as high as the brain stem, causing nausea and vomiting, sedation, and respiratory depression. When an agent that has high lipid solubility, such as fentanyl, is used, much of it is absorbed by the substance of the spinal cord and rostral spread to the brain stem is less likely.

Respiratory depression, delayed for 3–6 hours after intrathecal morphine, is the most serious complication of this technique. It is particularly serious and frequent if the dose of morphine is increased beyond 0.5 mg. Therefore, frequent monitoring of respiratory function is mandatory (see "Safety Considerations" below). The side effect of nausea and vomiting can be particularly severe and can be treated with metoclopramide, 10 mg, intravenously every 6 hours or other antiemetics. In addition, urinary retention requiring catheterization is not uncommon. Generalized itching is another annoyance that can be treated with diphenhydramine, 25 mg, given intravenously every 6 hours as needed. If the pruritis is refractory to diphenhydramine, incremental doses of naloxone, 50 μg, can be given intravenously by titration to the point at which pruritis is relieved but analgesic action is not antagonized.

A major disadvantage of intrathecal opioids is a lack of flexibility, and repeated dural puncture cannot be justified in long-term care. Delivery of epidural opioids via an indwelling epidural catheter is more practical.

Epidural Opioids

The epidural space is highly vascular, and the kinetics of opioids deposited into this space depends on the lipid solubility of the agent. When morphine, an agent of low lipid solubility, is injected into the epidural space, much of it is absorbed into the systemic circulation and only a small amount crosses the dural barier to reach the cerebrospinal fluid. Once it is in the cerebrospinal fluid, it is free to spread rostrally as with intrathecal morphine. Therefore, morphine injected into the epidural space sited in the lumbar region can be used to relieve pain originating in the lower extremities and the abdominal and chest walls. The time of onset is 30 minutes, the time to peak action is 60–90 minutes, and the duration of action is up to 12 hours. The long duration of action of epidural morphine makes it suitable for intermittent administration. The dose should be adjusted according to age: 5 mg for those up to 50 years old, 4 mg for those up to 60, and 3 mg for those older.

When the lipophilic agent fentanyl is injected into the epidural space, a relatively smaller amount is absorbed into the systemic circulation. That which crosses into the cerebrospinal fluid is also quickly taken up by neural tissue and does not spread as far rostrally as morphine. Therefore, the site of action of epidural fentanyl is more segmental in nature and the epidural catheter should be introduced at a level consistent with the dermatomes of the wound involved. The onset of action of epidural fentanyl is only 5 minutes, the time to peak action is 20 minutes, and the duration of action is 2–3 hours. Because of this short duration of action, fentanyl is more suitable for continuous epidural infusion at a rate of 0.5–1 µg/kg/hr.

The side effects of epidural opioids (respiratory depression, nausea and vomiting, urinary retention, and pruritis) are similar to those of intrathecal opioids. They should be treated accordingly.

Neural Blockade Analgesia

Epidural Neural Blockade

Continuous infusion of bupivacaine, 0.25%, at 5–8 ml/hr into the epidural space predates epidural opioids as a method of postoperative pain relief. In this technique, the epidural catheter is introduced near the dermatomes of the wound involved. Some degree of motor and sympathetic blockade is always present; therefore, ambulation of the patient is difficult and hemodynamic instability is a problem. In order to minimize motor and sympathetic blockade, more dilute solutions (e.g., 0.0625–0.125% bupivacaine) have been tried with varying success. Some authors recommend a combination of low-dose bupivacaine and fentanyl as an alternative (e.g., bupivacaine, 1 mg/ml, and fentanyl, 10 µg/ml, at a rate of 4–8 ml/hr). In this way, both the complications of motor and sympathetic blockade and the side effects of epidural opioid can be minimized.

Interpleural Neural Blockade

Instillation of local anesthetic into the pleural space has met with varying success in treating pain associated with thoracic surgery, rib fractures, and abdominal surgery through a subcostal incision. The local anesthetic drug acts by diffusing across the parietal pleura to act on intercostal nerves. The epidural-type catheter can be left in place before chest wall closure in surgery on the thorax or introduced into the pleural space via a Tuohy needle in the seventh intercostal space at the midaxillary line in closed-chest procedures. The recommended dose is 20 ml of 0.5% bupivacaine every 4–6 hours as required. If a chest drain is present, it should be clamped before instillation of the anesthetic solution and for half an hour after. A potential complication of this technique is pneumothorax caused by insertion of the catheter.

Peripheral Neural Blockade

Infiltration of the wound and simple nerve blocks using bupivacaine can contribute to pain relief for several hours. In addition, continuous sciatic and femoral nerve blocks and axillary brachial plexus block can be managed with an indwelling catheter. These methods should be considered even if the surgical procedure is performed under general anesthesia. They will not only provide postoperative analgesia but also will reduce the intraoperative requirement of anesthetic drugs.

Epidural Alpha$_2$-Agonists

The discovery of a descending adrenergic pain control pathway terminating in the substantia gelatinosa region of the spinal cord has spawned the application of adrenergic drugs epidurally to treat pain. Clonidine, an alpha$_2$-agonist, is the first drug to be tried in this novel technique, with good results and no respiratory depression. However, there is a high incidence of hypotension and bradycardia associated with this technique, probably through preganglionic sympathetic inhibition. Other more specific alpha$_2$-agonists, including dexmeditomidine and tizanidine, are on the horizon, but the usefulness of this technique in treating acute postoperative pain is still being defined.

Other Modalities

In addition to the pharmacologic treatments of acute postoperative pain, there are several nonpharmacologic modalities that are being used with varying degrees of success. They include transcutaneous electrical nerve stimulation (TENS), acupuncture, and cognitive and behavioral manipulations.

In TENS, a pulsatile electric current is used to relieve pain by stimulating a site over peripheral nerves supplying the painful area. In acupuncture, needles are inserted into specific points related to distant organs and regions of the body, and are then manipulated to obtain pain relief in those organs or regions. Both may have a neurophysiologic basis for their action. If Aβ fibers are activated by TENS or acupuncture, both of these modalities can inhibit the transmission of pain impulses from C fibers presynaptically to short interneurons in the substantia gelatinosa as described under "Segmental Pain Modulation Pathways" (see Fig. 19−1*B*). If Aδ fibers are stimulated, TENS and acupuncture can activate enkephalinergic inhibitory neurons and inhibit the relay function of the interneurons (see Fig. 19−1*B*). Furthermore, it has been shown that acupuncture can cause the release of endogenous opioids, pointing to a neuropharmacologic basis of its action.

Cognitive and behavioral manipulations refer to techniques in which the patient is conditioned to exercise control over the perception of pain. Cognitive manipulations include distraction, dissociation, and diversion of attention from the painful event (e.g., focusing on pleasant personal events); behavioral manipulations involve activities that reinforce the patient's sense of control over the painful event (activating the demand control in IV-PCA is a perfect example).

All the nonpharmacologic techniques mentioned above require intensive preparation and education of the patient. Although there are advocates, these modalities are more useful in treating chronic than acute pain.

Safety Considerations

There is always the risk of respiratory depression when opioids are given by continuous infusion or the IV-PCA, intrathecal, and epidural routes. Every effort should be made to safeguard against this potentially lethal complication and to treat it promptly if it occurs. Although patients can be nursed in general wards, personnel capable of managing the airway and supporting ventilation should be available in the hospital at all times, nursing staff should be educated with respect to the monitoring and management of these patients, and physicians from the acute pain management team should be available for consultation. A printed protocol describing the technique being used, the level of monitoring required, and the management of complications should accompany the patient. Details of the protocol may differ from institution to institution, but it should contain the following common elements:

1. Clear identification of the technique, the drug, the dose, the dose interval, and the infusion rate where applicable.

2. Orders to monitor the intensity of pain while the patient is awake. (This is best done by using a digital scale of 0 to 10, with 0 representing no pain and 10 excruciating pain.)

3. Orders to monitor the patient's respiratory rate and level of sedation hourly at the beginning but at longer intervals if the patient has been stable for at least 12 hours. The patient's blood pressure and pulse rate as well as the level of sensory and motor block should be monitored if local anesthetic is given epidurally. (Increasing level of sedation may appear before overt signs of respiratory depression.)

4. Prescribed treatments for breakthrough pain. (In general, no opioids or other central nervous system depressants by another route are allowed, but an additional loading dose of opioid by IV-PCA or additional fentanyl given epidurally is permissible. NSAIDs have the potential to act synergistically with opioids without causing respiratory depression and should be added when necessary. The acute pain management team should be consulted if pain is refractory.)

5. Prescribed treatments for respiratory depression (respiratory rate less than 8 per minute) or inability to rouse patient. (They should include oxygen supplementation, support for the airway and ventilation, administration of naloxone intravenously, and calling for the acute pain management team.)

6. Prescribed treatments for other complications, including nausea and vomiting, pruritis, and urinary retention.

Special Considerations in Surgical Outpatients

20

Ambulatory care offers the opportunity to treat patients at a reduced cost and without separating them from family. This concept is gaining popularity in the practice of surgery, and as many as 60% of the surgical procedures nationwide are done on an outpatient basis today. Most procedures that do not affect the function of major organ systems and do not interfere with the patient's ability to participate in self-care can be done in well-equipped outpatient surgical facilities. In order to provide these outpatients with the same high quality of care enjoyed by inpatients, special considerations should be given to their assessment and management.

Assessment of the Patient

Candidates for outpatient surgery should receive the same intensive preanesthetic assessment recommended for inpatients (see Chapter 12). Although full assessment can be done by the anesthesiologist only on the day of surgery, the patient's surgeon or family physician should be recruited to participate in preoperative screening of the patient. Alternatively, screening can be done through a telephone interview. Adequate information should be sought during the screening process to determine the patient's health, curent medications, adequacy of treatment, allergy to drugs, past anesthetic experience and complications, family history of anesthetic complications, physical and mental capacity to participate in self-care, and suitability of environment for home care (e.g., availability of responsible adult at home to take care of patient). With carefully formatted questions, it is usually possible to separate patients into those who are suitable for outpatient surgery with no preconditions and those who need further investigation and preparation. Patients in the second group should be referred to an anesthesia consultation clinic for follow-up evaluation.

■ Selection Criteria for Outpatient Surgery

Care exercised in selecting patients and procedures in outpatient surgery will decrease the number of unanticipated admissions resulting from unforeseen complications. These criteria should be set according to sound judgment, and all the factors should be taken into consideration together in arriving at a decision.

Physical Status

All patients in Class I and II of the American Society of Anesthesiologists' Classification of Physical Status are acceptable for outpatient surgery, but only medically stable patients in Class III whose systemic illness or its treatment is not affected by the anesthetic or the operation are suitable candidates. For instance, a stable diabetic treated with an oral hypoglycemic agent or insulin is suitable whereas a brittle diabetic is not, particularly if the surgery is going to upset dietary intake. Some anesthesiologists argue that even a stable Class IV patient (a patient with an incapacitating systemic illness that is a constant threat to life) is acceptable for outpatient surgery. However, no hard and fast ruling can be made on this count. Such a patient may be acceptable if there is adequate support within the surgical facility, in the community, and in the patient's home.

Concurrent Illnesses

In addition to having an acceptable physical status, a patient who has concurrent illnesses is acceptable only if treatment received is optimal and the disease state is stable. If the disease is unstable despite treatment, the patient should be referred for further investigation. For example, a patient who has stable angina on therapy is an acceptable candidate, but one who has new symptoms of nocturnal pain is not.

Age

Both healthy seniors and young infants are acceptable candidates. Whereas chronologic age is not a determining factor in outpatient surgery, physiologic age is. Geriatric patients can become confused and disoriented when dislocated from their home environment. In this respect, they will benefit most from surgery in an outpatient setting. As for infants born prematurely, care should be exercised because they are prone to have apneic spells for 12–24 hours after general anesthesia. There is no universal agreement on when an ex-premature infant outgrows this complication. It varies between a postconception age (gestional age plus postnatal age) of 44 and 60 weeks. The best guide to selection is the infant's postnatal development. If the infant has caught up with nonpremature peers in development, then he or she is likely free from this complication.

Mental and Physical Capacity

For an adult patient to have surgery on an outpatient basis, he or she must be willing to participate and capable of participating in self care. The degree of participation depends on the degree of help available at home. Patients living in nursing homes will face minimal demands, whereas those only staying with friends may receive minimal support.

Socioeconomic Profile

The patient's socioeconomic profile is also an important factor in determining suitability. There must be a responsible adult at home to care for the patient, and this guardian must be capable of following and carrying out instructions. The distance between the patient's home and health care facilities is another consideration. Although it may not be acceptable for a patient to have surgery and return to an isolated farmhouse, it is perfectly acceptable for a patient to have surgery in an urban center and return to a rural community that has hospital and ambulance service.

Type of Surgery

The list of procedures acceptable for outpatient surgery is being expanded constantly, partly through accumulated experience and also a result of the current trend toward "minimally invasive" surgery (e.g., laparoscopic instead of open cholecystectomy). With the availability of short-acting drugs, "home readiness" even after a long procedure under general anesthesia is no long a problem. Nevertheless, certain generalizations can be made to guide selection. A procedure should not be performed on an outpatient basis if

1. The procedure on part of an organ system causes incapacity in the entire system from which the patient must recover (e.g., an intra-articular operation on the knee that causes incapacity is only one leg is acceptable; resection of even a short segment of bowel causes generalized ileus and is unacceptable).

2. The procedure causes external fluid or internal fluid shift that requires prolonged observation and intravenous replacement in the postoperative period (e.g., a massive liposuction procedure).

3. The procedure interferes with the medical treatment of a major concurrent illness (e.g., when coumadin given to a patient who has a prosthetic valve must be stopped or when oral medication before surgery in the mouth must be replaced by parenteral medication).

4. The procedure prevents the patient from receiving oral intake and intravenous therapy is necessary to maintain fluid balance.

5. The procedure causes enough pain to warrant repeated administration of an opioid parenterally for relief, be it intramuscular, intravenous, intrathecal, or epidural.

6. The procedure gives rise to the necessity for administering drugs regularly by the parenteral route (e.g., antibiotics intravenously for infection or heparin subcutaneously for antithrombotic prophylaxis).

7. The procedure gives rise to the necessity for regular visits by other health care professionals in the immediate postoperative period (e.g., regular physiotherapy).

Physical Facility

Facilities offering outpatient surgery can be a hospital-associated unit, a free-standing center, or a surgeon's clinic. How these facilities function is an important determining factor in the selection of patients and procedures. A hospital unit offers the advantage of readily available inpatient support, although no outpatient surgical center should be allowed to operate without such support. In addition, some outpatients need a longer period of observation after certain types of procedures without the necessity for full admission. Obviously a nine-to-five unit should not take on these types of patients or procedures, whereas one that has extended hours can.

■ Preoperative Fasting and Premedication

Aspiration of gastric contents is a potential complication of general anesthesia; it can also happen in accidents associated with regional anesthesia (e.g., toxic reactions or inadvertently high spinal block). Previous recommendation of nothing by mouth from midnight before surgery has proved to be over-zealous, particularly if the operation is scheduled for the afternoon. Most authorities now recommend

1. Abstinence from solid food for a minimum of 5 hours on the day of surgery
2. Unrestricted clear fluid intake up to 3 hours before the scheduled operation
3. Oral medication (including the patient's own for concurrent illness) with not more than 30 ml of water up to 1 hour before the scheduled surgery

There is evidence to suggest that more than 85% of adult surgical outpatients have gastric content over 25 ml and gastric pH less than 2.5, both of which would increase the risk of acid pneumonitis if aspirated. Therefore, many authors recommend the use of one or more of the following measures to decrease gastric content volume and acidity:

1. Cimetidine, 600 mg, or ranitidine, 150 mg, orally 90 minutes before the scheduled operation or cimetidine, 300 mg, or ranitidine, 50 mg, intravenously 45 minutes before the scheduled operation. (These two H_2-receptor antagonists decrease both gastric content volume and gastric acidity by suppressing gastric acid secretion.)
2. Metoclopramide, 20 mg, orally 90 minutes before or metoclopramide, 10 mg, intravenously 45 minutes before the scheduled operation. (Metoclopramide, a dopamine antagonist, increases gastric emptying and lower esophageal sphincter tone. Both actions can contribute to lowering the risk of regurgitation.)
3. One-third molar sodium bicitrate, 30 ml, orally within 30 minutes before the induction of anesthesia. (Sodium bicitrate is a nonparticulate antacid.)

With respect to preoperative sedatives or anxiolytics, they are usually not necessary. The level of anxiety can be minimized by settling the patient in a pleasant waiting area and allowing the patient to stay with companions until the operating room is ready. If necessary, 10–15 mg of diazepam may be given orally to relieve anxiety. Unlike lorazepam, an anxiolytic dose of diazepam will not prolong the recovery stage of anesthesia.

■ Anesthetic Considerations

Local and Regional Anesthesia

Local or regional anesthesia is an excellent choice for outpatient surgery. These techniques are associated with no clouding of sensorium, little or no nausea and vomiting, and good pain relief that persists well into the postoperative period. Local infiltrations, peripheral nerve blocks, brachial plexus block, and intravenous regional anesthesia are popular techniques; epidural anesthesia using a short-acting agent (chloroprocaine) may be considered; and spinal anesthesia gives better muscle relaxation than epidural anesthesia. If spinal anesthesia is employed, a 24-gauge or finer pencil-point needle (see Fig. 17–5) should be used to minimize the risk of postdural puncture (spinal) headache.

Conscious Sedation

Originally practiced by dental surgeons in their offices, this technique is used to supplement local or regional anesthesia in patients in whom general anesthesia is inappropriate and yet local or regional anesthesia by itself is inadequate. In this technique, an intravenous sedative or hypnotic and an opioid are given in small increments until the patient is sedated and amnesic and yet able to maintain his or her own airway and respond to simple commands. Because verbal response requires a higher degree of cortical arousal than motor response, the patient's level of consciousness is best evaluated by instructions to perform a simple act (e.g., open your eyes, take a deep breath, squeeze my hand). The most appropriate agents for this technique are those that have a short duration of action, such as midazolam, propofol, and alfentanil. Because the margin between conscious sedation and loss of consciousness is narrow, these drugs should be given slowly by titration and the patient should receive comprehensive monitoring as described under "Basic Intraoperative Monitoring" in Chapter 14. It must be stressed that conscious sedation should not be "pushed" beyond its limit so that a failed regional technique will work. When the basic regional technique does not provide complete anesthesia, either the procedure should be postponed or the patient given a general anesthetic if it is appropriate.

General Anesthesia

If general anesthesia is elected, techniques associated with a short recovery time and minimal residual sedation should be employed. Therefore, methohexital or propofol is more appropriate than thiopental for induction; desflurane or sevoflurane is superior to the other volatile agents for maintenance; fentanyl or alfentanil is more suitable than morphine as an analgesic supplement; and atracurium, vecuronium, rocuronium, and mivacurium are better choices among nondepolarizing muscle relaxants. Outpatient anesthesia is not a contraindication to tracheal intubation and controlled ventilation; however, if succinylcholine is used to facilitate intubation of the trachea, precurarization is recommended to minimize muscle pain.

Combined Techniques

Even when general anesthesia is the technique of choice, it is worthwhile considering supplementing it with regional anesthesia. A combined technique reduces the requirement of general anesthetic agents and speeds recovery. The regional anesthesia supplement will also provide the patient with excellent analgesia in the postoperative period. Even simple infiltration of the wound with bupivacaine is beneficial.

Postoperative Care

The surgical outpatient should be allowed to recover from the effects of anesthesia just as inpatients. The topic of recovery is fully discussed in Chapter 18. However, the surgical outpatient faces problems that require special consideration. They include management of postoperative pain, the treatment of nausea and vomiting, and the establishment of "home readiness."

Postoperative Pain

Many new techniques of treating acute postoperative pain have been developed in the last decade and are described in detail in Chapter 19. However, IV-PCA and neuroaxial analgesic techniques are not suitable and some of the other techniques must be modified for the surgical outpatient.

The advantage of combined general and regional anesthetic techniques was touched on in the previous section of this chapter. It should be encouraged where applicable. The "pre-emptive" technique of treating pain is also an excellent strategy to be used on outpatients. This involves the administration of a potent opioid analgesic at induction of anesthesia and during the surgical procedure so that the patient will emerge from the anesthetic smoothly at the end without experiencing pain. This technique can be reinforced with the administration of a NSAID given intramuscularly or rectally soon after induction. With this approach, most patients will feel little pain in the recovery phase, and only acetaminophen with codeine will need to be prescribed on an "as necesary" basis. For those who need a potent opioid for pain relief during recovery, incremental doses should be given by the nurse-dispensed intravenous method. The intravenous route has the advantage of flexibility and predictability over the intramuscular route, which will add up to a smaller total dose required by the end of the stay (see Chapter 19 for the appropriate drugs and their doses).

Nausea and Vomiting

Refractory nausea and vomiting following surgery under general anesthesia is a common reason for unanticipated postoperative admission of the surgical outpatient. Therefore, all the measures mentioned under "Nausea and Vomiting" in Chapter 18 should be exercised to reduce this complication. Unrelieved pain itself can cause nausea and should be treated aggressively. For patients who are susceptible (those who have a positive history), the strategy of "pre-emptive" treatment should be tried (give a potent antiemetic with induction of anesthesia). Ondansetron, a $5HT_3$-receptor (serontonin) antagonist, is expensive, but if it is effective and can keep the patient out of the hospital, then it is cost-effective.

Home Readiness

In addition to meeting the criteria for discharge from the PACU discussed in Chapter 18, surgical outpatients should meet specific criteria before they are discharged home. Details of such criteria may vary from institution to institution, but they all have the following common elements:

1. Vital signs are within 20% of preanesthesia level and stable for at least half an hour. (Blood pressure should be checked with patient both lying supine and sitting up in bed to rule out orthostatic hypotension.)

2. Patient is oriented with respect to person, time, and place. (For patients who are mentally infirm, mental status must have returned to the preoperative level.)

3. Symptoms of minor complaints (e.g., drowsiness, sense of fatigue) are stable.

4. There is no sign of bleeding at the site of surgery.

5. Circulation of the limb or digit that was operated on is normal.

6. Pain is controlled with oral analgesics only.

7. Patient can tolerate clear fluids by mouth without nausea or vomiting. (Patients who cannot keep down clear fluids should not be discharged.)

8. Patient is able to void. (This is particularly important after epidural or spinal anesthesia. It is a sign of recovery of autonomic function.)

9. Both sensory and motor function have returned to the limb or limbs after regional, epidural, or spinal anesthesia.

10. Patient is not dizzy and is able to ambulate with assistance. (Trial of ambulation after epidural or spinal anesthesia should be done in three progressive steps: sit up in bed only, dangle legs by the bedside, and bear weight with assistance. Dizziness associated with sitting up and dangling legs implies orthostatic hypotension and incomplete recovery of sympathetic function.)

When all is well, the patient is ready to be discharged home in the company of a responsible adult. The attending anesthesiologist or his or her deputy should make a final visit to assess the patient's home readiness and to sign the discharge order.

Because the residual effect of anesthetic and sedative drugs can last 24 hours or more, the ambulatory surgical outpatient should be instructed not to perform any tasks that require quick reflexes or judgment (e.g., operating a motor vehicle or machinery or signing a business contract) for at least 24 hours after recovering from anesthesia. The residual effect of anesthetics and sedatives produces poor tolerance for central nervous system depressants, so the patient should be instructed not to take any alcoholic beverages or tranquilizers for the next 24 hours. In addition, the patient should be warned of the common side effects of general anesthesia (nausea or vomiting, sore throat, muscle pain). The patient should also be given the telephone number of a responsible physician (e.g., the anesthesiologist or surgeon on call) and told to report any untoward complications immediately. In order to ensure that there is no misunderstanding, these postoperative instructions should be handed out in printed form and reviewed with the accompanying adult.

Fluid and Electrolyte Requirements of Surgical Patients

21

All surgical patients are required to abstain from oral intake for several hours before and after an operation, and in some cases for even longer periods. Maintenance of fluid and electrolyte homeostasis with intravenous fluid is therefore critical for these patients' well-being. Not only should basal requirements be met, but pre-existing deficits and ongoing losses should be replaced; that is,

$$\text{Total requirement} = \underset{\text{requirement}}{\text{Basal}} + \underset{\text{deficit}}{\text{Pre-existing}} + \underset{\text{losses}}{\text{Ongoing}}$$

In this chapter, a practical approach to fluid and electrolyte therapy is set forth. A discussion on the use of blood and plasma products is reserved for Chapter 22.

Basal Requirements

Water

A healthy adult consumes approximately 2500 ml of water per day, of which 1500 ml is ingested as liquid, 800 ml is part of solid food, and 200 ml is derived from oxidation of carbohydrate and fat. Normal daily losses are 1500 ml as urine and another 1000 ml as insensible loss (800 ml via the skin and respiratory tract and 200 ml in feces). Thus intake and output are in balance. With fluid deprivation, the body can conserve water by increasing urinary concentration of solutes and decreasing urine volume; however, the normal kidney can concentrate urine only to a maximum specific gravity of 1.035. Approximately 500–600 ml of urine is still required to excrete 600 mOsm of solute each day. Although fluid retention is part of the metabolic response to injury, it is normally safe to calculate the basal water requirement of the patient undergoing surgery according to these guidelines:

4 ml/kg/hr for the first 10 kg body weight
2 ml/kg/hr for the second 10 kg body weight
1 ml/kg/hr for each additional kilogram of body weight

Sodium

The salt intake of a normal person is 50–100 mEq/day. Sodium homeostasis is maintained mainly by excretion in urine; a small amount is lost through skin in sweat and some is lost through the intestine. Under conditions of reduced intake, the kidneys can conserve sodium and excrete urine that is practically free of sodium, but the surgical patient benefits from receiving the normal daily requirement. If all of the basal fluid intake is given as 0.3% saline and 3.3% dextrose in water, the daily requirement of sodium will be met.

Potassium

The ability of the kidneys to conserve potassium is poor. In order to avoid a deficit, a daily basal requirement of 30–60 mEq of potassium must be met. However, during the operation and in the early postoperative phase, tissue catabolism is accompanied by mobilization of a large amount of potassium. Therefore, administration of potassium in the first 2 postoperative days usually is not necessary unless a deficit can be demonstrated. Thereafter, a maintenance dose of 0.5–1 mEq/kg/day should be given intravenously if the patient has not resumed oral feeding.

Pre-existing Deficits

Owing to the nature of the surgical illness, many patients present with pre-existing deficits of water and salt. A mild degree of fluid loss produces no symptoms, but a 5% loss of body weight in fluid is reflected in poor skin turgor, dry oral mucous membranes, longitudinal furrowing of the tongue, decreased intraocular tension, oliguria, tachycardia, and orthostatic hypotension. Collapsed peripheral veins, sunken eyeballs, cold extremities, frank hypotension, and clouded sensorium are signs of more severe volume depletion. An acute drop in body weight is an accurate reflection of the amount of fluid lost externally. Similarly, frequency of vomiting or diarrhea, biochemical changes (see below), and measurement of central venous or pulmonary capillary wedge pressure can be used to estimate the magnitude and character of fluid loss.

Water and Sodium Deficits

Many patients who require surgery have combined water and sodium deficits. For convenience, these deficits can be classified into three categories, according to the amount of sodium in the fluid: (1) loss of isotonic water and sodium, (2) loss of excess water, or (3) loss of excess sodium.

In general, *isotonic losses of water and salt* occur through the gastrointestinal tract, by vomiting, diarrhea, nasogastric suction, and so forth. Other losses include fluids sequestered in the lumen of the bowel and at the site of injury (so-called third-space losses). As fluid is lost, contraction of plasma volume leads to hemoconcentration, decreased renal blood flow, prerenal azotemia, metabolic acidosis, hyperkalemia, and eventually circulatory collapse. Urinary sodium concentration is often less than 10 mEq/L, but serum sodium concentration is normal. Weight lost acutely is the best estimate of the amount of external fluid loss. Otherwise, central venous or pulmonary capillary wedge pressure measurement should be used as a guide to replacement therapy. If plasma sodium concentration is normal, the ideal replacement fluid is a balanced salt solution such as lactated Ringer's solution.

The most common cause of *excess water loss* is inadequate water intake. Dehydration may be aggrevated by excessive insensible loss in a hot climate or during febrile illness, and it is frequently observed in patients who are debilitated and living alone. Diuresis resulting from glycosuria and diabetes insipidus is a less common cause of excess water loss; in addition to hypovolemia, affected patients have hypernatremia. Because normal serum sodium concentration is approximately 140 mEq/L, the volume of deficit can be estimated according to the equation

$$\text{Volume deficit} = \left(\frac{\text{Measured serum Na conc.}}{140} - 1 \right) \times \text{Total body water}$$

(Total body water is approximately 50% of body weight in women and 60% in men.) This volume deficit should be replaced with 5% dextrose. However, in hypotensive patients, a hypotonic saline solution should be used instead (e.g., 0.3% saline in 3.3% dextrose).

Excess sodium loss is characterized by hyponatremia. Surgical causes of excess sodium loss are rare. Hyponatremia is usually the result of replacing isotonic deficits with a hypotonic solution. If serum concentration falls below 110 mEq/L, cerebral edema and convulsions (water intoxication) may occur. Normal serum sodium concentration is 140 mEq/L; the amount of deficit can be calculated according to the equation

Na deficit = (140 − Measured serum Na conc.) × Total body water

Isotonic saline, which has 154 mEq of sodium per liter, is the ideal replacement fluid when hyponatremia is mild. When water intoxication is imminent, 5% saline should be infused slowly until symptoms have abated. Hypertonic saline can cause rapid expansion of intravascular volume, leading to pulmonary congestion. Rapid or prolonged infusion of 5% saline is never indicated.

If volume deficit is a common complication of many surgical illnesses, volume overload is a complication of overzealous fluid therapy. Clinical signs of fluid overload include tachycardia, hypertension, breathlessness, dependent edema, and jugular venous distention. The end result of fluid overload is pulmonary edema. When symptoms of fluid overload are mild, sodium and fluid restriction is usually adequate treatment; when symptoms are severe, a diuretic is indicated. If volume overload is associated with heart failure, digitalis or vasodilator therapy should be considered.

Potassium Deficits

Clinical signs of *hypokalemia* are muscle weakness, paralytic ileus, U-wave or other changes on the ECG, and ventricular irritability. Furthermore, hypokalemia can enhance the action of nondepolarizing muscle relaxants.

More common causes of potassium deficiency are prolonged parenteral fluid therapy with no added potassium, excessive gastrointestinal losses with inadequate replacement, and diuretic therapy. In the absence of acid-base disturbance, concentration of potassium in serum can be used as a guide to estimate potassium deficits. Normal serum potassium concentration is 3.5−5 mEq/L. With a serum potassium concentration of 3 mEq/L, the total body deficit is approximately 100 mEq. Thereafter, another 200 mEq of potassium is lost from the body store for each 0.5-mEq/L drop in serum potassium concentration.

Treatment of hypokalemia should be directed toward elimination of the precipitating cause and replacement of known deficits. Normally, the amount of potassium added to intravenous fluids should be limited to 40 mEq/L and the rate of infusion should be limited to 20 mEq/hr. If a higher concentration

TABLE 21-1. Drugs Useful in Treatment of Hyperkalemia

DRUG	DOSE AND ROUTE
Sodium bicarbonate	Increments of 50 mEq IV
Insulin and glucose	10 U regular insulin in 500 ml of 10% dextrose IV over 1 hr
Sodium polystyrene sulfonate	15 g orally or 50 g rectally 1–4 times per day
Furosemide	40–80 mg IV or orally
Calcium chloride	1 g IV over 10–15 min with ECG monitoring

or a faster rate of infusion is desirable, electrical activity of the heart should be monitored continuously by ECG during infusion.

Overzealous replacement therapy, renal failure, and increased tissue catabolism (e.g., resulting from burns or crush injuries) can cause *hyperkalemia*. Symptoms and signs of hyperkalemia are nausea and vomiting, abdominal colic, and diarrhea; ECG signs are peaking of T wave, widening of QRS complex, ST segment depression, and asystole. Several methods are available for the treatment of hyperkalemia. Administration of sodium bicarbonate will, by inducing metabolic alkalosis, redistribute potassium to intracellular sites. Insulin added to a glucose infusion will promote movement of potassium into cells. The cationic exchange resin sodium polystyrene sulfonate will remove potassium from the gastrointestinal tract when it is given orally or rectally. Furosemide, by promoting urinary excretion of potassium, also can return serum potassium concentration toward normal. If myocardial depression is a complication, calcium chloride can be used to antagonize the depressant effect of potassium on the heart. The recommended doses of these drugs are listed in Table 21-1. When renal failure is the cause of hyperkalemia, peritoneal dialysis or hemodialysis is indicated.

Acid-Base Abnormalities

Abnormal fluid and electrolyte losses are almost always complicated by acid-base abnormalities. *Metabolic acidosis* may be due to excessive loss of alkali (e.g., diarrhea, ureterosigmoidostomy, and renal tubular acidosis); formation of lactic acid (e.g., severe dehydration and shock, hypoxemia); or presence of other organic acids (e.g., renal failure, diabetic ketosis, and methanol or salicylate intoxication). In metabolic acidosis caused by excess loss of bicarbonate, the anion gap is normal; with other causes, the anion gap exceeds 15 mEq/L. (The anion gap is obtained by subtracting the serum concentrations of chloride and bicarbonate from that of sodium.) Treatment directed at correcting the precipitating cause is all that is required when metabolic acidosis is mild. Severe metabolic acidosis, however, should be corrected with intravenous sodium bicarbonate. Hypertonic sodium bicarbonate solution can cause volume overload, and rapid correction of acidosis can lead to hypokalemia; therefore, it is usually not advisable to correct severe acidosis completely with a single dose. The following equation should be used to calculate the initial dose:

$$\begin{array}{l}\text{Sodium bicarbonate} \\ \text{required (mEq)}\end{array} = \text{Base deficit} \times \text{Body weight (kg)} \times 0.15$$

After this dose, the patient's condition should be reassessed and treatment revised accordingly.

Metabolic alkalosis may be due to excessive loss of acid (e.g., vomiting, continuous gastric suction, intestinal fistula) or ingestion of alkali (the mild-alkali syndrome). When circulating volume is contracted, renal conservation of sodium is accompanied by reabsorption of bicarbonate; when potassium depletion is severe, sodium is reabsorbed in exchange for hydrogen ions by the kidneys. Both are common causes of metabolic alkalosis in surgical patients. Treatment of metabolic alkalosis should include saline infusion to replace volume deficits and administration of potassium chloride.

Respiratory disturbance can also lead to acid-base abnormalities. Acute *respiratory acidosis* is always the consequence of hypoventilation (e.g., resulting from respiratory depression by anesthetic agents or splinting of chest and abdomen). Treatment of acute respiratory acidosis should be directed at correcting the precipitating cause. If necessary, tracheal intubation and controlled ventilation should be employed. Overzealous mechanical ventilation is the most common cause of acute *respiratory alkalosis*. Treatment should be aimed at reducing tidal volume and respiratory rate accordingly. Mechanical dead space can be used to reduce alveolar ventilation in cases in which a large tidal volume is desirable.

■ Ongoing Losses

Like pre-existing deficits, ongoing losses can be external and obvious or internal and occult. Ongoing external loss of fluid can be measured accurately by monitoring the patient's input and output. It is more difficult to estimate the volume sequestered around surgical wounds as edema fluid (third-space loss). This volume is only a few hundred milliliters after minor op-

TABLE 21-2. Electrolyte Contents of Alimentary Fluids*

ALIMENTARY FLUID	NA$^+$ (mEq/L)	K$^+$ (mEq/L)	Cl$^-$ (mEq/L)	HCO$_3^-$ (mEq/L)
Gastric fluid	60 (10–115)	10 (0–30)	130 (10–155)	
Pancreatic secretion	140 (115–185)	5	75 (55–95)	115
Bile	145 (130–165)	5	100 (90–180)	35
Duodenal fluid	140	5	80	
Ileal fluid	140 (80–150)	5	105 (40–140)	30
Colonic fluid	60	30	40	

*These are average values; the normal range is shown in parentheses.

erations (e.g., elective hernia repair or operation on head and neck), but it can be 3 liters or more after extensive dissections (e.g., pancreatectomy or repair of abdominal aortic aneurysm). Therefore, it is important to monitor urine output and central venous or pulmonary capillary wedge pressure when third-space loss is anticipated to be great.

Solutions used to replace ongoing losses from the intestine should be chosen to reflect the composition of the lost fluids. The electrolyte contents of intestinal and other alimentary fluids are listed in Table 21–2. Sequestered fluids, in contrast, have a composition similar to that of extracellular fluid. A balanced salt solution should be used to replace such losses.

■ General Guidelines for Replacement Therapy

In order to maintain fluid and electrolyte balance, it is important to administer basal requirements, replace existing deficits, and keep up with additional losses. Whether the patient is on the ward or in the operating room, it is only a matter of simple arithmetic to calculate the total amount of fluid and electrolytes required and to replace it with a combination of 5% dextrose and hypotonic or isotonic saline. The composition of some commonly used parenteral fluids is given in Table 21-3.

For the patient who is old and infirm or who has cardiac, renal, or hepatic disease, replacement of large pre-existing deficits should be more gradual. Only half the calculated deficit

TABLE 21–3. Electrolyte Contents of Parenteral Solutions*

SOLUTION	Na⁺ (mEq/L)	K⁺ (mEq/L)	Ca²⁺ (mEq/L)	Cl⁻ (mEq/L)	Lactate (mEq/L)
Lactated Ringer's	130	4	3	109	28
0.9% (Normal) saline	154			154	
M/6 sodium lactate	167				167
0.45% Saline	77			77	
0.3% Saline	51			51	
0.2% Saline	34			34	

*Hypotonic saline solutions usually come with dextrose to make them isotonic.

should be replaced initially. In order to prevent pulmonary congestion, it may be necessary to monitor central venous or pulmonary capillary wedge pressure while the deficit is being replaced. In these cases, the patient's clinical condition should be reassessed frequently and management should be revised accordingly.

Crystalloid or Colloid Solutions to Replace Blood Loss

Red cells and plasma are part of ongoing losses during surgery. All healthy patients with a normal preoperative hemoglobin concentration and hematocrit can tolerate a 30% loss of red cell volume, as long as plasma volume is kept normal. Whether plasma volume loss should be replaced with a crystalloid or colloid solution in blood loss of this magnitude is controversial. Without the benefit of the oncotic pressure inherent in plasma or other colloid solutions, crystalloid solutions such as normal saline or lactated Ringer's solution will move out of the intravascular compartment into the interstitial and intracellular compartments quickly, and three volumes of a crystalloid solution to one volume of blood loss is required to keep plasma volume normal. However, the movement of crystalloid solution into interstitial and intracellular compartments can cause tissue edema. In contrast, a 1:1 volume is sufficient if a colloid solution is used. This in theory will reduce the development of tissue edema. However, all synthetic colloid solutions (see dextran 40, dextran 70, 6% hetastarch, and 10% pentastarch in Table 21–4) can cause hypersensitivity reactions, interfere with coagulation, and hinder the process of cross-matching blood. Moreover, in the presence of capillary leakage, the use of colloids can actually lead to the development of more severe tissue edema. At present there is no clear evidence that colloid so-

TABLE 21–4. Colloid Solutions

	Na$^+$ (mEq/L)	Cl$^-$ (mEq/L)	OSMOLARITY (mOsm/L)	ONCOTIC PRESSURE (mm Hg)
5% Albumin	145	145	290	20
Dextran 40	154	154	310	40
Dextran 70	154	154	310	70
6% Hetastarch	154	154	310	30
10% Pentastarch	154	154	325	30

lution is better than crystalloid solution in maintaining plasma volume or vice versa. If blood loss is only moderate, it is not unreasonable to use a crystalloid solution alone (up to 3000 ml) initially to maintain plasma volume, after which the judicious use of a synthetic colloid solution up to 20 ml/kg is appropriate. If blood loss continues beyond 30%, then both red cells and plasma should be replenished as outlined in "To Replace Red Blood Cell Loss" and "To Replenish Plasma Volume" in Chapter 22.

> **Note:** Neither crystalloid nor colloid solutions have any oxygen-carrying capacity. When they are used to replace blood loss during the initial phase of resuscitation, it is important to maintain optimal oxygenation and cardiac output so that oxygen delivery to tissues is not compromised. If the patient is anemic, red cell replacement should begin earlier, before 30% of the red cell volume is lost.

Blood Transfusion 22 in Surgical Patients

Transfusion (of lamb's blood into humans) was pioneered by Richard Lower in 1667. Because of obvious dangers associated with heterologous transfusion, it was abandoned as a means of treating hemorrhagic shock until the 19th century, when James Blundell reintroduced the concept of human blood transfusion (both homologous and autologous) as a method of replacing blood loss of postpartum hemorrhage. Nevertheless, it took almost another 100 years for the technique to become safe, which it did after the discovery of ABO blood groups by Karl Landsteiner in 1900.

Homologous Blood Transfusion

In a modern blood bank, whole blood is seldom available for transfusion; it is separated into its components to meet specific needs: to replace red cell loss, to replenish plasma volume, and to correct coagulopathies. When whole blood continues to be lost, a combination of blood products may be required to replace deficits.

Common Blood Products and Their Components

Whole Blood. One unit of whole blood contains 450 ml of donor blood in citrate-phosphate-dextrose-adenine (CPDA-1) or citrate-phosphate–double dextrose (CP2D) anticoagulant. It has a hematocrit of 0.3–0.4 (30–40%). Whole blood can be stored at 1–6° C for 35 days if it is anticoagulated with CPDA-1 and for only 21 days if anticoagulated with CP2D. The levels of labile clotting factors V and VIII are reduced with storage.

Red Blood Cells. Also known as packed red blood cells or red cell concentrate, these are obtained from whole blood by removing approximately 200 ml of plasma. One unit has a volume of 240–340 ml and a hematocrit of about 0.75 (75%). It can be stored at 1−6° C for up to 35 days. AS-3 red blood cells are packed red blood cells suspended in Nutricel (an additive solution containing dextrose, adenine, citrate, phosphate, and sodium chloride). It has a hematocrit of 0.45−0.65 (45−65%) and can be stored at 1−6° C for 35 days.

Leukocyte-Poor Red Blood Cells.   Leukocyte-poor red blood cells are also known as buffy coat−poor packed red blood cells. In this preparation, the white cell fraction of packed red blood cells or AS-3 red blood cells is removed by centrifugation, sedimentation, washing, or filtering. One unit has a volume of about 200 ml. It can be stored for 35 days at 1−6° C if it is prepared in a closed system. Because of potential contamination, it should be infused within 6 hours of preparation (storage at 20 −24° C) or within 24 hours (storage at 1−6° C) if it is prepared in an open system. This product should be reserved for patients with a known transfusion reaction to white cells, for organ transplantation candidates, and for patients who require repeated transfusions.

Frozen Red Blood Cells.   Prepared from units of whole blood, packed red blood cells may be stored in the frozen state for 10 years after addition of the cryopreservative agent glycerol. After thawing, washing, and suspension in normal saline, 80% of the original red cell mass remains. After reconstitution, the cells should be stored at 1−6° C and transfused within 24 hours. This method of red cell preservation is usually reserved for autologous blood donated by individuals with rare blood types, those with multiple red cell alloantibodies, and those in whom homologous transfusion is contraindicated (e.g., bone marrow transplant patients).

Platelet Concentrate (from Whole Blood).   Prepared from a single unit of whole blood, each unit of platelet concentrate contains around 60×10^9 platelets suspended in 40−70 ml of plasma. It may be stored at 20−24° C for up to 5 days, but individual units that are pooled before transfusion should be infused promptly.

Platelet Concentrate (by Apheresis).   Another type of platelet concentrate is obtained by apheresis with intermittent or continuous-flow centrifugation from a human leukocyte antigen (HLA)-matched donor. It contains $300−400 \times 10^9$ platelets suspended in 200−300 ml of plasma. It is stored at 20−24° C and has a shelf life of 5 days if prepared in a closed system, but only 1 day if prepared in an open system. It is specifically indicated in patients who are refractory to platelet transfusion because of HLA incompatibility.

Leukocyte Concentrate.   Obtained from a single donor by apheresis, a unit of leukocyte concentrate contains around $10−20 \times 10^9$ granulocytes in 200−300 ml of plasma. HLA-matched and cytomegalovirus (CMV)-seronegative products are also available. These products are used in severely neutropenic patients who have septicemia refractory to antibiotic and other conservative therapy. They are usually given when prepared but may be stored for 24 hours at 20–24° C.

Plasma. Stored plasma is separated from whole blood by centrifugation or sedimentation within 72 hours of collection. One unit has a volume of approximately 200 ml. It contains all coagulation factors except V and VIII. Stored plasma has a shelf life of 24 months if frozen at −18° C; after thawing it should be stored at 1–6° C and used within 72 hours. Plasma can also be stored unfrozen at 1–6° C; in this instance its shelf life is 35 days.

Fresh Frozen Plasma. When plasma is separated from whole blood or prepared by apheresis and frozen within 8 hours of collection, it is called fresh frozen plasma. One unit has a volume of approximately 200 ml and contains all coagulation factors, including the labile factors V and VIII. Shelf life is 12 months at −18 to −30° C. (Factor VIII level is better preserved at −30° C.) It requires 20–30 minutes to thaw.

Cryoprecipitated Factor VIII. Also known as cryoprecipitated antihemophilic factor (cryoprecipitated AHF), cryoprecipitated factor VIII has approximately 80 or more units of factor VIII activity and 150 mg of fibrinogen in a volume of 5–15 ml per bag. In addition to factor VIII, it is a source of von Willebrand's factor, factor XIII, fibrinogen, and fibronectin. Shelf life is 1 year at −18 to −30° C. (Factor VIII is better preserved at −30° C or colder.) It requires 10 minutes to thaw.

Antihemophilic Factor. Also known as coagulation factor VIII, AHF is a lyophilized fractionated plasma product heat-treated to inactivate human immunodeficiency virus (HIV) and some hepatitis viruses. It must be reconstituted before being used.

Albumin. Albumin is available as 50–100 ml of 25% solution and as 250–500 ml of 5% solution. HIV and hepatitis viruses are eliminated during pasteurization. Shelf life is 5 years at 4° C and 3 years at room temperature.

Specialized Products. In addition to those mentioned above, specialized products are also available: irradiated red blood cells in which the donor lymphocytes are eliminated to prevent graft versus host reactions; CMV-seronegative red blood cells and platelets for immunocompromised recipients; recombinant factor VIII concentrate; prothrombin complex–activated preparation for hemophiliacs who have factor VIII inhibitors; and factor IX concentrate to treat Christmas disease.

Therapeutic Uses of Homologous Blood Products

To Replace Red Blood Cell Loss

Packed red blood cells in combination with plasma products have superseded whole blood for blood replacement. All healthy patients with a normal preoperative hemoglobin concentration and hemotocrit can tolerate a 30% loss of blood volume, as long as circulatory volume is maintained at a normal level with the infusion of a physiologic saline solution (lactated Ringer's solution, normal saline) or a colloid plasma expander (dextran 40, dextran 70, hetastarch, pentastarch). If loss of blood volume exceeds 30%, further blood loss should be replaced according to the clinical condition of the patient. Packed red cells should be used to replace red blood cell loss, and a physiologic saline solution, 5% albumin, plasma, or plasma expander to replace plasma volume loss (see "Crystalloid or Colloid Solutions to Replace Blood Loss" in Chapter 21 and "To Replenish Plasma Volume" below). Specially prepared products such as leukocyte-poor or irradiated red blood cells should be used only when indicated (e.g., in organ transplant recipients).

Packed red blood cells flow only slowly because of their high viscosity. The flow rate can be improved by adding 50–100 ml of normal saline (*not* lactated Ringer's solution or other solutions containing dextrose, dextran, or calcium) to the pack. AS-3 red blood cells have a lower hematocrit and flow faster, addition of normal saline is usually not necessary.

To Replenish Plasma Volume

As was pointed out in the previous section, infusion of a crystalloid solution and colloid plasma expander may be used to sustain normal plasma volume during the initial phase of hemorrhage. In general, the volume of physiologic saline to be used for this particular purpose should be limited to 3000 ml and the volume of synthetic colloid solution limited to 20 ml/kg (see "Crystalloid or Colloid Solutions to Replace Blood Loss" in Chapter 21). When these volumes are exceeded, 5% albumin can be used if replenishment of clotting factors is not necessary. Stored plasma is more appropriate if replenishment of clotting factors other than factors V and VIII is indicated, and fresh frozen plasma should be used if replenishment of the labile factors is also required. Plasma products are also used to replace protein and fluid loss in victims of extensive burns. In many ways 5% albumin has advantages over plasma; it is free of potential contamination by HIV and hepatitis viruses, is compatible with all blood groups, and has a long shelf life at room temperature.

To Correct Coagulopathies

Different blood products are used to correct specific coagulation defects. Stored plasma has all the plasma proteins except labile clotting factors V and VIII. It is indicated for replacing stable clotting factors and for rapid reversal of the anticoagulant effects of coumadin-like drugs. Fresh frozen plasma, in comparison, has all the clotting factors intact. During massive transfusion, when a volume equal to or greater than the patient's blood volume must be replaced in less than 24 hours, fresh frozen plasma and plasma may be transfused alternately to correct dilutional coagulopathy if it is confirmed.

Platelet concentrates are generally not indicated in thrombotic thrombocytopenia or idiopathic thrombocytopenia unless there is life-threatening hemorrhage. They should be used to treat dilutional coagulopathy during massive transfusion only if thrombocytopenia is proven. When platelet concentrate is used, a unit will increase the platelet count of an average adult patient by $5-10 \times 10^9/L$ ($5000-10,000/\mu L$), and one unit per 10 kg is enough to raise the platelet count above the hemostatic level of $50 \times 10^9/L$ ($50,000/\mu L$). Each unit of platelet concentrate contains a significant volume of donor plasma. Only platelet concentrates from donors whose plasma is ABO compatible with the recipient's red blood cells should be used. In some patients, HLA compatibility is an important consideration (e.g., in patients who have had repeated transfusions and in bone marrow transplant recipients). In these instances, platelet concentrates prepared by apheresis from HLA-matched donors should be used. One bag of platelet concentrate by apheresis is equivalent to six units of platelet concentrate prepared from whole blood; it can increase the platelet count of an average adult patient by $30-60 \times 10^9/L$ ($30,000-60,000/\mu L$).

Cryoprecipitated factor VIII is used to treat bleeding diathesis in hemophilia A (classic hemophilia) and von Willebrand's disease. The factor VIII activity of an adult patient is increased by approximately 2% for each bag of cryoprecipitated factor VIII administered. Enough should be given to raise the activity level to 30% of normal in order to treat or prevent minor hemorrhage, to 50% to prevent hemorrhage following minor operations, and to 75% to prevent hemorrhage following major procedures. Ideally, units from donors with the identical ABO blood group to that of the recipient should be used. Owing to its high fibrinogen content, this preparation can also be used for fibrinogen replacement. Unlike cryoprecipitated factor VIII, the AHF preparation does not have the von Willebrand's factor and is suitable for treating only hemophilia A. It is heat-treated to inactivate all the HIV and some of the hepatitis viruses. It is the preferred product for repeated transfusion in hemophiliacs.

Homologous Blood Transfusion Reactions

Despite advances in testing of blood groups and subtypes and in fractionation and storage of blood components, transfusion reactions still occur in approximately 3% of the units of blood transfused. The recipient can react to both the formed elements and the soluble proteins of the donor's blood. Although ABO-incompatible transfusion reactions are potentially fatal, reactions to other blood or plasma proteins are less serious.

Febrile Reactions

Febrile reactions occur in 1–2% of all transfusions. A transfusion-related fever may be due to lysis of incompatible red cells, reaction to white cells and other proteins, or cytokines released by white cells. The latter is more common and can be prevented by the use of leukocyte-poor red cells or washed red cells.

Allergic Reactions

Development of mild urticaria during transfusion is as common as febrile reactions. This can be treated or prevented with administration of an antihistamine (chlorpheniramine, 10 mg, given intravenously with each unit of blood but not exceeding 40 mg in 24 hours). On rare occasions bronchospasm, angioneurotic edema, and frank anaphylaxis are seen, particularly in recipients with strong anti–immunoglobulin A (IgA) antibodies. When an anaphylactic reaction occurs, the transfusion should be stopped and complications should be treated with epinephrine, bronchodilators, antihistamines, steroids, and other supportive measures as outlined under "Anaphylactic and Anaphylactoid Reactions" in Chapter 16. Washed red blood cells and IgA-deficient plasma should be requested for these persons in future transfusions.

Acute Hemolytic Transfusion Reactions

Acute hemolytic transfusion reactions are the consequence of lysis of the donor's red cells by the recipient's serum, as a result of ABO incompatibility. Renal failure and disseminated intravascular coagulation are the most serious complications of incompatible blood transfusion. The immediate clinical signs of a reaction are chills, pyrexia, headaches, paresthesia, restlessness, nausea and vomiting, chest pain, shortness of breath, tachycardia, and hypotension. Most of these signs are masked in the anesthetized surgical patient, except cyanosis, hypotension, and general oozing at the surgical site. Treatment should include the following measures:

1. Stop infusing the incompatible blood immediately and send the unused fraction back to the blood bank for examination. (If the patient still requires blood, use compatible blood when it becomes available.)
2. Increase the inspired oxygen fraction.

3. Treat bronchospasm.

4. Support the circulation.

5. Monitor urine output and induce diuresis with mannitol.

6. Consider alkalinizing the urine. (Renal failure following massive intravascular hemolysis is due to the precipitation of acid hematin in distal tubules, which can be minimized by increasing urine flow. Increasing urine pH may also be protective.)

7. Sample the patient's blood for antibody screening and direct antiglobulin test.

8. Monitor coagulation function and treat disseminated intravascular coagulation.

Delayed Hemolytic Transfusion Reactions

In patients who were exposed and sensitized to red cell antigen of minor subgroups in previous transfusions or pregnancy, the recipient's serum may be found to be compatible with donor red cells having these same antigens in a subsequent crossmatch. However, following transfusion, a rapid rise in antibody titer can develop in the next few days, leading to lysis of transfused red cells. This delayed reaction is usually mild. Some reactions cause few symptoms; others can present as fever or prehepatic jaundice.

Other Complications of Homologous Blood Transfusion

Dilutional Coagulopathy

Packed red blood cells are low in platelets and stored plasma low in labile factors V and VIII. In a massive transfusion, defined as one in which the patient's entire blood volume or more is replaced within 24 hours, depletion of these factors can cause a bleeding diathesis if only packed red cells and stored plasma are transfused. Although dilutational coagulopathy can be corrected by giving platelet concentrates and fresh frozen plasma (see "To Correct Coagulopathies" above), laboratory evidence of low platelet count or elevated prothrombin time and partial thromboplastin time should be sought before embarking on replacement therapy. Excessive bleeding may be the result of inadequate surgical hemostasis or disseminated intravascular coagulation caused by the underlying surgical illness or incompatible transfusion reaction. They should be ruled out.

Hepatitis

The incidence of viral hepatitis in recipients following massive transfusion of stored blood was as high as 32% until the practice of testing all donated blood for hepatitis B and C was introduced. Although the incidence of post-transfusional hepatitis has fallen dramatically, there is still a 1:200,000 chance of contracting hepatitis B and a 1:3300 chance of contracting hepatitis C from each unit of red blood cells or plasma transfused.

Human Retrovirus Infection

The human retroviruses HIV-1 and HIV-2 are responsible for AIDS and the retrovirus HTLV-1 is associated with T-cell leukemia and myelopathy. (The pathogenicity of HTLV-2 retrovirus is unknown, and no simple test can differentiate HTLV-1 from HTLV-2.) Currently all blood banks have instituted procedures to eliminate blood products as a source of these infections by

1. Encouraging persons from high-risk groups to refrain from donating blood
2. Testing all donated blood for HIV and HTLV antibodies
3. Subjecting all factor VIII and IX preparations to heat treatment to kill any AIDS virus that may be present

Because of the latency between exposure and appearance of antibodies, it is conceivable that an occasional unit of contaminated blood will escape detection. It is estimated that the chances of a patient's contracting HIV and HTLV infections following a single unit transfusion are 1 in 225,000 and 1 in 60,000, respectively. This risk will decrease, or even disappear, when testing for the presence of the antigens (instead of the antibodies) in donated blood becomes routine.

Because bank blood is a potential medium for transmission of AIDS and other infectious diseases, the anesthesiologist can help to reduce the incidence of transfusion-related infections by

1. Choosing techniques that limit blood loss in certain types of surgery (e.g., epidural or spinal anesthesia in pelvic and hip surgery and controlled hypotension in radical cancer surgery)
2. Considering the use of procoagulants (aprotinin, epsilon-aminocaproic acid, tranexamic acid, or desmopressin), particularly in cardiac or transplant surgery
3. Prescribing blood products judiciously in the perioperative period
4. Using autologous blood or autotransfusion techniques to decrease dependence on bank blood, as described below

Other Infectious Diseases

In addition to hepatitis B and C, HIV-1 and -2, and HTLV-1, all donated blood is screened for syphilis infection. Nevertheless, banked blood is a potential medium for transmission of infectious diseases, including CMV and Epstein-Barr virus infections, malaria, brucellosis, toxoplasmosis, and Colorado tick fever. However, these incidents are relatively uncommon if donors are carefully selected.

Potassium Intoxication

Potassium diffuses out of red cells as stored blood ages. The potassium concentration of 35-day-old stored blood may be as high as 25 mEq/L. These potassium ions are recaptured by the red cells when they have regained their metabolic function. Therefore, hyperkalemia is not seen in the recipient even after transfusion of a large volume of stored blood. During rapid transfusion, this high potassium concentration of stored blood can cause myocardial depression and cardiac standstill during its first pass through the coronary circulation. Furthermore, stored blood is low in calcium ion concentration and is cold; these characteristics can aggravate the myocardial depressant effect of a high potassium concentration.

Citrate Intoxication

Stored blood is prevented from coagulating by the addition of a citrate and phosphate—containing solution to remove calcium ions. Owing to an excess of citrate, hypocalcemia is a potential complication following massive transfusion of whole blood or plasma. Fortunately, citrate is metabolized rapidly by the liver. A large drop in serum calcium ion concentration is unlikely, unless whole blood or plasma is administered at a rapid rate or the recipient is hypothermic. It is recommended that 500 mg of calcium gluconate or chloride should be given for every two units of whole blood or plasma transfused if it is given at a rate of one unit every 5 minutes or faster.

Acid-Base Abnormalities

Thirty five—day-old banked blood has a pH of 6.9 or lower. It is acidotic because of added citrate anticoagulant and accumulation of lactate from anaerobic metabolism of stored red cells. Patients who have received a massive transfusion may become acidotic initially, but the acidosis is never serious if plasma volume, cardiac output, and body temperature are maintained at normal levels. With time, the citrate is metabolized to pyruvate and bicarbonate and metabolic acidosis will give way to metabolic alkalosis.

Hypothermia

Rapid transfusion of a large volume of cold stored blood can cause a large drop in body temperature, particularly in the anesthetized patient. Hypothermia involving the body core or the myocardium locally is a contributing factor in many reported cases of cardiac arrest associated with massive transfusion; it can also slow the enzymatic cascade of normal coagulation and contribute to the development of coagulopathy. These complications can be alleviated by warming stored blood as it is being infused.

A Practical Guide to Clinical Transfusion

Before giving blood products to a patient, certain procedures should be strictly followed, so that an incompatible transfusion can be avoided. These procedures include determining the recipient's blood group, selecting donor blood that is compatible, testing for compatibility between the donor's red cells and recipient's serum, and verifying the identity of the recipient before transfusion. Because blood and plasma products deteriorate rapidly at room temperature, they should be stored properly before use.

Blood Group Testing and Cross-match

Determination of blood group involves testing the recipient's red cells for A, B, and Rh antigens and screening the serum for most, but not all, of the irregular blood group antibodies. Cross-matching implies checking compatibility of the donor's red cells against the recipient's serum. A full cross-match requires 45 minutes. A short cross-match requires only 15 minutes, but the test is less sensitive. In most situations a full cross-match should be routine, but an abbreviated cross-match can be requested if blood is required urgently. In some life-threatening situations, blood transfusion may be necessary without a cross-match. In the face of such a grave emergency, the patient's blood group and type should be determined, and group- and type-specific blood (i.e., group- and type-identical blood) can be used for immediate transfusion. When group- and type-specific blood is transfused, the chance of a hemolytic transfusion reaction (acute or delayed) is 1 in 1000 per unit transfused in patients who have not had a previous transfusion and 1 in 100 in someone who has. In both instances, transfusing group- and type-specific blood can be made almost as safe as transfusing cross-matched blood, if the recipient's serum is screened for irregular antibodies and donor red blood cells with the correspondent antigens are avoided.

Another common practice in dire emergencies is to transfuse un-cross-matched group O red cells. Whole blood contains nearly 300 ml of plasma per pack, and group O *whole blood* can contain potent anti-A and anti-B antibodies in its plasma that can destroy the red cells of recipients whose blood group is A, B, or AB. Therefore, use of group O whole blood in emergency transfusion is discouraged. Group O *packed red blood cells* contains only 50 ml of plasma in each unit and can be used to replace red cell loss in an emergency until cross-matched units are available. (Plasma loss can be replaced with physiologic saline or a plasma expander.) Having no antigens on the cell stroma, O-negative packed red blood cells from so-called universal donors is ideal. However, because of a shortage of group O-negative blood, group O-positive packed red cells are used in male patients and postmenopausal female patients while group O-negative packed red cells are reserved for potentially fertile female patients in many trauma centers. Rh-negative recipients who are given Rh-positive red cells usually exhibit only delayed hemolytic transfusion reactions that are not serious. Nevertheless, after a massive transfusion of group O packed red cells, passively acquired anti-A and anti-B hemolysin levels in the recipient can become high enough to lyse A, B, or AB donor red cells subsequently transfused. (The recipient's own A, B, or AB red cell mass would be extremely low after a massive transfusion; lysis of these red cells would not present any problem.) Therefore, it is important to continue with group O red blood cell transfusion in group A, B, or AB recipients if more than 1.5 units/10 kg body weight has been used in the initial phase of resuscitation. Transfusion using red blood cells that match the patient's own blood group should not begin until the acquired anti-A and anti-B antibody titers have fallen to safe levels.

Identifying the Recipient

Incompatible transfusions are usually the result of clerical rather than technical error. Properly identifying both blood products to be used and the recipient is the only way to avoid a mistake. The patient's name, birth date, and hospital number on the label of the blood or plasma pack should match those on the patient's chart and identification bracelet; group and type of donor's blood should match the recipient's. This checking procedure should be witnessed by one other responsible hospital staff member. Only properly labeled blood or plasma products should be accepted.

Storage of Blood Products

Blood products are expensive, even with a voluntary donor service. In order to avoid deterioration, whole blood, red cell concentrates, and plasma should be stored at 1−6° C in a nearby thermostatically regulated refrigerator until used. If the container bag of the product has been entered during preparation, it is potentially contaminated and should be infused when processed. Activity of labile clotting factors in thawed fresh frozen plasma as well as that of cryoprecipitated factor VIII preparations, and function of platelets in pooled concentrates, deteriorate rapidly. These products should be infused as soon as they are prepared.

Infusion Sets and Filters

A disposable infusion set with an in-line filter should be standard equipment for infusing blood or plasma products. When whole blood or red cell preparations are infused, use of an 18-gauge or larger intravenous cannula is recommended so that an acceptable infusion rate can be achieved. Before and after the infusion of blood, the infusion set should be flushed with normal saline. Not all intravenous solutions are compatible with stored blood. The calcium in lactated Ringer's solution can promote clotting, and solutions containing glucose or dextran can cause rouleau formation.

An in-line filter has a pore size of 80−175 μm. It removes larger cellular debris and clots and should be used for infusion of all blood and plasma products. A new set should be used for platelet concentrate transfusion; trapped debris in a used set can cause platelet aggregation. Because fibrinous clots trapped by the filter provide a good culture medium for bacteria, the infusion set and its filter should be discarded after transfusion is complete.

Several disposable microfilters with pore sizes of 10−40 μm are available that remove microscopic cellular aggregates believed to be the cause of post-transfusion respiratory insufficiency. Because these filters trap a significant amount of platelets, they should not be used during platelet transfusion. Furthermore, the ability of these filters to reduce the incidence of post-transfusion respiratory insufficiency is largely unproved. These filters are indicated only for high-volume transfusions or for patients with pre-existing pulmonary disease.

Blood Warmers

Incorporation of a blood-warming device in the infusion line eliminates complications associated with the use of cold stored blood during massive and rapid transfusion. Warming of blood can be achieved with a thermostatically controlled water bath or dry bath. In order to avoid damage to red cells and plasma proteins, the temperature of the bath should be kept at 37° C. The practice of prewarming blood in an oven is not recommended.

Infusion Rate

Infusion rate is largely determined by the nature of the problem that necessitates the transfusion. In most cases, transfusion of a unit of blood or its components should be completed within 4 hours, but patients with cardiac disease may not tolerate transfusion of blood even at this slow rate. In order to avoid fluid overload in these patients, pretreatment with a diuretic should be considered.

Transfusion under pressure to increase the infusion rate is necessary for patients who are bleeding actively. This can be achieved by applying pressure to the plastic bag with an inflatable compressor or by using a hand pump in the infusion set. Injection of air into the container to achieve pressurization is absolutely contraindicated. It should be remembered that a large-bore intravenous cannula will do more to improve infusion rate than high pressure.

■ Autologous Blood Transfusion

Autologous blood transfusion involves collecting the patient's blood and reinfusing it when required. Three methods, practiced independently or in combination with one another, are available to surgical patients: predeposition of blood before elective surgery, preoperative phlebotomy and hemodilution, and intraoperative blood salvage. Autologous transfusion is complementary to but does not supplant the use of homologous blood products.

Predeposition of Blood

Most blood bank facilities will accept predeposition of autologous blood for use in elective surgical procedures provided that significant blood loss is anticipated and that the patient-donor meets the following criteria:

1. Has a hemoglobin concentration of at least 110 g/L (11 g/dl) and a hematocrit of 0.33 (33%) before each phlebotomy.

2. Is free of cardiorespiratory, neurovascular, or other systemic disease that makes blood donation unsafe.

3. Does not have sepsis and has not been on antibiotics in the last 72 hours.

4. Tests negative for hepatitis B and C, HIV-1 and -2, HTLV-1, and syphilis. (To accept seropositive blood would expose blood bank personnel and hospital staff to the risk of infection and the possibility of contaminating homologous products inadvertently.)

Arrangements can also be made for designated donors to deposit homologous blood based on the same criteria. No age criterion is set for predeposition of blood. A volume of 450 ml is collected from candidates weighing 50 kg or more, and a proportionately smaller volume from subjects weighing less.

Because blood anticoagulated with CPDA-1 has a shelf life of 35 days at 1–6° C, weekly phlebotomy for 4 weeks up to 72 hours before the operation will make available four units of whole blood at the time of surgery. In the perioperative period, predeposited units are given as required in the order of collection. All patient-donors in such a program are given oral iron supplements daily. That and the stimulus of repeated phlebotomy "prime" the bone marrow to produce red cells at an accelerated rate. This is an added advantage of blood predeposition before surgery.

Preoperative Phlebotomy and Hemodilution

In this technique, phlebotomy is performed immediately before surgery, either before or after induction of anesthesia. Up to two units of whole blood is collected from adults, and circulating volume is maintained at a normal level by a continuous infusion of physiologic saline or plasma expander as blood is withdrawn. Like bank blood, the phlebotomized blood should be anticoagulated with CPDA-1 or CP2D solution, not heparin. In the perioperative period, the collected blood is returned to the patient as required. The unit of diluted blood collected last is infused first. Unused units should not be redirected to the homologous supply.

Preoperative phlebotomy and hemodilution can be practiced on all healthy surgical patients with normal preoperative hemoglobin concentrations and hematocrits if significant blood loss is anticipated during the procedure. This technique has several advantages:

1. Hemodilution decreases blood viscosity and improves microcirculation and tissue perfusion.

2. Loss of red cell mass is reduced during intraoperative bleeding.

3. Blood collected is fresh and all clotting factors are intact.

Intraoperative Blood Salvage

This technique involves collecting shed blood for reinfusion. The collected blood is simply filtered before retransfusion in one system, and the red cells are separated, washed, and resuspended in saline before reinfusion in another. The former is simple to operate but carries the risk of infusing cellular debris, platelet aggregates, activated coagulation factors, anticoagulants, free hemoglobin, and air into the patient with the salvaged blood. While the latter system is free of the above complications, it requires expensive automated equipment and the attention of a full-time technologist. The time required to process salvaged blood also means some delay in returning red cells to the patient. Neither method is suitable for salvage of blood in areas contaminated by sepsis or malignant cells.

Anesthetic Mishaps, Quality Assurance, and Risk Management

23

The frequency of litigation associated with medical practice has increased sharply in recent years, both in North America and in Western Europe. The awards in many of the cases settled also have escalated dramatically, sometimes to amounts that were unthinkable just a few years ago. There are many reasons for these changes. Society today is better educated and has a greater abundance of material wealth than ever before. Not only is the general public increasingly aware of the progress in modern medicine, but many regard these advances as assurance of abundance in health. With rising expectations, demands for perfection in the results of care and treatment are only natural.

Administration of an anesthetic is a complex and demanding pursuit fraught with pitfalls and hazards. Anesthesia is a high-risk specialty, not least with regard to the potential for litigation. The anesthesiologist, being a member of the surgical team, may also be named in suits in which he or she has no direct responsibility. This chapter is not a dissertation on medical jurisprudence but focuses instead on safely conducted anesthesia, which reduces the opportunities for mishaps and thus the frequency of litigation.

Anesthetic Mishaps

It has been estimated that perioperative mortality attributable to anesthesia occurs at a rate of 1 in 10,000 anesthetic procedures. However, there are no data on the prevalence of anesthetic accidents or the incidence of nonfatal anesthetic injuries. All anesthetic accidents have the potential to cause harm. Of all "critical incidents," 6.5% can be expected to be associated with unfavorable outcomes (death, cardiac arrest, canceled procedure, and extra stay in recovery room, intensive care unit, or hospital).

When mishaps in the operating room are analyzed, certain recurring problems are identified:

1. Mistaken identity of the patient leading to incorrect operation or mismatched transfusion.

2. Incorrect position of the patient on the operating table leading to nerve palsy or cardiovascular and respiratory embarrassment (see "Positioning the Patient on the Operating Table" in Chapter 15).

3. Misuse or malfunction of anesthetic equipment leading to asphyxia, barotrauma of the airway, and other injuries (Table 23–1).

4. Misuse or malfunction of electrical instruments leading to burns or electrocution.

5. Complications associated with the use of intravenous equipment leading to misplaced catheters, embolization of catheter fragments, air embolism, and so forth.

TABLE 23–1. Mishaps Associated with Use of Anesthetic Equipment

EQUIPMENT	POSSIBLE MALFUNCTION OR MISUSE
Anesthetic Machine	
Gas supply	Incorrect connection, leaks, empty cylinders, total disruption of pipeline supply
Flowmeters	Incorrect settings, leaks
Vaporizers	Wrong agent, leaks, toxic dose through malfunction or malposition, errors in calibration
Anesthetic Circuit	Disconnection, leaks, improper connection (especially with the circle system), improper setting of APL valve and pressure-limiting device leading to high airway pressure
Ventilator	Disconnection, leak, failure of changeover mechanism, loss of power
Ancillary Equipment	
Laryngoscope	Damage to teeth and lips, failure of light source (especially in an emergency such as rapid-sequence induction)
Endotracheal tube	Bronchial or esophageal intubation, leakage, rupture of cuff, disconnection, accidental extubation, obstruction (caused by kinking, compression, herniated cuff)
Malleable stylet	Perforation of airway
Laryngeal spray	Systemic toxicity of local anesthetics
Suction apparatus	Failure (especially during an emergency)

6. Improper labeling of drugs leading to administration of the wrong drug or gross overdose.

7. Improper monitoring of the patient's condition and failure to recognize signs of impending danger.

It is rare that an isolated incident results in catastrophe. Although equipment malfunction appears to be involved in a large number of these accidents, there is almost always some degree of additional human error that compounds the problem. The human factor is commonly related to a lack of vigilance resulting from haste, fatigue, or distraction. Inexperience or inadequate knowledge about the equipment, technique, or procedure also has been found to contribute to disaster.

Prevention of Mishaps

It is agreed that many of the incidents described are avoidable. A concerted effort to reduce their occurrence requires that attention be focused on the patient, on the proper care and use of anesthetic and ancillary equipment, and on maintaining vigilance. The importance of properly identifying the patient and nature and site of the operation and of assessing the patient's medical condition has been discussed in previous chapters.

Proper Care and Use of Equipment

In a specialty such as anesthesiology, where there is a broad interface between sophisticated technology and clinical methods, it is mandatory that practitioners understand the principles and workings of the equipment they use. Only equipment that meets current safety standards should be installed. When new standards are issued or old ones revised, anesthesiologists have the responsibility of upgrading the equipment in their own institutions. All incidents of malfunction or potential misuse should be reported immediately so that they can be acted on and rectified without delay.

Although the function of all electrical instruments and anesthetic equipment is checked periodically by the technical staff of the hospital, it is the duty of the anesthesiologist to ensure that these devices are in satisfactory condition and functioning properly every time they are used. To do so, the anesthesiologist should develop a checklist somewhat similar to those used by aircraft pilots for routine preflight equipment checks. The checklist should be comprehensive enough for safe practice yet convenient enough for frequent use. Procedures for checking the anesthetic machine, the anesthetic circuit, the ventilator, and intubation equipment have been discussed in previous chapters. The following scheme can easily be incorporated into routines that include checking the patient and drugs:

1. *Patient:* identity, nature and site of operation, consent, availability of blood (if applicable)

2. *Anesthetic machine:* gas supply (pipelines and cylinders), flowmeters, vaporizers oxygen flush control, oxygen analyzer, alarm

3. *Anesthetic circuit:* connection to machine, reservoir bag, APL (or relief) valve, safety pop-off valve, leaks, specific components of individual circuits (e.g., soda lime canister of the circle system, inner tubing of the Bain circuit)

4. *Ventilator:* bellows, inspiratory phase, changeover from inspiration to expiration, expiratory phase, changeover from expiration to inspiration, leaks

5. *Endotracheal equipment:* laryngoscope (type and size of blade, light source); endotracheal tube (size, length, integrity of cuff); ancillary equipment (intubation forceps, malleable stylet, laryngeal spray, lubricant, cuff inflator)

6. *Suction apparatus:* source, tubing, and catheter

7. *Intravenous drugs:* anesthetics, relaxants, narcotic analgesics, other drugs (e.g., vasopressors), correct labels

In many ways the working environment of anesthesiologists is not conducive to safety. Unlike airplane pilots, they have yet to benefit from the consideration of ergonomic design in the operating room, but they can position themselves and their equipment to obtain a convenient view of the anesthetic machine, the monitors, and the patient, and they should allow themselves sufficient space to operate efficiently. The work table and top of the anesthetic machine should be kept tidy. A neatly organized working environment minimizes distraction and decreases fatigue.

Vigilance and Diligence

Vigilance is the key to successful monitoring. Although it is customary to record vital signs only every 5 minutes, it must be remembered that cerebral dysfunction and death can occur within 10 seconds and 4 minutes, respectively, after the onset of cerebral anoxia. Therefore, some form of continuous monitoring of oxygenation (e.g., color of skin or shed blood and pulse oximetry) and cardiac output (e.g., heart sounds) is mandatory. (Pulse oximetry will do both.)

Unfortunately, eternal vigilance is not a human characteristic. It is often during the calm of the maintenance phase that distraction and fatigue become more evident and attention lapses. It is therefore not surprising that over half of reported mishaps occur during this period. In recognition of this problem, automated monitoring instruments with alarms have been introduced (see Chapter 14). Although these devices are undeniably useful, they are only aids, not substitutes for the discipline of vigilance. The diligence of the anesthesiologist is still required.

In the Event of Mishaps

The operating room environment is a critical area for mishaps. Most anesthesiologists will admit that they have experienced minor mishaps more than once in their careers. How, then, should these mishaps be handled?

First and foremost, the situation should be corrected as rapidly and completely as possible and assistance should be summoned if the need arises. All that has taken place should then be documented very thoroughly at the earliest opportunity, although this may be difficult in the heat of the moment. A thorough documentation made at the time of the incident is of paramount importance if the anesthesiologist is unfortunate enough to be involved in litigation as a result of the misadventure. Memory for details is notoriously short.

At the postoperative visit, the anesthesiologist should explain to the patient, as fully as possible, the circumstances of the occurrence. This should be a complete and truthful explanation, with due respect and sympathy, so that the patient can understand exactly what has befallen him or her and yet have some insight into the anesthesiologist's difficulties. In most cases patients are not hostile, and they may even volunteer information concerning previously unrecognized predisposing factors that may absolve the anesthesiologist. The anesthesiologist can gain the respect of the patient by discussing the matter frankly.

If there is any possibility that legal action will follow, the anesthesiologist should contact his or her medical defense organization or the insurance carrier as soon as possible. The serving of a writ and a statement of claim outlining the complaints of the injured party (the plaintiff) may be the first intimation that legal action is being taken. In this situation, it is imperative that the defense organization or insurance carrier be contacted immediately because the defendant's position may be jeoparadized if this first action is not taken at the earliest opportunity.

The defense organization or insurance carrier will no doubt require complete details of the incident. The most important rule to follow in any episode is to be complete, in content and veracity, in the information that is given. It should be remembered that the legal process may move very slowly, so it may be years before a case comes before the courts. The parties concerned are rarely able to remember the details required of them if records are not available. If the details of a mode of treatment are not recorded, it may be assumed erroneously that the treatment was not given. Therefore, impeccable record keeping can assist the defense considerably.

■ Quality Assurance and Risk Management

It is obvious from previous sections that all health care institutions should set standards for anesthesia practice and direct efforts to prevent mishaps. The Joint Commission on Accreditation of Healthcare Organizations has ruled that all health care facilities should establish quality assurance/risk management programs in clinical departments.

Quality assurance in the health care industry refers to a dynamic process by which standards of services in an institution are defined and achievement of these standards is assured by assessment of outcome. The goal of *risk management* is to prevent accidents and injuries and to cope with the consequences should they occur. These two processes are necessarily related: both involve detection, evaluation, and resolution of problems as well as follow-up re-evaluation of the effect of the process. While quality asssurance defines the quality of care, risk management removes the potential to cause harm. Through prevention, risk management improves the quality of care.

To establish a quality assurance and risk management program, the department should establish policy and credential criteria for members of its staff, draw up procedural manuals and guidelines of safe practice, and set up audit and review committees. These committees should be concerned with issues in three areas: structure, process, and outcome. In anesthesia practice, *structure* refers to all physical facilities and their utilization (e.g., availability of capnographs and pulse oximeters, policies on their utility in the operating suite). *Process* is the way anesthesia is practiced by members of the staff (e.g., compliance with monitoring guidelines, completeness of record). *Outcome* in anesthesia practice is measured by prevalence of critical incidents and anesthetic complications (e.g., accidental extubation, intraoperative hypotension and hypovolemia, perioperative deaths). Problems in all three areas can be identified by the reporting of untoward events (called indicators) and audits of these events. When a problem is identified, its implications should be thoroughly assessed, corrective procedures recommended and implemented, and progress followed up and re-evaluated at a later date.

A quality assurance and risk management program can be carried out successfully by a department only with the full cooperation of its staff. In order to encourage and foster honesty, the program must be nonthreatening to its participants. It should be made clear that documentations collected for the purpose of quality assurance cannot be used as evidence in a lawsuit. (In some countries, including the United States, such data are protected by peer review legislation.) Quality assurance activities should be directed to improve the performance of staff members. They should not be used as a yardstick for promotion evaluation, nor should disciplinary actions result directly from them.

Further Reading I

General

Aldrete JA, Kroulik D: A postanesthetic recovery score. Anesth Analg 49:924, 1970.

Berry AJ, Greene ES: The risk of needlestick injuries and needlestick-transmitted diseases in the practice of anesthesiology. Anesthesiology 77:1007, 1992.

Ellis H, Felman S: Anatomy for Anaesthetists. Oxford, England, Blackwell Scientific Publications, 1993.

Guedel AE: Inhalational Anesthesia. A Fundamental Guide. New York, MacMillan, 1937.

Lubin MF, Walker HK, Smith RB (eds): Medical Management of the Surgical Patient, ed 3. Philadelphia, Lippincott, 1995.

Martin JT (ed): Positioning in Anesthesia and Surgery, ed 2. Philadelphia, WB Saunders Company, 1988.

Nunn JF: Applied Respiratory Physiology, ed 4. Oxford; Boston: Butterworth-Heinemann, 1993.

Rao TL, Jacobs KH, El-Etr AA: Reinfarction following anesthesia in patients with myocardial infarction. Anesthesiology 59:499, 1983.

Smith G, Rowbotham DJ (eds): Supplement on Postoperative Nausea and Vomiting. Br J Anaesth 69: Supp 1, 1992.

Steen PA, Tinker JH, Tarhan S: Myocardial reinfarction after anesthesia and surgery. JAMA 239:2566, 1978.

Stoelting RK, Dierdorf SF (eds): Anesthesia and Co-existing Disease, ed 3. New York, Churchill-Livingstone, 1993.

Tarhan S, Moffit EA, Taylor WF: Myocardial infarction after general anesthesia. JAMA 220:1451, 1972.

Airway Management

American Society of Anesthesiologists Task Force on Management of the Difficult Airway: Practice guideline for management of the difficult airway. Anesthesiology 78:597, 1993.

Benumof JL (ed): Airway Management: Principles and Practice. St. Louis, Mosby—Year Book, 1995.

Cormack RS, Lehane J: Difficult tracheal intubation in obstetrics. Anaesthesia 39:1105, 1984.

Finucane BT, Santora AH: Principles of Airway Management, ed 2. St. Louis, Mosby—Year Book, 1995.

Knill RL: Difficult laryngoscopy made easy with "BURP." Can J Anaesth 40:798, 1993.

Mallampati SR, Gatt SP, Gugino LD, et al: A clinical sign to predict difficult tracheal intubation: A prospective study. Can J Anaesth 32: 429, 1985.
Ovassapian A: Fiberoptic Airway Endoscopy in Anesthesia and Critical Care. New York, Raven Press, 1990.

Anesthesia Equipment

Dorsch JA, Dorsch SE: Understanding Anesthesia Equipment: Construction, Care and Complications, ed 3. Baltimore, Williams & Wilkins, 1994.
Ehrenwerth, J, Eisenkraft JB (eds): Anesthesia Equipment: Principles and Applications. St. Louis, Mosby—Year Book, 1993.
U.S. Food and Drug Administration: Anesthesia apparatus checkout recommendations, 1993. Federal Register (59 FR 35373), July 11, 1994.

History of Anesthesia

Atkinson RS, Boulton TB: The History of Anaesthesia. Pearl River, Parthenon Publishing Group, 1989.
Duncum BM: The Development of Inhalation Anaesthesia. Oxford, England, Oxford University Press, 1947.
Keys TE: The History of Surgical Anesthesia. New York, Schuman, 1945.
Rupreht J, van Lieburg MJ, Lee JA, Erdmann W (eds): Anaesthesia: Essays on its History. Berlin, Springer-Verlag, 1985.
Sykes WS: Essays on the First Hundred Years of Anaesthesia, vols I, II and III. Edinburgh, Churchill-Livingstone, 1982.

Malignant Hyperthermia

Kaplan RF: Malignant hyperthermia. In: Refresher Course Manual. American Society of Anesthesiologists, 1992.
Levitt RC, Olckers A, Meyers S, et al: Evidence of the localization of malignant hyperthermia susceptibility locus (MHS2) to human chromosome 17q. Genomics 14:562, 1992.
Littleford JA, Patel LR, Bose D, et al: Masseter muscle spasm in children: Implications of continuing the triggering anesthetic. Anesth Analg 72:151, 1991.
MacLennan DH: The genetic basis of malignant hyperthermia. Trends Pharmacol Sci 13:330, 1992.
MacLennan DH, Duff C, Zorzato F, et al: Ryanodine receptor gene is a candidate for predisposition to malignant hyperthermia. Nature 343: 559, 1990.
McCarthy TV, Healy JMS, Hefron JJA, et al: Localization of the malignant hyperthermia susceptibility locus to human chromosome 19q12-13.2. Nature 343:563, 1990.

Mechanical Ventilation

Marini JJ, Ravenscraft SA: Principles and Practice of Mechanical Ventilation. Baltimore, Williams & Wilkins, 1994.

Tobin MJ (ed): Principles and Practice of Mechanical Ventilation: New York, Health Profession Division, McGraw-Hill, 1994.

Mechanism of Anesthetic Drug Action

Bowman WC, Prior C, Marshall IG: Presynaptic receptors in the neuromuscular junction. Ann N Y Acad Sci 604:69, 1990.

Chang KJ, Cooper BR, Hazum E, Cuatrecasas P: Multiple opiate receptors: Different regional distribution in the brain and differential binding of opiates and opioid peptides. Molec Pharmacol 16:91, 1979.

Changeux JP, Giraudat J, Dennis M: The nicotinic acetylcholine receptor: Molecular architecture of a ligand-regulated ion channel. Trends Pharmacol Sci 8:459, 1987.

Costa E, Guidotti A: Molecular mechanisms in the receptor action of benzodiazepines. Annu Rev Pharmacol Toxicol 19:531, 1979.

Franks NP, Lieb WR: Do general anesthetics act by competitive binding to specific receptors? Nature 310:599, 1984.

Franks NP, Lieb WR: Molecular mechanisms of general anesthesia. Nature 300:487, 1982.

Gage PW: Generation of end-plate potentials. Physiol Rev 56:117, 1976.

Gasic GP, Hollman M: Molecular neurobiology of glutamate receptors. Annu Rev Physiol 54:507, 1992.

Ho IK: Mechanism of action of barbiturates. Annu Rev Pharmacol Toxicol 21:83, 1981.

Kobilka B: Adrenergic receptors as models for G protein-coupled receptors. Annu Rev Neurosci 15:87, 1992.

Ling GSF, Pasternak GW: Spinal and supraspinal opioid analgesia in the mouse: The role of subpopulations of opioid binding sites. Brain Res 271:152, 1983.

Martin D, Lodge D: Ketamine acts as a non-competitive N-methyl-D-aspartate antagonist on frog spinal cord in vitro. Neuropharmacology 24:999, 1985.

Millar SL: A theory of gaseous anesthetics. Proc Natl Acad Sci (USA) 47:1515, 1961.

Miller RJ, Cuatrecasas P: Neurobiology and neuropharmacology of the enkephalins. Adv Biochem Psychopharmacol 20:187, 1979.

Narahashi T: Drug-ionic interactions: Single-channel measurements. Ann Neurol 16:S39, 1984.

Nicoll RA, Malenka RC, Kauer JA: Functional comparison of neurotransmitter receptor subtypes in mammalian central nervous system. Physiol Rev 70:513, 1990.

Olsen RW: Drug interactions at the GABA receptor-inophore complex. Annu Rev Pharmacol Toxicol 22:245, 1985.

Pasternak GW: Pharmacological mechanisms of opioid analgesics. Clin Neuropharmacol 16:1, 1993

Pauling L: A molecular theory of general anesthesia. Science 134:15, 1961.

Roth SH, Miller KW: Cellular and Molecular Mechanisms of Anesthetics. New York, Plenum Press, 1986.

Seeman P: The membrane actions of anesthetics and tranquillizers. Pharmacol Rev 24:583, 1972.

Sieghart W: GABA$_A$ receptors: Ligand-gated Cl$^-$ ion channels modulated by multiple drug-binding sites. Trends Pharmacol Sci 13:446, 1992.

Strichartz G: Molecular mechanisms of nerve block by local anesthetics. Anesthesiology 45:421, 1976.

Trudell JR: A unitary theory of anesthesia based on lateral phase separations in nerve membrane. Anesthesiology 46:5, 1977.

Monitoring

Blitt CD: Monitoring in Anesthesia, ed 3. New York, Churchill Livingstone, 1994.

Smith NT, Saidman LJ: Monitoring in Anesthesia. Newton, Butterworth-Heinemann, 1993.

Standards for Basic Anesthetic Monitoring. American Society of Anesthesiologists, October 25, 1995.

Outpatient Surgery

Chung F: Recovery pattern and home-readiness after ambulatory surgery. Anesth Analg 80:896, 1995.

McGoldrick KE: Ambulatory Anesthesiology: A Problem Oriented Approach. Baltimore, Williams & Wilkins, 1995.

Ong BY, Palahniuk RJ, Cumming M: Gastric volume and pH in outpatients. Can J Anaesth: 25:36, 1978.

Pain Management

American Society of Anesthesiologists Task Force on Pain Management, Acute Pain Section: Practice guidelines for acute pain management in the perioperative setting. Anesthesiology, 82:1071, 1995.

Ferrante FM, VadeBoncouer TR (eds): Postoperative Pain Management. New York, Churchill Livingstone, 1993.

Heath M, Thomas VJ: Patient-Controlled Analgesia: Confidence in Postoperative Pain Control. New York, Oxford University Press, 1993.

Melzack R, Wall PD: Pain mechanism: A new theory. Science 150:971, 1965.

Pharmacology

Bevan DR, Bevan JC, Donati F: Muscle Relaxants in Clinical Anesthesia. Chicago, Year Book Medical Publishers, 1988.

Bowdle TA, Horita A, Kharasch ED (eds): The Pharmacologic Basis of Anesthesiology. New York, Churchill Livingstone, 1994.

Freye E, Coleman WA: Opioid Agonists, Antagonists and Mixed Narcotic Analgesics: Theoretical Background and Consideration for Practical Use. New York, Springer-Verlag, 1987.

Griffith HR, Johnson GE: The use of curare in general anesthesia. Anesthesiology 3:148, 1942.

Morgan M, Vickers, MD: Drugs in Anesthetic Practice. Newton, Butterworth-Heinemann, 1991.

Practice Guidelines

Basic Standards for Preanesthesia Care. American Society of Anesthesiologists, October 14, 1987.
Guideline for Ambulatory Surgical Facilities. American Society of Anesthesiologists, October 12, 1988.
Guidelines for the Ethical Practice of Anesthesiology. American Society of Anesthesiologists, October 25, 1995.
Guidelines for Patient Care in Anesthesiology. American Society of Anesthesiologists, October 16, 1985.
Guidelines to the Practice of Anaesthesia. Canadian Anesthetists' Society, 1995.
Standards for Postanesthesia Care. American Society of Anesthesiologists, October 19, 1994.

Quality Assurance

Angran DM: Selecting, developing and evaluating indicators. Am J Hosp Pharm 48:1931, 1991.
Cooper JB, Cullen DJ, Eichhorn JH, et al: Administrative guides for response to an adverse anesthesia event. J Clin Anesth 5:79, 1993.
Cooper JB, Newbower R, Kitz RJ: An analysis of major errors and equipment failures in anesthesia management: Considerations for prevention and detection. Anesthesiology 60:34, 1984.
Deasy TL: Quality improvement: The gurus and their approaches. Int Anesthesiol Clin 30:1, 1992.
Donabedian A: The role of outcomes in quality assessment and assurance. Qual Rev Bull 18:356, 1992.
Everett WD: An epidemiological approach to quality assurance in the hospital. Health Care Manage Rev 18:91, 1993.

Regional Anesthesia

Brown DL: Atlas of Regional Anesthesia. Philadelphia, W.B. Saunders Company, 1992.
Hahn MB, McQuillan PM: Regional Anesthesia: An Atlas of Anatomy and Techniques. St. Louis, Mosby—Year Book, 1995.

Transfusion Medicine

Ali A (ed): Clinical Guide to Transfusion, ed 3. Canadian Red Cross Society, 1993.
Mollison PL, Engelfriet CP, Contreras M: Blood Transfusion in Clinical Medicine, ed 9. Oxford, England, Blackwell Scientific Publications, 1993.
Salem MR (ed): Blood Conservation in the Surgical Patient. Baltimore, Williams & Wilkins, 1995.
Walker RH (ed): Technical Manual, ed 11. Bethesda, MD, American Association of Blood Banks, 1993.
Widmann FK (ed): Standards for Blood Banks and Transfusion Services, ed 15. Bethesda, MD, American Association of Blood Banks, 1993.

Index

Note: Page numbers in *italics* indicate figures; page numbers followed by t indicate tables.

Absorption, of local anesthetic, 86
Acetaminophen, 270
Acetylcholine. See *Neuromuscular blockade.*
Acetylcholine-gated ion channel, 60–62, *61*
Acid pneumonitis, 229–230
Acid-base balance, abnormalities in, 294–295
   transfusion-induced, 307–308
   in liver disease, 142
   muscle relaxants and, 71
Acidosis, local anesthetic in, 85
   metabolic, 292
      causes of, 294–295
      treatment of, 295
   respiratory, 295
Acquired immunodeficiency syndrome (AIDS), drug abuse and, 151
   transfusion-induced, 306
Action potential, 61–62
Addiction, to heroin, addisonian crisis in, 151
   anesthesia in, 151
   withdrawal in, 258
   to morphine, 49
Addisonian crisis, 151
Adhesive arachnoiditis, 248
Adrenaline, 249
Adrenocortical insufficiency, anesthesia in, 146–147
   in heroin addict, 151
Adrenocorticotropic hormone, release of, 48
Agonist(s), 45, 51–55. See also specific drug, e.g., *Meperidine.*
   competitive, 46
   partial, 45, 55–57
Agonist-antagonist(s), 46, 55–57

Air, color codes for, 98
Airway, carbon dioxide waveform in, *204*, 204–206
   closure of, ventilation-perfusion inequality and, 130
   emergency, 183–185, *184*
   in cocaine intoxication, 151
   obstruction of, during anesthesia, 224–225
      in recovery, 254
   preoperative assessment of, 155–157, *156*
   resistance in, during anesthesia, 133
      in mechanical ventilation, 120
   trauma to, during intubation, 186
Airway management, in anesthetized patient, BURP maneuver in, 181
   Combitube in, 182
   cricothyrotomy airway in, *184*, 184–185
   direct laryngoscopy in. See *Laryngoscopy.*
   emergency airways in, 183–185, *184*
   face mask for, 169t, 215–216
      with satisfactory airway, 181–182
      with unsatisfactory airway, 182–183
   head tilt-jaw thrust maneuver in, 162, *163*
   laryngeal mask airway in, *165*, 165–168, 166t, *167*, 169t, 182–183
   pharyngeal airway in, 163–165, *164*, 179–180, 216
   tracheal intubation in. See *Tracheal intubation.*

Airway management (*Continued*)
transtracheal jet ventilation in,
185
Airway pressure. See also *Pressure*
entries.
monitoring of, 196–198, *197*
Alarm(s), in anesthetic machine,
105–107
in mechanical ventilation, 123–
124
Albumin, collection and storage of,
301
Alcohol, withdrawal from, 258
Alcoholism, anesthesia in, 150
Alcuronium, 66
in renal failure, 144
Aldosteronism, 142
Alfentanil, 53–54
Alimentary fluid, 296t
Alkalosis, metabolic, 295
respiratory, 295
Alkylphenol(s). See also specific
drug, e.g., *Propofol.*
intravenous, 20–21
Allergic reaction. See also
Histamine release.
management of, 231–233
physiology of, 230
preoperative assessment of, 154–
155
to blood transfusion, 304
to colloid solution, 297
to epinephrine, 86
to intravenous anesthetic, 231
to latex, 231
to local anesthetic, 86, 231
to morphine, 49, 231
to muscle relaxant, 231
to opioid, 231
to succinylcholine, 76
Alpha phase, *12*, 12–16, *15*
Alphaprodine, 55
Alveolar concentration, 31t, 31–
32
Alveolar uptake, 32–36, *33*
Alveolar ventilation, carbon
dioxide pressure and, 133
dead space in, 127, 130, 132
inhalation anesthetic and, 34,
128
morphine and, 47
oxygen pressure in, 135
Alveolar-mixed venous tension
gradient, 35
Ambulatory surgery. See
Outpatient surgery.

American Society of
Anesthesiologists, physical
status classification of, 158–
159, 282
Aminoester(s), 87–88
Aminoglycoside(s), 73
Aminophylline, 232
Ammonia, elevated, 142
Analgesia, in ether anesthesia, 9
in general anesthesia, 9–10
narcotic. See *Narcotic*
analgesic(s).
Anaphylactic/anaphylactoid
reaction, 230–233. See also
Allergic reaction; Histamine
release.
Anatomic dead space, 127
Anatomic shunt, 134
Anemia, anesthesia in, 142, 147–
148
in arthritis, 149
in chronic renal failure, 143–
144
Anesthesia, definition of, 3
general. See *General anesthesia.*
history of, 1–3
molecular action mechanisms of,
3–8, *5*, *7*
personnel involved in, 3
regional. See *Regional*
anesthesia.
spinal. See *Spinal anesthesia.*
Anesthesiologist, definition of, 3
Anesthetic(s). See specific drug,
e.g., *Curare*; specific drug
type, e.g., *Inhalation*
anesthetic(s).
Anesthetic circuit, 109–118
adjustable pressure-limiting
valve in, 109–110, *110*, 113,
113, *115*
Ayre's T-piece as, *115*, 115–116
Bain circuit as, *115*, 116
checking of, 117–118, 316–317
circle system as, 112–114, *113*
classification of, 111–112
components of, 109–111
for child, 114
Magill circuit as, 114, *115*
mishaps in, 315t
pressure alarms in, 123
pressure gauge in, 111
reservoir bag in, 110–111, *113*,
115
scavenging devices and, 109
tubing in, 109

Anesthetic circuit (*Continued*)
  Waters to-and-fro circuit as, 116, *117*
  with nonrebreathing valves, 116, *117*
Anesthetic machine, 92–108. See also *Anesthetic circuit.*
  alarms in, 105–107
  back-pressure check valve of, 104, *105*
  checking of, 107–108, 316–317
  color codes for, 98
  common gas outlet of, 97
  components of, 92–97, *93*, *95–96*
  diameter-index safety system of, 101, *101*
  flowmeter of, 94–95, *95*, *102*, 102–103
  gas cylinders of, 98–100, *99–100*
  gas sources for, 93
  mishaps with, 315, 315t
  oxygen control by, analyzer with alarm in, 106–107
    checking of, 107–108
    emergency flush valve in, 97
    failure alarm in, 105–106
    failure safety valve in, 105
    flowmeter for, *102*, 102–103
    minimum flow-ratio controller in, 106
  pin-index safety system of, 100, *100*
  pipeline connections of, *101*, 101–102
  pressure gauges of, 93–94
  pressure regulators of, 94
  quick-mount system of, *101*, 101–102
  safety features of, 97–107, *99–103*, *105*
  safety pressure-relief valve of, *100*, 100–101
  vaporizers of, 95–97, *96*
    agent-specific filling system for, *103*, 103–104
    exclusive control of, 104
Anesthetic mishaps, correction of, 316
  incidence of, 314
  litigation and, 314, 318–319
  prevention of, 316–318
  quality assurance and risk management and, 319–320
  types of, 315t, 315–316

Anesthetist, definition of, 3
Ankylosing spondylitis, 149
Antagonist(s), 57–58. See also specific drug, e.g., *Naloxone.*
Antibiotic(s), 73
Anticholinesterase(s), muscarinic side effects of, 69
  muscle relaxant reversal with, 63–64, 68–70
Anticonvulsant(s), benzodiazepines as, 22
  muscle relaxant interaction with, 73
  propofol as, 21
  thiopental as, 20
Antidiuretic hormone, morphine-induced release of, 48
  pain and, 266
Antiemetic, 161, 259
Antihemophilic factor (factor VIII), 301
Antihistamine, preanesthetic, 161
Anxiety relief, preoperative, 160, 237, 285–286
Aortic regurgitation, 149
Apheresis, leukocyte concentrate from, 300–301
  platelet concentrate from, 300
Apnea, fentanyl-induced, 54
  peripheral nerve stimulation in, 209
Arachnoiditis, adhesive, 248
Areflexia, 9–10
Arrhythmia, during anesthesia, 228–229
  from intubation, 186–187
  succinylcholine-induced, 74
  ventricular, from intubation, 186–187
Arterial pressure, alveolar ventilation and, 135
  direct monitoring of, 193, 232
  in breathing control, 129
  measurement of, 198–199
Arthritis, 149–150
Aspiration, consequences of, 229
  extubation and, 222
  preoperative prevention of, 160–161, 229–230
Asthma, ketamine in, 25
  propofol in, 21
Asystole, 228
Atopy, 154–155
Atracurium, 67
Atrial fibrillation, during anesthesia, 228

Atrial flutter, during anesthesia, 228

Atropine, for lower than normal heart rate, 228
  prophylactic, 69
  sinus tachycardia from, 228
  to reverse muscle relaxant action, 69

Autologous blood patch, 247–248

Autologous blood transfusion. See *Blood transfusion, autologous.*

Automatic breathing, 189

Awake intubation, 177–178

Axillary approach, to brachial plexus block, *242*, 243–244

Ayre's T-piece, *115*, 115–116

Back-pressure check valve, 104, *105*

Bain circuit, *115*, 116

Baralyme, in anesthetic circuit, 112–113, *113*
  sevoflurane and, 43–44, 112

Barbiturate(s). See also specific drug, e.g., *Thiopental.*
  anesthesia depth from, 188
  intravenous, 17–20

Barbiturate coma, 18

Barbotage, 246

Baroreceptor reflex, 21

Behavioral manipulation, 279

Bellows, in mechanical ventilation, 122

Benzodiazepine(s). See also specific drug, e.g., *Diazepam.*
  at GABA-gated ion channel, 5, *5*
  intravenous, 21–24

Beriberi heart disease, 150

Berman intubating airway, *164*, 165, 179–180

Beta phase, *12*, 16–17

Beta-adrenergic antagonist, adrenaline interaction with, 249
  anesthetic interaction with, 138–139

Biochemical abnormality, 142

Blood, albumin from, 301
  components and products of, 299–301
    storage of, 310–311
  cryoprecipitated factor VIII from, 301

Blood (*Continued*)
  intraoperative salvage of, 313
  leukocyte concentrate from, 300
  plasma from, 301
  platelet concentrate from, 300
  red cells in. See *Red blood cell(s).*
  whole, 299

Blood gas, analysis of, 198–200, *199*

Blood loss, measurement of, 194
  replacement of, with crystalloid or colloid solution, 297–298, 298t
    with packed red blood cells, 301–302

Blood patch, autologous, 247–248

Blood pressure. See also *Hypertension; Hypotension.*
  monitoring of, 190–192, 232

Blood sugar, monitoring of, 212
  wound healing and, 146

Blood transfusion, autologous, indications for, 311
  intraoperative blood salvage in, 313
  predisposition of blood for, 311–312
  preoperative phlebotomy and hemodilution for, 312
  for immunocompromised patient, 301
  history of, 299
  homologous, acid-base abnormalities from, 307–308
    blood group testing and cross-matching for, 303, 308–309
    blood product storage in, 310–311
    blood products and components in, 299–301
    blood warmers for, 310–311
    citrate intoxication from, 307
    coagulopathy in, 305
    disease transmission in, 306–307
    guidelines for, 308–309
    hypothermia from, 308
    in anemic surgical patient, 148
    infusion rate in, 311
    infusion sets and filters for, 310
    mishaps in, 315
    potassium intoxication from, 307

Blood transfusion (*Continued*)
  reactions to, 303–305
  recipient identification in, 309, 315
  uses of, 301–303
  to correct coagulopathy, 302–303
  to replace red blood cell loss, 301–302
  to replenish plasma volume, 302
Blood warmer, 310–311
Body temperature. See also
      Hyperthermia; *Hypothermia*;
      Malignant hyperthermia.
  monitoring of, 211–212
Brachial plexus block, 84–85, 240–241
  approaches to, axillary, *242*, 243–244
    interscalene, 241–242, *242*
    supraclavicular, *242*, 242–243
Bradycardia, during anesthesia, 228
  during spinal anesthesia, 246
  morphine-induced, 47
Breath holding, 224
Breathing. See also *Respiratory*
      entries.
  automatic, 189
  physiology of, 128–129
  anesthetics and, 129
Bromsulphalein, 143
Bronchial constriction, 47–48
Bronchial intubation, 187
Bronchospasm, airway carbon
      dioxide waveform in, 204,
      204, 205
  during anesthesia, 226
  from intubation, 186–187
  in allergic reaction, 232
Brucellosis, 307
Bupivacaine, absorption of, 86
  cardiotoxicity of, 90
  clearance of, 87
  in epidural neural blockade, 277
  in lumbar epidural anesthesia, 250
  in spinal anesthesia, 245–246
  pharmacokinetics of, 90
Buprenorphine, 56–57, 271
BURP (backward, upward,
      rightward pressure)
      maneuver, 181
Butorphanol, 56, 271

Butyrophenone(s), 26–27. See also
      specific drug, e.g.,
      Droperidol.

Caffeine, for spinal headache, 247
  malignant hyperthermia and, 234
Calcium channel blocker, 138–139
Calcium chloride, 294, 294t
Capnograph, *203–204*, 203–206, 226, 234
  in recovery room, 253
Carbamazepine, 73
Carbohydrate metabolism, 145
Carbon dioxide, analyzers of, *203–204*, 203–206, 226, 234, 253
  as anesthetic, 1
  color code for, 98
  elimination of, 133, 195
  end-tidal plateau of, *204*, 204–205
  in hypoventilation, 226
Carbon dioxide absorbent, 43–44
Carbon dioxide pressure, arterial,
      alveolar ventilation and, 133
  in breathing control, 129
  measurement of, 198
Carbon dioxide waveform,
      expiratory, 176
  in airway, *204*, 204–206
Carbon monoxyhemoglobin, in
      smoker, 141
Cardiac. See also *Heart.*
Cardiac arrest, during spinal
      anesthesia, 246
  hyperkalemic, succinylcholine
      and, 75–76
Cardiac arrhythmia. See
      Arrhythmia.
Cardiac output, during anesthesia,
      134, 134–135
  inhalation agents and, 35
  measurement of, 194
  monitoring of, 298
Cardiomyopathy, 150
Cardiovascular function,
      bupivacaine and, 90
  enflurane and, 41
  halothane and, 40
  isoflurane and, 39
  local anesthetic and, 85
  meperidine and, 51
  morphine and, 47
  NSAIDs and, 270
  pain and, 266
  sevoflurane and, 43

Cardioversion, 228
Ceiling effect, 50, 56, 271
Central nervous system,
    descending pain control
    pathways in, 165
  droperidol and, 27
  flumazenil and, 23–24
  in cocaine intoxication, 151–
    152
  local anesthetic and, 85
  morphine and, 46–47
  thiopental and, 18–19
  toxicity in, 85
    from local anesthetic, 250
Central venous pressure, fluid loss
    and, 292
  measurement of, 193–194
  monitoring of, 232
Cerebral protection,
    benzodiazepines for, 22
  ketamine for, 25
  thiopental for, 18
Cerebrovascular function, 41
Certified registered nurse
    anesthetist, definition of, 3
Cervical spine, preoperative
    assessment of, 156
Chest wall spasm, intubation, 186–
    187
Child. See also *Infant.*
  anesthetic circle system for, 114
  inhalation anesthetic in, 28
  laryngeal mask airway for, 166t
  malignant hyperthermia in, 233
Chloral, intravenous, history of, 2
Chloride channel, GABA-gated, 5,
    5
Chloroprocaine, 88
Chlorpheniramine, 161
Cholinesterase, 77–78
Christmas disease, 301
Cimetidine, for allergic reaction,
    232
  for obese surgical patient, 149
  to prevent aspiration, 285
Circle system, 112–114, *113*
Circulatory function, complications
    in, 227–229
  in heroin addict, 151
  local anesthetic toxicity and, 251
  monitoring of, 190–194
Cirrhosis, anesthesia in, 142
  in alcoholic, 150
  vecuronium in, 67
Cis-atracurium, 67

Citrate intoxication, transfusion-
    induced, 307
Clindamycin, 73
Coagulation, NSAIDs and, 270
  pain and, 267
Coagulopathy, blood transfusion
    for, 302–303
  dilutional, 305
  in liver disease, 142
Cocaine, action mechanism of, 87
  history of, 79
  intoxication from, anesthesia in,
    151–152
  uses of, 87
Codeine, dosage of, 55
    oral, 270–271
  for postoperative pain, 270–271
  pharmacokinetics of, 54
Cognitive manipulation, 279
Cold, common, 140
Colistin, 73
Colloid solution, 297–298, 298t
Colonic fluid, 296t
Color code(s), for gases, 98
Colorado tick fever, 307
Combitube, 182–184, *184*
Concentration, of inhalation
    anesthetic, 28–29, *29–30*,
    37
Concentration effect, *33*, 33–34
Conscious sedation, 286–287
Consciousness, spontaneous
    breathing and, 132, *132*
Constant-flow generator, *120*, 120–
    121
Constant-pressure generator, *120*,
    120–121
Copper kettle vaporizer, 95–96, *96*
Coughing, 223–224
Crash induction. See *Rapid-
    sequence induction.*
Creatine kinase, 234
Cricothyrotomy airway, *184*, 184–
    185
Croup, 187
Cryoprecipitated antihemophilic
    factor, 301, 303
Crystalloid solution, 297–298
Curare, 2–3. See also
    Precurarization.
Cyanosis, detection of, 223
  in recovery, 255
Cyclophosphamide, 78
Cytomegalovirus, 307
Cytotoxic agent(s), 78

Dantrolene, as diuretic, 236
  preanesthetic, 161
  to prevent malignant
      hyperthermia, 234–235
Dead space, in alveolar ventilation,
      127, 130, 132
Death, from morphine overdose, 47
  impending, in ether anesthesia, 9
Decamethonium, 144–145
Deep vein thrombosis, 149
Dehydration, 292
Delirium, 258
Dentition. See Teeth.
Depolarizing neuromuscular
      blockade, 63–64. See also
      Muscle relaxant(s); specific
      drug, e.g., Succinylcholine.
  Phase I, 63–64
    in myasthenia gravis, 72
  Phase II, 64
Desensitization block, 64
Desflurane, color code for, 98
  MAC of, 31t, 42
  muscle relaxant interaction with,
      72–73
  pharmacokinetics of, 42
Dextran(s), 297, 298t
Diabetes insipidus, 292
Diabetes mellitus, 145–146
Diameter-index safety system, of
      anesthetic machine, 101,
      101
Diazemuls, 23. See also Diazepam.
Diazepam, convulsion threshold
      and, 250
  dosage of, 22
  for awake intubation, 178
  for central nervous system
      toxicity, 250
  for delirium, 258
  indications for, 22
  pharmacokinetics of, 22–23
Dibucaine number, 77
Digital nerve block, 238, 238–239
Digitalis, hypokalemia and, 138
  indications for, 228
Dilutional coagulopathy, 305
Dilutional hyponatremia, 142
Dimenhydrinate, for nausea, 259
Diphenhydramine, for allergic
      reaction, 232
Diuresis, diabetes-induced, 292
Diuretic(s), alcohol as, 150
  hypokalemia from, 138
  in malignant hyperthermia, 236
Dobutamine, 227

Dopamine, 227
Doxacurium, 66
  in renal failure, 144–145
Dräger volumeter, 195–196, 196
Droperidol, dosage of, 26
  for nausea, 259
  pharmacokinetics of, 26
  side effects of, 27
Drug abuse, anesthesia in, 151–
      152
Drug intoxication, diagnosis of,
      258
Dual block, 64
Dubucaine, 89
Duodenal fluid, 296t

Eaton-Lambert syndrome, 72
Echothiophate, 78
Edrophonium, 69
Elderly person, atrial flutter or
      fibrillation in, 228
  fluid and electrolyte replacement
      therapy in, 296–297
  muscle relaxants in, 70
  outpatient surgery on, 283
  somnolence in, 257
  spinal anesthesia in, 244–245,
      245
  d-tubocurarine in, 65
Electrocardiogram, monitoring
      with, 192–193
  in recovery room, 253
Electroencephalogram, anesthetic
      depth on, 189–190
Electrolyte(s). See also Fluid(s) and
      electrolyte(s); specific
      electrolyte, e.g., Sodium.
  in alimentary fluid, 296t
  in parenteral solution, 297t
Elimination, Hoffman, 67
  of carbon dioxide, 133, 195
  of inhalation anesthetic, 36–37,
      37, 257
  of intravenous anesthetic, 12,
      16–17
  of local anesthetic, 86–87
  of morphine, 50
Embolization, 11, 315
Emergence. See also Recovery.
  from general anesthesia, 221–222
  from ketamine anesthesia, 21,
      258
Emergency, airway in, 183–185,
      184
  laryngospasm in, 254

Encephalopathy, alcohol-induced, 150

Endocrine system, pain and, 267

Endotracheal intubation. See *Tracheal intubation.*

End-plate potential, 61, *61*

End-tidal carbon dioxide plateau, *204*, 204–205
  in hypoventilation, 226

End-tidal nitrogen concentration, 207

Enflurane, color code for, 98
  induction of, 217
  MAC of, 31t, 41
  muscle relaxant interaction with, 72–73
  nephrotoxicity of, 144
  pharmacokinetics of, 41–42
  side effects of, 41, 42

Epidural analgesia/anesthesia, *245*, *247*, 248–250
  alpha₂-agonist in, 278
  neural blockade in, 277
  opioids in, 276–277

Epidural hematoma, 248

Epinephrine, for allergic reaction, 231–232
  halothane interaction with, 40
  hypersensitivity to, 86
  local anesthetic with, 86

Epstein-Barr virus, 307

Erythrocyte(s). See *Red blood cell(s).*

Esophageal intubation, 187
  expiratory carbon dioxide waveform and, 176

Esophageal varice(s), 142

Ether anesthesia, history of, 2
  stages of, 8–9

Etidocaine, clearance of, 87
  pharmacokinetics of, 90

Etomidate, at GABA-gated ion channel, 5, *5*
  dosage of, 25
  pharmacokinetics of, 25–26
  side effects of, 26

Excitement stage, of ether anesthesia, 9

Excretion, of inhalation agent, 36–37, *37*
  of intravenous anesthetic, *12*, 17
  of morphine, 50

Expiration to inspiration changeover, in mechanical ventilation, 122

Expiratory flow, in mechanical ventilation, 121

Extubation, after tracheal intubation, 185–186
  laryngospasm from, 187
  inadvertent, 219
  laryngeal reflex and, 222

Eyelash reflex, 188
  in intravenous induction, 215

Face mask ventilation, characteristics of, 169t
  for shivering patient, 256–257
  in intravenous induction, 215–216
  with satisfactory airway, 181–182
  with unsatisfactory airway, 182–183

Factor VIII (antihemophilic factor), 301

Factor IX, 301

Fasting, preanesthesia, 159, 285–286

Febrile transfusion reaction, 304

Fentanyl, dosage of, 52–53
  epidural, 277
  for awake intubation, 178
  heart rate and, 228
  intrathecal, 276
  pharmacokinetics of, 52–53
  respiratory function and, 54
  droperidol with, 26

Fiberoptic laryngoscopy, 178–180

Fibrillation, atrial, 228

Fitness for anesthesia, preoperative assessment of, 157–158

Flow cycling, in mechanical ventilation, 121

Flowmeter, mishaps with, 315t
  of anesthetic circuit, 94–95, *95*
  of anesthetic machine, *102*, 102–103

Pilot-tube, 196, *197*

Fluid and electrolyte(s), acid-base abnormality and, 294–295
  basal requirements for, 290–291
  in chronic renal failure, 144
  muscle relaxant action and, 71
  ongoing losses of, 295–296, 296t
  presurgical deficits in, 291–295
  replacement therapy in, 296–298, 297t, 298t

Fluid overload, clinical signs of, 293
  intravenous injection and, 11
  treatment of, 293
Flumazenil, as competitive antagonist, 22
  dosage of, 23–24
  for somnolence, 257
  pharmacokinetics of, 23
Fluoride-resistant variant, of cholinesterase, 78
Flutter, atrial, 228
Forceps, intubating, 172, *173*
Fracture hematoma, infiltration of, 239
Fresh frozen plasma, 303
Frozen red blood cell(s), 300
Functional residual capacity, 34
  in obesity, 148
  PEEP and, 136
  ventilation-perfusion inequality and, 130–131
Furosemide, 294, 294t

GABA-gated ion channel. See *Gamma-aminobutyric acid-gated ion channel.*
Gallamine, 66–67
  in renal failure, 144
  sinus tachycardia from, 228
  succinylcholine interaction with, 76
Gallbladder disease, 48
Galvanic fuel cell oxygen analyzer, 200, *201*, 202
Gamma-aminobutyric acid-gated ion channel, intravenous anesthetic at, 4–5, *5*
  protein interaction hypothesis and, 8
Gas(es). See also *Anesthetic machine*; *Inhalation anesthetic(s)*; specific gas, e.g., *Nitrous oxide.*
  color codes for, 98
  cylinders for, 98–100, *99–100*
  in blood, analysis of, 198–200, *199*
Gas machine. See *Anesthetic machine.*
Gastric contents, aspiration of. See *Aspiration.*
  emptying of, timing of, 159
Gastric fluid, 296t

Gastrointestinal tract, meperidine and, 51
  morphine and, 48
  NSAIDs and, 269
  pain and, 267
  pressure in, succinylcholine and, 75
Gate control hypothesis, *263*, 265–266
General anesthesia. See also specific drug, e.g., *Propofol*; specific drug type, e.g., *Intravenous anesthetic(s).*
  complication(s) during, 223–236
    airway obstruction as, 224–225
    anaphylactic and anaphylactoid reactions as, 230–233
    arrhythmias as, 228–229
    aspiration of gastric contents as, 229–230
    breath holding as, 224
    bronchospasm as, 226
    circulatory, 227–229
    coughing as, 223–224
    hypertension as, 227–228
    hypoventilation as, 225–226
    laryngospasm as, 225
    malignant hyperthermia as, 233–236
    respiratory, 223–226
  components of, 9–10
  controlled ventilation in, 221
  definition of, 1
  depth of, in maintenance phase, 220
    monitoring of, 188–190
  emergence from, 221–222
  for outpatient surgery, 287
  hepatic function in, 142–143
  history of, 1–3
  in heroin addict, 151
  induction of, by tracheal intubation, 217. See also *Tracheal intubation.*
    inhalational, 216–217, 224
    intravenous, 215–216
    rapid-sequence, 217–219
  ion channels and, 4–6, *5*
  lipid solubility hypothesis and, 6–8, *7*
  maintenance of, 220–221
  Meyer-Overton rule in, 6
  patient positioning for, 219, 224
  preparation for, 214–215
  principles of, 3–10

General anesthesia (*Continued*)
  protein interaction hypothesis
      and, 8
  spontaneous ventilation in, 220–
      221
  techniques of, 214–222
Genitourinary system, morphine
      and, 48
  pain and, 267
Gentamicin, 73
Glaucoma, 78
Glottis, exposure of, *180*, 180–181
Glucagon, 232
Glucose, blood level of, monitoring
      of, 212
  wound healing and, 146
Glycogen storage disease, 142
Glycopyrrolate, prophylactic, 69
  to reverse muscle relaxant ac-
      tion, 70
Glycoside(s), cardiac, 138
Glycosuria, 292
Graft *versus* host reaction, 301

Hallucinogen intoxication, 258
Halothane, cardiac effects of, 228–
      229
  color code for, 98
  epinephrine interaction with, 40
  hepatotoxicity of, 41, 143
  induction of, 216–217
  MAC of, 31t, 40
  malignant hyperthermia and, 234
  pharmacokinetics of, 40–41
  physical properties of, 40
  repetition of, 154
  shivering after, 256–257
  side effects of, 40–41
Head, position of, for rapid-se-
      quence induction, 218
  for tracheal intubation, 174–
      175, *175*
Head tilt-jaw thrust maneuver, 162,
      163
Headache, after spinal anesthesia,
      246–248, *247*
Heart. See also *Cardiac*; *Cardio-*
      entries.
  disease of, beriberi, 150
      ischemic, 25, 137–139
Heart rate, lower than normal, 228
Helium, color code for, 98
Hematologic abnormality, 142. See
      also *Coagulopathy.*

Hematoma, fracture, infiltration of,
      239
  from spinal anesthesia, 248
Hemodialysis, succinylcholine in,
      78
Hemodilution, preoperative, for au-
      tologous blood transfusion,
      312
Hemodynamic monitoring, inva-
      sive, 193–194, 253
Hemoglobin, monitoring of, 212
Hemolytic transfusion reaction,
      acute, 304–305
  delayed, 305
Hemophilia, cryoprecipitated fac-
      tor VIII in, 303
  prothrombin complex-activated
      blood transfusion in, 301
Henderson-Hasselbalch equation,
      13
Hepatitis. See also *Liver* entries.
  drug abuse and, 151
  halothane-induced, 41
  transfusion-induced, 306
Heroin, addiction to, addisonian
      crisis in, 151
  anesthesia in, 151
  withdrawal from, 258
Hexobarbital, 2
  history of, 2
Histamine H_2-receptor antagonist,
      for allergic reaction, 232
  for obese surgical patient, 149
Histamine release. See also *Aller-
      gic reaction.*
  morphine-induced, 47
  thiopental-induced, 19
  d-tubocurarine-induced, 65
History, anesthetic, in preoperative
      assessment, 153–154
  medical, in preoperative assess-
      ment, 154–155
HIV infection, 306
Hoarseness, 187
Hoffman elimination, 67
Homologous blood transfusion. See
      *Blood transfusion,
      homologous.*
HTLV infection, 306
Human retrovirus infection, 306
Hydrocodone, 55
Hydrocortisone, 161
Hyperbaric solution, 245–246
Hyperbilirubinemia, 142
Hypercapnia, 205, 223
  in malignant hyperthermia, 234

Hypercapnia (*Continued*)
  local anesthetic in, 85
  morphine-induced, 48
  sinus tachycardia from, 228
Hyperglycemia, 146
Hyperkalemia, causes of, 294
  in malignant hyperthermia, 235
  local anesthetic in, 85
  treatment of, 235, 294, 294t
Hypersensitivity. See *Allergic reaction*; *Histamine release.*
Hypertension, anesthesia-induced, 227
  from intubation, 186–187
  in chronic renal failure, 143
  in recovery, 256
  ketamine and, 25
  management of, 228
  preexisting, anesthesia in, 139–140
  preoperative prevention of, 227–228
Hyperthermia, 211–212
  malignant. See *Malignant hyperthermia.*
Hypnosis, 9
Hypoalbuminemia, 142
Hypocapnia, 205
Hypokalemia, anesthesia during, 138
  clinical signs of, 293
  in liver disease, 142
  treatment of, 293–294
Hyponatremia, causes of, 293
  dilutional, 142
Hypotension, arterial, metocurine-induced, 66
    d-tubocurarine-induced, 65
  during anesthesia, 227
  in heroin addict, 151
  in lumbar epidural anesthesia, 250
  in recovery, 256
  in spinal anesthesia, 246
  management of, 246
Hypothermia, 211
  muscle relaxants and, 70–71
  transfusion-induced, 308
Hypothyroidism, 19
Hypoventilation, 225–226
  in recovery, 254–255
  pain-induced, 266
Hypovolemia, 228
Hypoxemia, in recovery, 255
  local anesthetic and, 85, 250–251

Hypoxemia (*Continued*)
  malignant hyperthermia and, 234
  respiratory complications of, 223
  sinus tachycardia and, 228
Hypoxia, during emergence, 222
  pulmonary vasoconstriction and, 131

Ibuprofen, 269
Ileal fluid, 296t
Illness, systemic, adrenocortical insufficiency as, 146–147
  alcoholism as, 150
  anemia as, 147–148
  anesthesia in, 137–152
  arthritis as, 149–150
  biochemical abnormalities as, 142
  chronic obstructive lung disease as, 140–141
  common cold as, 140
  concurrent, in outpatient selection, 282
  preoperative assessment of, 157, 282
  diabetes mellitus as, 145–146
  drug abuse as, 151–152
  hematologic abnormalities as, 142
  hypertension as, 139–140
  ischemic heart disease as, 137–139
  liver disease as, 141–143
  obesity as, 148–149
  renal insufficiency as, 143–145
Imidazole(s), 25–26. See also specific drug, e.g., *Etomidate.*
Immune system, pain and, 267
Impending death, in ether anesthesia, 9
Indomethacin, 269
Induction. See anesthesia type, e.g., *General anesthesia, induction of.*
  rapid-sequence. See *Rapid-sequence induction.*
Infant. See also *Child.*
  laryngeal mask airway for, 166t
  neonatal, laryngoscope for, 170
  outpatient surgery on, 283
Infusion sets and filters, for blood transfusion, 310

Inhalation anesthetic(s), 28–44.
 See also *Anesthetic circuit*;
 Anesthetic machine; specific
 drug, e.g., *Nitrous oxide*.
 alveolar concentration of, 31t,
  31–32
 alveolar uptake of, 32–36, *33*
 alveolar ventilation and, 34,
  128
 alveolar-mixed venous tension
  gradient and, 35
 anesthesia depth from, 189
 cardiac output and, 35
 color codes for, 98
 concentration of, 28–29, *29, 37*
 coughing and, 223–224
 distribution of, 36
 elimination of, 36–37, *37*, 257
 excretion of, 36–37, *37*
 for outpatient surgery, 287
 functional residual capacity and,
  34
 history of, 1–3
 indications for, 28
 induction of, 216–217
  breath holding in, 224
 inspired concentration of, *33*,
  33–34
 lipid solubility hypothesis and,
  6–8, *7*
 malignant hyperthermia and,
  234
 metabolism of, 37
 Meyer-Overton rule in, 6
 monitoring of, 200, *201*, 202–
  208, *203–204, 207*
 morphine and, 49
 muscle relaxant interaction with,
  72–73
 partial pressure of, 29–30, *30*
 protein interaction hypothesis
  and, 8
 second gas effect of, 35–36
 solubility of, 34–35
 tidal volume and, 128
 tissue uptake of, 36
Innovar, 26. See also *Droperidol*.
Inspiration-expiration ratio, in mechanical ventilation, 126
Inspiratory flow, in mechanical
  ventilation, 119–121, 126
Inspired concentration, *33*, 33–34
Insulin, anesthesia and, 145–146
 for hyperkalemia, 294, 294t
Interscalene approach, to brachial
  plexus block, 241–242, *242*

Intoxication. See specific agent,
  e.g., *Cocaine, intoxication
  from*.
Intracranial pressure, 75
Intraocular pressure, 75
Intrathecal opioid(s), 275–276
Intravenous anesthetic(s), 11–27.
 See also specific drug, e.g.,
 Propofol.
 advantages of, 11
 allergic reaction to, 231
 alpha phase of, 12–16, *15*
 at GABA-gated channel, 4–5, *5*
 beta phase of, *12*, 16–17
 distribution of, 12–16, *15*
 elimination of, *12*, 16–17
 for outpatient surgery, 287
 history of, 2–3
 in liver disease, 141
 induction of, 215–216
 ion trapping and, 14
 ionization state of, 13–14
 lipid solubility of, 13
 mishaps with, 315t
 molecular size of, 13
 overdose of, 13, 18
 peak concentration of, 11–12, *12*
 pharmacokinetics of, 11–17, *12*,
  15
 physical characteristics of, 13–
  14
 protein binding of, 13
 side effects of, 11
 tissue uptake of, 14–16, *15*
Intravenous narcotic analgesia,
  postoperative, *272*, 273–274
Intravenous regional anesthesia,
  239–240, *240*
Intubation, bronchial, 187
 endotracheal. See *Tracheal
  intubation*.
 esophageal, 187
  expiratory carbon dioxide
   waveform and, 176
Ion channel(s). See also *Nerve conduction*; *Neuromuscular
  transmission*.
 acetylcholine-gated, 60–62, *61*
 GABA-gated, intravenous anesthetic at, 4–5, *5*
  protein interaction hypothesis
   and, 8
 ligand-gated, 4, 60
 metabotropic receptor-gated, 4–
  5, *5*
 NMDA-gated, ketamine at, 6

Ion channel(s) (*Continued*)
  protein interaction hypothesis and, 8
  voltage-gated, 4–5, *5*, 60–61, *61*, 81, *81*
Ion trapping, 14
Ionization, of intravenous anesthetic, 13–14
Irradiated red blood cell(s), 301
Ischemic heart disease, 25, 137–139
Isoflurane, advantages of, 39
  color code for, 98
  concentration of, *29–30*
  induction of, 217
  MAC of, 31t, 39
  muscle relaxant interaction with, 72–73
  oxytocin and, 39
  pharmacokinetics of, 38–39
  physical properties of, 38
  side effects of, 39
Itching, 276

Jaundice, obstructive, 142

Kanamycin, 73
Ketamine, anesthesia depth from, 188–189
  at NMDA-gated ion channel, 6
  contraindications to, 25
  dosage of, 24–25
  emergence from, 21, 258
  pharmacokinetics of, 24–25
  sinus tachycardia from, 228
Ketorolac, 269
Kidney. See also *Renal* entries.
  intravenous anesthetic clearance by, *12*, 17
  morphine clearance by, 50
Korotkoff's sounds, 191

Labetalol, 256
Laboratory testing, preoperative, 157
Laryngeal mask airway, advantages of, 165–166, 169t, 183
  components of, 165, *165*
  disadvantages of, 166, 169t
  indications for, 182
  positioning of, 166–168, *167*
  removal of, 168
  selection guide for, 166t

Laryngeal spray, for intubation, 173, *173*
  systemic toxicity of, 315t
Laryngoscopy, equipment for, 170, *170–171*
  extubation after, 185–186
  flexible fiberoptic, 178–180
  glottis exposure in, *180*, 180–181
  mishaps in, 315t
  under local anesthesia, 178
Laryngospasm, after extubation, 187
  detection of, 225
  from surgical stimulation, 189
  in recovery, 254
  management of, 225
Latex hypersensitivity, 231
Leg pain, after spinal anesthesia, 248
  lidocaine-induced, 89
Leukocyte concentrate, from apheresis, 300–301
Leukocyte-poor red blood cell(s), 300
Levallorphan, 57
Lidocaine, absorption of, 86
  advantages of, 88
  cardiovascular function and, 85
  clearance of, 87
  for awake intubation, 177–178
  for premature ventricular beat, 229
  in intravenous regional anesthesia, 239–240
  in lumbar epidural anesthesia, 249–250
  in spinal anesthesia, 245–246
  leg pain after, 89
  pharmacokinetics of, 88–89
Ligand-gated ion channel, 4, 60
Lincomycin, 73
Lip(s), trauma to, during intubation, 186
Lipid solubility, of fentanyl, 52
  of intravenous anesthetic, 13
  of meperidine, 52
Lipid solubility hypothesis, 6–8, *7*, 83
Litigation, anesthetic mishaps and, 314, 318–319
Liver, halothane effects on, 41
  inflammation of. See *Hepatitis*.
  intravenous anesthetic elimination by, *12*, 16–17
  morphine clearance by, 50

Liver disease, anesthesia in, 141–143
  anesthetic agent hepatotoxicity in, 142–143
  biochemical abnormalities in, 142
  cirrhosis as. See *Cirrhosis.*
  fluid and electrolyte replacement therapy in, 296–297
  hematologic abnormalities in, 142
  protein binding of drug in, 13, 18
  succinylcholine in, 78
Local anesthetic(s), 79–91. See also specific drug, e.g., *Mepivacaine.*
  absorption of, 86
  action mechanism of, 82–84
  allergic reaction to, 231
  aminoamides as, 88–91
  aminoesters as, 87–88
  anxiety management and, 237
  cardiovascular effects of, 85
  central nervous system and, 85
  contraindications to, 237
  elimination of, 86–87
  epidural, 277
  epinephrine with, 86
  for outpatient surgery, 286
  history of, 79
  hypersensitivity to, 86
  in digital nerve block, *238*, 238–239
  in fracture hematoma infiltration, 239
  in heroin addict, 151
  in intravascular space, 237
  in pleural space, 277–278
  lipid solubility hypothesis and, 83
  local infiltration of, 238, *238*
  membrane expansion hypothesis and, 83
  membrane receptor hypothesis and, 83
  nerve conduction and, 80–82, *81*, 84–85
  pathogenic organisms in, 237
  peripheral nerve anatomy and, 79–80, *80*
  surface charge hypothesis and, 83–84
  systemic effects of, 84–86
  systemic toxicity of, 250–251
  tachyphylaxis and, 85–86

Local anesthetic(s) (*Continued*)
  tracheal intubation under, 177–178
Lubricant, for tracheal intubation, 174
Lumbar epidural anesthesia, *245*, *247*, 248–250
Lung. See *Pulmonary* entries.

MAC (minimum alveolar concentration), 31t, 31–32
MacIntosh laryngoscope blade, 170, *170*
Magill circuit, 114, *115*
Magill intubating forceps, 172, *173*
Magill laryngoscope blade, 170, *170*
Magnesium, 73
Maintenance phase, 220–221
  breath holding in, 224
Malaria, 307
Malignant hyperthermia, causes of, 233
  diagnosis of, 234
  incidence of, 233
  management of, 235–236
  masseter spasm and, 75, 233–234
  mortality rate from, 234–235
  preanesthetic dantrolene in, 161
Mallampati pharyngeal classification, 156, *156*
Mandibular hypoplasia, 155–156
Mapleson A circuit, 114, *115*
Mass spectrometer, respiratory and anesthetic monitoring with, 206–207, *207*
Masseter spasm, malignant hyperthermia and, 75, 233–234
  succinylcholine-induced, 74–75
Mechanical ventilation, airway resistance and, 120
  alarms in, 123–124
  bellows design in, 122
  checking ventilator in, 124–125
  constant-flow, *120*, 120–121
  constant-pressure, *120*, 120–121
  expiration to inspiration changeover in, 122
  expiratory flow in, 121
  in breath holding, 224
  in laryngospasm, 225
  in paralyzed person, 132, *132*
  indications for, 220

Mechanical ventilation (*Continued*)
inspiration to expiration change-over in, 121
inspiration to expiration ratio in, 126
inspiratory flow in, 119–121, 126
mishaps in, 315t, 316–317
PEEP in, 121
phases of, 119–122, *120*
pressure alarms in, 123
pressure control devices in, 120, 123
pressure monitoring in, 122–123
respiratory rate in, 126
safety features in, 122–124
spirometer in, 123–124
tidal volume in, 125–126
ventilation-perfusion inequality and, 132, *132*
Membrane expansion hypothesis, 83
Membrane fluidization hypothesis, 7, 7–8
Membrane receptor hypothesis, 83
Mendelson's syndrome, 229
Meperidine, dosage of, 52
intramuscular, 271
intravenous, 273
oral, 271
for shivering patient, 257
pharmacokinetics of, 52
systemic effects of, 51–52
Mepivacaine, clearance of, 87
pharmacokinetics of, 90
Metabolic acidosis, 292
causes of, 294–295
treatment of, 295
Metabolic alkalosis, 295
Metabotropic receptor-gated ion channel, 4
Metaproterenol, 232
Methadone, 151, 258
Methemoglobinemia, 89–90
Methohexital, 19–20
Methoxyflurane, 43, 144
Methoxyfluruane, 144
N-Methyl-D-aspartate-gated ion channel, ketamine at, 6
protein interaction hypothesis and, 8
Methylene blue, 90
Methylphenidate, 257
Metoclopramide, 259, 285
Metocurine, 66, 144
Meyer-Overton rule, 6

Micrognathia, 155–156
Midazolam, 22–23
Miller laryngoscope blade, 170, *170*
Minimum alveolar concentration (MAC), 31t, 31–32
Mivacurium, 68, 72
Molecular size, of intravenous anesthetic, 13
Monitoring, 188–213
anesthetic vapor measurement in, 206
blood gas analysis in, 198–200, *199*
capnograph in, *203–204*, 203–206, 226, 234, 253
clinical signs in, anesthesia depth and, 188–189
neuromuscular function and, 208–209
respiratory function and, 194–195
direct arterial, 232
during patient positioning, 219
electrocardiogram in, 192–193, 253
electroencephalogram in, 189–190
guidelines for, 212–213
in obesity, 149
in recovery room, 253–254
invasive hemodynamic, 193–194, 253
mass spectrometer in, 206–207, *207*
mishaps in, 317–318
of airway pressure, 196–198, *197*
of anesthesia depth, 188–190
of blood loss, 194
of blood pressure, 190–192, 232
of blood sugar, 212
of body temperature, 211–212
of cardiac output, 298
of central venous pressure, 232
of circulatory function, 190–194
of hemoglobin concentration, 212
of neuromuscular function, 208–211, *210*
of nitrous oxide, 206
of oxygenation, 253
during crystalloid/colloid replacement therapy, 298
of pulmonary artery pressures, 232

Monitoring (*Continued*)
  of pulse, 190–191
  of renal function, 208
  of respiratory and anesthetic
      gases, 200, *201*, 202–208,
      203–204, *207*
  of respiratory function, 194–200,
      196–197, *199*
  of urine output, 296
  of ventilatory volume, 195–196,
      196–197
  oxygen analyzers in, galvanic
      fuel cell, 200, *201*, 202
    paramagnetic, 202–203, *203*
    polarographic, *201*, 202
  peripheral nerve stimulation in,
      209–211, *210*
  pulse oximetry in, *199*, 199–200,
      234
  Raman photospectrometer in,
      207, 207–208
  sphygomomanometry in, 191–
      192
  transfer of duty in, 212–213
Morphine, action mechanism of,
      45–46
  addiction to, 49
  allergic reaction to, 49, 231
  as agonist, 45
  distribution of, 50
  dosage of, intramuscular, 271
    intravenous, 273
    oral, 271
  drug interactions with, 49
  elimination of, 50
  heart rate and, 228
  history of, 2
  idiosyncratic reactions to, 49
  in neurosurgery, 48
  intrathecal, 276
  overdose of, 47
  systemic effects of, 46–48
  tolerance to, 48–49
  uptake of, 50
  uses of, 50–51
Motor unit, 59
Mouth opening, preoperative as-
      sessment of, 155
Muscle(s), pain in, 74
  relaxation of. See also *Muscle
      relaxant(s)*.
    in general anesthesia, 10
  spasm of, chloroprocaine-in-
      duced, 88
    malignant hyperthermia and,
      75, 233–234

Muscle(s) (*Continued*)
    peripheral nerve stimulation
      and, 209–211, *210*
Muscle relaxant(s), 59–78. See also
    specific drug, e.g., *Curare*.
  allergic reaction to, 231
  depolarizing, 63–64
    in myasthenia gravis, 72
  for outpatient surgery, 287
  history of, 2–3, 59
  indications for, 208–209
  intravenous induction of, 215–
      216
  neuromuscular blockade and,
      62–64
  neuromuscular transmission and,
      59–62, *60–61*
  nondepolarizing, 62–63
    acid-base balance and, 71
    age and, 70
    digitalis and, 138
    drug interaction with, 72–73
    Eaton-Lambert syndrome and,
      72
    electrolyte imbalance and, 71
    hypokalemia and, 138
    hypothermia and, 70–71
    intermediate-acting, 66–68
    long-acting, 64–66
    myasthenia gravis and, 72
    priming dose and, 70
    renal failure and, 66–67, 71–
      72, 144–145
    reversal of, 63, 68–70
    short-acting, 68
    succinylcholine and, 65, 73, 76
  peripheral nerve stimulation
      characteristics in, 209–211,
      210
Myasthenia gravis, 72, 77
Myotonia, 77

Nalbuphine, 56, 271
Naloxone, as antagonist, 57
  buprenorphine and, 57
  for hypoventilation, 255
  for morphine-induced biliary
      colic, 48
  for somnolence, 257
  indications for, 57
  overshoot phenomenon with,
      57–58
  structure of, 56
  systemic effects of, 57

Naltrexone, 58

Naproxen, 269

Narcotic analgesic(s), 45–58. See also specific drug, e.g., *Morphine.*
  action mechanism of, 45–46, 46t
  ceiling effect of, 50, 271
  continuous infusion of, 275, 279–280
  epidural, 276–277, 279–280
  for somnolence, 257
  history of, 2–3, 45
  in liver disease, 141
  indications for, 45
  intramuscular, 271, *272,* 273
  intrathecal, 275–276, 279–280
  intravenous, *272,* 273–274
    patient-controlled, *272,* 274–275, 279–280
  oral, 270–271
  postoperative, 270–271, *272,* 273–277, 279–280
  safety considerations in, 279–280

Nasopharyngeal airway, 163–165, *164*

Nasotracheal intubation, flexible fiberoptic, 179
  techniques of, 176–177

Nausea, after outpatient surgery, 288
  in recovery, 258–259
  morphine-induced, 47–48
  prevention and treatment of, 151, 259

Neck, posture of, in tracheal intubation, 174–175, *175*

Neonate. See also *Child; Infant.*
  laryngoscope for, 170

Neostigmine, 69
  succinylcholine interaction with, 78
  to reverse muscle relaxant action, 69

Nephrotoxicity, of anesthetics, 144

Nerve(s), peripheral, anatomy of, 79–80, *80*
  stimulation of, 209–211, *210*

Nerve block, recovery from, 259–260

Nerve cell membrane, ion channels of, anesthetic action on, 4–6, *5*

Nerve conduction. See also *Ion channel(s).*
  in ankylosing spondylitis, 149

Nerve conduction (*Continued*)
  local anesthetic and, 84–85
  physiology of, 80–82, *81*

Nerve stimulation, peripheral, 209–211, *210*
  transcutaneous electrical, 278–279

Neuromuscular blockade. See also *Muscle relaxant(s).*
  controlled ventilation in, 221
  depolarizing, 63–64, 72
  digital, *238,* 238–239
  nondepolarizing, 62–63
  peripheral nerve stimulation characteristics in, 209–211, *210*
  Phase I depolarizing, 63–64
  Phase II depolarizing, 64
  residual, 255

Neuromuscular function, after spinal anesthesia, 248
  clinical signs of, 208–209
  peripheral nerve stimulation in, 209–211, *210*

Neuromuscular transmission. See also *Ion channel(s).*
  physiology of, 59–62, *60–61*

Neurosurgery, morphine in, 48

Nifedipine, 256

Nitrogen, color code for, 98
  end-tidal concentration of, 207

Nitroglycerin, 48

Nitrous oxide, color code for, 98
  concentration of, 28–29
  control/delivery of. See *Anesthetic machine.*
  history of, 1–2
  indications for, 38
  MAC of, 31t, 38
  monitoring vapor of, 206
  physical properties of, 37–38
  side effects of, 38
  storage of, 38

NMDA-gated ion channel. See *N-Methyl-D-aspartate-gated ion channel.*

Nodal rhythm, slow, 228–229

Nondepolarizing neuromuscular blockade, 62–63. See also *Muscle relaxant(s), nondepolarizing.*

Nonopioid analgesic(s), for postoperative pain, 269–270

Nonsteroidal antiinflammatory drugs (NSAIDs), contraindications to, 270

Nonsteroidal antiinflammatory
        drugs (NSAIDs) (*Continued*)
    for postoperative pain, 269
    side effects of, 269–270
Nystagmus, 217

Obesity, anesthesia in, 148–149
    endocrine abnormalities in, 148–
        149
    rapid-sequence induction in,
        217–218
Opioid(s). See *Narcotic analge-
        sic(s)*; specific drug, e.g.,
        Morphine.
    allergic reaction to, 231
Opioid receptor(s), 46t
Oral contraceptive(s), 78
Oropharyngeal airway, 163–165,
        164
Orotracheal intubation. See also
        Tracheal intubation.
    contraindications to, 176
    techniques of, *175*, 175–176,
        179–180
Outpatient surgery, conscious seda-
        tion for, 286–287
    fasting before, 285–286
    general anesthesia for, 287
    home readiness after, 288–289
    local and regional anesthesia for,
        286
    medication before, 285–286
    nausea and vomiting after, 288
    pain management after, 287–288
    physical facility for, 284–285
    preoperative assessment in, 281–
        282
    procedures suitable for, 283–284
    selection criteria for, age as, 283
        concurrent illness as, 282
        mental capacity as, 283
        physical facility as, 284–285
        physical status as, 282
        socioeconomic profile as, 283
Ovassapian airway, 165
Oxycodone, 55–56
Oxygen, alarms for, 105–107
    analyzers of, galvanic fuel cell,
        200, *201*, 202
        paramagnetic, 202–203, *203*
        polarographic, *201*, 202
    color codes for, 98
    control/delivery of. See *Anes-
        thetic machine.*
    flowmeter for, *102*, 102–103

Oxygen (*Continued*)
    minimum flow-ratio controller
        for, 106
    safety valve for, 105
Oxygen pressure, arterial, alveolar
        ventilation and, 135
    in breathing control, 129
    measurement of, 198–199
Oxygen saturation, measurement
        of, 199–200
Oxygenation, during anesthesia,
        133–135, *134*, 195
    measurement of, 198–200, *199*
    monitoring of, during crystal-
        loid/colloid replacement
        therapy, 298
    in recovery room, 253

Packed red blood cell(s). See *Red
        blood cell(s), packed.*
Pain, control of, descending path-
        way for, 165
    gate hypothesis of, *263*, 265–
        266
    in recovery, 259
    modulation of, segmental path-
        way for, 265–266
    pathophysiology of, 266–267
    pathways of, parietal, 262–264,
        263
        somatic, 262–264, *263*
        visceral, 264
    postoperative management of,
        cognitive and behavioral ma-
            nipulation in, 279
        epidural alpha$_2$-agonists in,
            278
        general measures in, 267–269
        in outpatient surgery, 287–
            288
        narcotic analgesics in, 270–
            271, *272*, 273–277
        neural blockade analgesia in,
            277–278
        nonopioid analgesics in, 269–
            270
        NSAIDs in, 269–270
        safety considerations in, 279–
            280
        transcutaneous electrical nerve
            stimulation in, 278–279
    referred, 264
Paleospinothalamic tract, 264
Pancreatic secretion, electrolyte
        contents of, 296t

Pancuronium, 65
  in liver disease, 141
  in renal failure, 71
  sinus tachycardia from, 228
  succinylcholine interaction with, 76
Papaveretum, 51
Paralysis, after spinal anesthesia, 248
  mechanical ventilation in, 132, *132*
  partial, signs of, 209
Paramagnetic oxygen analyzer, 202–203, *203*
Parenteral solution, 297t
Parietal pain pathway, 262–264, *263*
Parkinsonism, 27
Paromomycin, 73
Partial pressure, 29–30, *30*
Patient, positioning of, airway obstruction and, 224
  for general anesthesia, 219, 224
  mishaps in, 315t
  respiratory function and, 220
Patient identification, for blood transfusion, 309, 315
Patient-controlled intravenous narcotic analgesia, *272*, 274–275, 279–280
PEEP. See *Positive end-expiratory pressure (PEEP)*.
Peñaz technique, 192
Pentastarch, 297, 298t
Pentazocine, 271
  dosage of, 56
    oral, 271
  drug interactions with, 56
  history of, 55
  systemic effects of, 55–56
  uses of, 56
Perfusion. See also *Ventilation-perfusion inequality*.
Peripheral nerve(s), anatomy of, 79–80, *80*
  stimulation of, 209–211, *210*
Pharyngeal airway, 163–165, *164*, 179–180
  in intravenous induction, 216
Pharynx, preoperative assessment of, 156, *156*
Phencyclidine(s), 24–25. See also specific drug, e.g., *Ketamine*.
Phenothiazine(s), 49
Phenytoin, 73
Phlebotomy, preoperative, 312

Photospectrometer, Raman, *207*, 207–208
Physical status, of outpatient, 282
  preoperative assessment of, 158–159
Physiologic dead space, 127
Physostigmine, for delirium, 258
  for somnolence, 257
Pickwickian syndrome, 148–149
Pilot-tube flowmeter, 196, *197*
Pin-index safety system, 100, *100*
Pipecuronium, 66
  in renal failure, 71, 144–145
Pipeline connection(s), on anesthetic machine, *101*, 101–102
Plasma, collection and storage of, 301
  fresh frozen, 303
  volume of, replenishment of, 302
Platelet concentrate, for coagulopathy, 303
  from apheresis, 300
  from whole blood, 300
Platelet transfusion, 142
Pleural space, local anesthetic instillation in, 277–278
Pneumonitis, aspiration, 160–161, 229–230
Pneumotachometer, 196, *197*
Polarographic oxygen analyzer, *201*, 202
Polymyxin, 73
Porphyria, 19
Positive end-expiratory pressure (PEEP), functional residual capacity and, 136
  in mechanical ventilation, 121
Postanesthesia care unit. See also *Emergence*; *Recovery*.
  arrival in, 253
  discharge from, 260, 261t
    after outpatient surgery, 288–289
  monitoring in, 253–254
  problem management in, 254–259
  transportation to, 252
Post-tetanic facilitation, 210
Potassium, basal requirement for, 291
  presurgical deficit in, 293–294
  serum concentration of, succinylcholine and, 75–76

Potassium channel. See *Ion channel(s)*.
Potassium intoxication, 307
Precurarization, for tracheal intubation, 217
    succinylcholine action after, 76
Prednisone, 147
Pregnancy, local anesthetic in, 85
    spinal anesthesia in, 246
    succinylcholine in, 78
Premedication, 159–161
Preoperative assessment, 153–159
    anesthetic history in, 153–154
    for outpatient surgery, 281–285
    laboratory tests in, 157
    medical history in, 154–155
    of age, 283
    of airway, 155–157, *156*
    of allergies and atopy, 154–155
    of cervical spine mobility, 156
    of concurrent illness, 157, 282
    of dentition, 155
    of fitness for anesthesia, 157–158
    of medication and treatment, 154
    of mental capacity, 283
    of mouth opening, 155
    of pharynx, 156, *156*
    of physical capacity, 283
    of physical status, 158–159, 282
    of socioeconomic profile, 283
    of thyrometal distance, 155–156
Preoperative preparation, anxiety relief in, 160, 237, 285–286
    drug interaction in, 161
    fasting in, 159, 285–286
    for outpatient procedure, 285–286
    gastric aspiration protection in, 160–161, 229–230, 285–286
    premedications in, 159–161, 285–286
Pressure, arterial. See *Arterial pressure.*
    monitoring of, in mechanical ventilation, 122–123
Pressure cycling, in mechanical ventilation, 121
Pressure gauge, in anesthetic circuit, 111, 122–123
    of anesthetic machine, 93–94
Pressure-limiting device, failure of, 198
    in anesthetic circuit, 109–110, *110*, 113, *113*, *115*

Pressure-limiting device (*Continued*)
    in anesthetic machine, 94
    in mechanical ventilation, 123
Prilocaine, clearance of, 87
    methemoglobinemia from, 89–90
    pharmacokinetics of, 89–90
Priming dose, of muscle relaxant, 70
Procainamide, 235–236
Procaine, 87–88
Prochlorperazine, for nausea, 259
    preanesthetic, 161
Propofol, anesthesia depth from, 188
    at GABA-gated ion channel, 5, *5*
    dosage of, 20
    pharmacokinetics of, 20–21
    side effects of, 21
Protein binding, of intravenous anesthetic, 13
    of thiopental, 18
Protein interaction hypothesis, 8
Pulmonary arterial pressure, monitoring of, 232
Pulmonary capillary wedge pressure, fluid loss and, 292
    measurement of, 194
Pulmonary compliance, 133
Pulmonary disease, chronic obstructive, 140–141
Pulmonary fibrosis, 149
Pulmonary vasoconstriction, hypoxic, 131
Pulse, monitoring of, 190–191
Pulse oximetry, *199*, 199–200, 234
Pupillary constriction, meperidine-induced, 51
    morphine-induced, 47
Pyridostigmine, 69

Quality assurance, 319
Quick-mount system, *101*, 101–102

Raman photospectrometer, *207*, 207–208
Ranitidine, for obese surgical patient, 149
    to prevent aspiration, 285
Rapid-sequence induction, in obese surgical patient, 149
    indications for, 217
    precurarization in, 219
    technique of, 218

Recovery. See also *Emergence.*
  airway obstruction in, 254
  delirium in, 258
  from regional anesthesia, 259–
      260
  hypertension n, 256
  hypotension in, 256
  hypoventilation in, 254–255
  hypoxemia in, 255
  monitoring in, 253–254
  nausea and vomiting in, 258–259
  pain in, 259
  scoring of, 261t
  shivering in, 256–257
  somnolence in, 257
Recovery room. See *Postanesthesia
    care unit.*
Red blood cell(s), frozen, 300
  irradiated, 301
  leukocyte-poor, 300
  packed, 299–300
    dilutional coagulopathy from,
        305
    indications for, 301–302
Referred pain, 264
Reflex tachycardia, 186–187
Regional anesthesia, anxiety man-
      agement and, 237
  brachial plexus block as, 240–
      244, *242*
  contraindications to, 237
  for outpatient surgery, 286
  in intravascular space, 237
  intravenous, 239–240, *240*
  lumbar epidural, *245, 247,* 248–
      250
  pathogenic organisms in, 237
  recovery from, 259–260
  spinal. See *Spinal anesthesia.*
Regurgitation, aortic, 149
  rapid-sequence induction and,
      217–218
Remifentanil, 54
Renal. See also *Kidney.*
Renal azotemia, 292
  chronic, anemia in, 143
    anesthetic agent nephrotoxic-
        ity in, 144
    fluid and electrolyte abnormal-
        ities in, 144
    hypertension in, 143
    muscle relaxants in, 66–67,
        71–72, 144–145
  fluid and electrolyte replacement
      therapy in, 296–297

Renal function, enflurane and, 42
  monitoring of, 208
  NSAIDs and, 270
Reservoir bag, 110–111, *113, 115*
Respiratory acidosis, 295
Respiratory alkalosis, 295
Respiratory function. See also *Air-
    way* entries.
  alveolar ventilation in. See *Alve-
      olar ventilation.*
  benzodiazepines and, 22
  breathing control and, 128–129
  carbon dioxide elimination in,
      133, 195
  clinical signs of, 194–195
  complications in, 223–226
  control of, guidelines for, 135–
      136
  fentanyl and congener effects on,
      54
  in smoker, 141
  intraoperative patient position
      and, 220
  intrathecal morphine and, 276
  isoflurane and, 39
  monitoring of, 194–200, *196–
      197, 199.* See also *Respira-
      tory gas(es), monitoring of.*
  morphine and, 47–48
  narcotic analgesics and, 279–280
  oxygenation in, 133–135, *134,*
      195
  pain and, 266
  pentazocine and, 55
  propofol and, 21
  pulmonary compliance in, 133
  thiopental and, 19
  ventilation-perfusion inequalities
      and, 129–132, *132*
  ventilatory flow and volume and,
      195–196, *196–197*
Respiratory gas(es), monitoring of.
      See also *Respiratory func-
      tion, monitoring of.*
  anesthetic vapor monitor in,
      206
  capnograph in, 203–206, *204*
  galvanic fuel cell oxygen ana-
      lyzer in, 200, *201,* 202
  mass spectrometer in, 206–
      207, *207*
  nitrous oxide vapor monitor
      in, 206
  paramagnetic oxygen analyzer
      in, 202–203, *203*

Respiratory gas(es) (*Continued*)
polarographic oxygen analyzer in, *201*, 202
Raman photospectrometer in, *207*, 207–208
Respiratory rate, in mechanical ventilation, 126
Ringer's lactate, electrolyte content of, 297t
indications for, 297
Riva-Rocci technique, 191
Rocuronium, 68
in liver disease, 141
in rapid-sequence induction, 218
in renal failure, 71
Ropivacaine, clearance of, 87
pharmacokinetics of, 90–91

Safety pressure-relief valve, of anesthetic machine, *100*, 100–101
Salbutamol, 232
Salivation, 74
Scavenging device, 109
Schwann cell, 79–80, *80*
Second gas effect, 35–36
Sedation, conscious, 286–287
Self-taming, 77
Selick's maneuver, 218
Sevoflurane, carbon dioxide absorbent interaction with, 43–44, 112
color code for, 98
MAC of, 31t, 42
muscle relaxant interaction with, 72–73, 144
nephrotoxicity of, 144
pharmacokinetics of, 42–43
side effects of, 43–44
Shivering, postoperative, 51, 256–257
Single-twitch stimulus, of peripheral nerve, 209–211, *210*
Sinus tachycardia, during anesthesia, 228
gallamine-induced, 67
in malignant hyperthermia, 235–236
pancuronium-induced, 65
Smoker, anesthetic complications in, 141
Socioeconomic profile, of outpatient, 283
Soda lime, in anesthetic circuit, 112–113, *113*
sevoflurane and, 43–44, 112

Sodium, basal requirement for, 291
presurgical deficit in, 291–293
Sodium bicarbonate, for allergic reaction, 232
for hyperkalemia, 294, 294t
for malignant hyperthermia, 235
for metabolic acidosis, 295
Sodium bicitrate, to prevent aspiration, 285
Sodium channel. See *Ion channel(s)*.
Sodium polystyrene sulfonate, 294, 294t
Solubility, of inhalation agent, 34–35
Somatic pain pathway, 262–264, *263*
Somatic response, to surgical stimulation, 189
Somnolence, 257
Sore throat, 187
Sphygmomanometry, 191–192
Spinal anesthesia, adhesive arachnoiditis after, 248
agents used in, 245–246
cardiac arrest in, 246
headache after, 246–248, *247*
hematoma from, 248
hepatic function in, 142–143
hypotension in, 246
in pregnancy, 246
leg pain after, 248
needles for, 247, *247*
neurological deficit after, 248
number of segments affected in, 246
paralysis from, 248
techniques in, 244–245, *245*
Spirometer, 123–124
Steroid therapy, anesthesia and, 146–147
in arthritis patient, 150
preanesthetic hydrocortisone in, 161
Streptomycin, 73
Stridor, 187
Stylet, malleable, 173, *173*, 315t
Succinylcholine. See also *Depolarizing neuromuscular blockade*.
cardiac rhythm and, 190
factors affecting action of, 76–78
for outpatient surgery, 287
for tracheal intubation, 217
in liver disease, 141
in myasthenia gravis, 77

Succinylcholine (*Continued*)
  in myotonia, 77
  in rapid-sequence induction, 218–219
  nondepolarizing blockade and, 65, 73, 76
  pharmacokinetics of, 73
  plasma cholinesterase and, 77–78
  precurarization and, 76
  recovery from, 222
  self-taming and, 77
  side effects of, 74–76
Sufentanil, 53
Supraclavicular approach, to brachial plexus block, *242*, 242–243
Surface charge hypothesis, 83–84
Surgical anesthesia, planes of, 9
Swan-Ganz catheter, 194
Sympathetic response, to surgical stimulation, 189
Syphilis, 307
Systemic illness. See *Illness, systemic.*

Tachycardia, from intubation, 186–187
  sinus, during anesthesia, 228
    in malignant hyperthermia, 235–236
Tachyphylaxis, of local anesthetic, 85–86
Tachypnea, airway carbon dioxide waveform in, 204, *204*
Teeth, preoperative assessment of, 155
  trauma to, during intubation, 186
Tetracaine, 88, 245–246
Tetracycline, 73
Thiamylal, 19
Thiopental, at GABA-gated ion channel, 5, *5*
  contraindications to, 19
  distribution of, *15*, 15–16
  dosage of, 18
  histamine release and, 19
  history of, 2, 17–18
  in liver disease, 141
  in rapid-sequence induction, 218
  induction of, 215–216
  pharmacokinetics of, *15*, 15–16, 18–19
  to induce barbiturate coma, 18

Third-space loss, of water and salt, 292
Threshold potential, 61, *61*
Thrombocytopenia, 303
Thrombosis, deep vein, 149
Thyromental distance, 155–156
Tidal volume, in mechanical ventilation, 125–126
  inhalation anesthetic and, 128
Time cycling, in mechanical ventilation, 121
Tissue uptake, of inhalation agents, 36
  of intravenous anesthetic, 14–16, *15*
Tolerance, to morphine, 48–49
Toxoplasmosis, transfusion-induced, 307
Tracheal intubation, advantages of, 169, 169t
  anesthesia induction by, 217
  awake, 177–178
  BURP maneuver in, 181
  characteristics of, 169t
  Combitube in, 182–184, *184*
  complications of, 186–187, 315, 315t, 317
  cricothyrotomy airway in, *184*, 184–185
  emergency airway in, 183–185, *184*
  extubation after, 185–186
    laryngospasm from, 187
  for outpatient surgery, 287
  forceps for, 172, *173*
  glottis exposure in, *180*, 180–181
  head and neck posture in, 174–175, *175*
  history of, 169
  impossible, incidence of, 181
  in intravenous induction, 216
  in obese surgical patient, 149
  laryngeal spray for, 173, *173*, 315t
  lubricant for, 174
  malleable stylet for, 173, *173*, 315t
  mishaps in, 315t
  nasotracheal route for, 176–177, 179
  orotracheal route for, *175*, 175–176, 179–180
  satisfactory airway in, face mask ventilation during, 181–182
  techniques of, 174–180, *175*

Tracheal intubation (*Continued*)
transtracheal jet ventilation in, 185
tubing for, 171–172, *172*
kink in, 205, 224, 315t
mishaps with, 315t
under local anesthesia, 177–178
unexpected difficulties in, *180*, 180–185, *184*
unsatisfactory airway in, face mask ventilation during, 182–183
Train-of-four stimulus, of peripheral nerve, 209–211, *210*
Transcutaneous electrical nerve stimulation, 278–279
Transfusion. See *Blood transfusion*; *Platelet transfusion.*
Transportation, to recovery room, 252
Transtracheal jet ventilation, 185
Tubing, endotracheal, 171–172, *172*
kink in, 205, 224, 315t
mishaps with, 315t
in anesthetic circuit, 109
d-Tubocurarine, 64–65
in liver disease, 141
in rapid-sequence induction, 219
in renal failure, 71
succinylcholine interaction with, 76

Unconsciousness, depth of, 188–190
in general anesthesia, 9
Urine output, monitoring of, 296
Uterus, gravid, halothane and, 41
isoflurane and, 39

Valium, 22–23. See also *Diazepam.*
Valve(s), in anesthetic circuit, adjustable pressure-limiting, 109–110, *110*, 113, *113*, *115*
nonrebreathing, 116, *117*
in anesthetic machine, backpressure checking, 104, *105*
emergency flushing, 97
failure safety, 105
safety pressure-relief, *100*, 100–101
safety, for oxygen, 105
Vapor, anesthetic, monitoring volume of, 206

Vaporizer, agent-specific filling system for, *103*, 103–104
copper kettle, 95–96, *96*
exclusive control of, 104
measured-flow, 95, *96*
mishaps with, 315t
of anesthetic machine, 95–97, *96*, *103*, 103–104
variable-bypass, *96*, 96–97
Vasopressin. See *Antidiuretic hormone.*
Vecuronium, 67
in liver disease, 141
in renal failure, 72
Venous admixture, 134
Venous thrombosis, deep, 149
Ventilation. See also *Airway management, in anesthetized patient.*
alveolar. See *Alveolar ventilation.*
controlled, 221
fentanyl/congeners and, 54
measuring flow and volume of, 195–196, *196–197*
mechanical. See *Mechanical ventilation.*
spontaneous, 220–221
Ventilation-perfusion inequality, 129–130
airway carbon dioxide waveform in, *204*, 204–206
airway closure and, 130
anesthesia effects on, 131
functional residual capacity and, 130–131
hypoxic pulmonary vasoconstriction and, 131
mechanical ventilation and, 132, *132*
pain-induced, 266
Ventricular arrhythmia. See also *Cardiac arrhythmia.*
from intubation, 186–187
Ventricular premature beat, during anesthesia, 229
Viomycin, 73
Visceral pain pathway, 264
Voltage-gated ion channel, 4–5, *5*, 60–61, *61*, 81, *81*
Volume cycling, in mechanical ventilation, 121
Volume expansion hypothesis, 6–7
Volumeter(s), mechanical, 195–196, *196–197*

Vomiting, after outpatient surgery, 288
  in recovery, 258–259
  morphine-induced, 47–48
von Willebrand's factor, 303

Water, basal requirement for, 290–291
  presurgical deficit in, 291–293
Waters to-and-fro circuit, 116, *117*

Williams intubating airway, *164*, 165, 179–180
Withdrawal, delirium in, 258
  from alcohol, 258
  from cocaine, 151
  from heroin, anesthesia during, 151
  from morphine, 49
Wound healing, hyperglycemia and, 146
  steroid therapy and, 147
Wright respirometer, 195, *196*